Disaster
Preparedness
and Response

What Do I Do Now?: Emergency Medicine

SERIES EDITOR-IN-CHIEF

Catherine A. Marco, MD, FACEP
Professor, Emergency Medicine & Surgery
Wright State University Boonshoft School of Medicine
Dayton, Ohio

OTHER VOLUMES IN THE SERIES

Disaster Preparedness and Response

By Paul P. Rega, MD, FACEP
Assistant Professor, School of Population Health in the College
of Health and Human Services, University of Toledo; Founder, Ohio-1
Disaster Medical Assistance Team, National Disaster Medical System

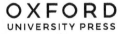

OXFORD
UNIVERSITY PRESS

OXFORD
UNIVERSITY PRESS

Oxford University Press is a department of the University of Oxford. It furthers
the University's objective of excellence in research, scholarship, and education
by publishing worldwide. Oxford is a registered trade mark of Oxford University
Press in the UK and certain other countries.

Published in the United States of America by Oxford University Press
198 Madison Avenue, New York, NY 10016, United States of America.

CIP data is on file at the Library of Congress
Names: Rega, Paul P., author.
Title: Disaster preparedness and response / Paul P. Rega.
Other titles: What do I do now?: Emergency medicine.
Description: New York, NY : Oxford University Press, [2022] |
Series: What do I do now?
Emergency medicine | Includes bibliographical references and index.
Identifiers: LCCN 2021054099 (print) | LCCN 2021054100 (ebook) |
ISBN 9780197577516 (paperback) | ISBN 9780197580172 (epub) |
ISBN 9780197580189
Subjects: MESH: Disasters | Disaster Planning | Emergency Medical Services |
Emergency Medicine | Case Reports
Classification: LCC HV553 (print) | LCC HV553 (ebook) | NLM WA 295 |
DDC 363.34/8—dc23/eng/20211124
LC record available at https://lccn.loc.gov/2021054099
LC ebook record available at https://lccn.loc.gov/2021054100

DOI: 10.1093/med/9780197577516.001.0001

9 8 7 6 5 4 3 2 1

Printed by Marquis, Canada

This book is dedicated to

Churton Budd, RN, EMT-P, the heart and soul of the OH-1 Disaster Medical Assistance Team

and to

Donald McConnaughy, Chief (retired), Maumee Fire and Rescue, a mentor, a partner, and a friend for life.

Contents

Preface

Disaster medicine has occupied an increasingly important niche within the specialty of emergency medicine over the latter half of the 20th century. Our specialty has been intimately involved with both national and international crises during that time. Regardless of whether an event was natural, anthropogenic, or a combination of both, emergency medicine was and is the ideal discipline to develop the human resources, the strategies, the tactics, and the evidence-based research to elevate the field of disaster medicine. It began, organizationally speaking, with Hurricane Hugo in 1989 and it is continuing through the 2019 COVID-19 pandemic and beyond.

Now that we are well into the 21st century, we must steady our footing as a specialty on the 20th century's foundation so that we can wrestle with the more intricate challenges of the future. For example, due to the omnipresent threat of national and global terrorism, there has been a discussion among disaster medical experts about emphasizing "counter-terrorism medicine" within the disaster medicine framework. Indeed, while preparing for and responding to myriad acts of terrorism remain vital aspects within our specialty's lexicon, allow me to posit that this scope is too narrow.

The past two decades have been a crystal ball into the future. Our global populations have experienced sectarian violence, wars, genocide, migration, terrorism, emerging infectious diseases, and pandemics. These natural and anthropogenic events will only worsen exponentially as we become intrinsically trapped by the effects of climate change. The United Nation's Intergovernmental Panel on Climate Change has recently concluded that regardless of how we try to reverse the effects of global warming, what we are experiencing now in terms of hurricanes, floods, and droughts will continue to worsen over the next 30 years. Should we, as a species, continue to equivocate and as global temperatures climb by 2100 to more than 3°C higher than pre-Industrial Revolution times, these events will become more frequent and more catastrophic. "Catastrophic" may even be too mild a term. It is possible that over the next few years, the academic arm of emergency medicine may need to consider developing a curriculum devoted to "Cataclysmic Medicine."

To confront these possibilities, there first needs to be a knowledge of disaster medicine and disaster management at its most basic level. It begins with crisis leadership, command and control, communications, and coordination. When all these pieces of the jigsaw puzzle are fitted together properly and enclosed by a proper ethical frame, then the best and most ethical and moral disaster medical can will be provided to the patient and to the community.

The intent of this book is to introduce these concepts using diverse viewpoints and scenarios. Readers are challenged to cogitate, create, and layer their own set of building blocks upon the preexisting foundation, thereby reinforcing and sustaining their own capacity to prepare for and respond to any adverse eventuality, mass casualty or otherwise. I hope that the experiential and evidence-based contents of this book will inspire readers to delve deeper into the nuances of disaster medicine and will serve as an impetus for a more profound quest for knowledge and a desire to serve those who will be experiencing the worst moments of their lives.

Further reading

Court M, Edwards B, Issa F, Voskanyan A, Ciottone G. Counter-terrorism medicine: Creating a medical initiative mandated by escalating asymmetric attacks. *Prehosp Disaster Med*. 2020;35(6):595–598.

Intergovernmental Panel on Climate Change. *Climate Change 2021: The Physical Science Basis. Contribution of Working Group I to the Sixth Assessment Report of the Intergovernmental Panel on Climate Change*. United Nations; 2021.

Rega PP. The ethics of disasters. In: Marco C, Shears RM, eds. *Ethical Dilemmas in Emergency Medicine*. Cambridge University Press; 2015:249–265. ISBN-13: 978-1107438590.

Roth PB, Vogel A, Key G, Hall D, Stockhoff CT. The St. Croix disaster and the National Disaster Medical System. *Ann Emerg Med*. 1991;20(4):391–395.

Tin D, Hart A, Ciottone GR. A decade of terrorism in the United States and the emergence of counter-terrorism medicine. *Prehosp Disaster Med*. 2021;36(4):380–384.

Acknowledgments

This book exists because of two individuals.

First, my gratitude goes to Catherine A. Marco, MD, FACEP, editor-in-chief of the *What Do I Do Now?: Emergency Medicine* series. This very accomplished physician and educator contacted me and asked me if I would consider writing a book on disaster medicine at its most elemental and pragmatic level—a distillation of all my experiences and research on the topic. Thank you, Catherine, for allowing me to write in the same style that I have used to teach my students in the classroom.

Second, my thanks to my project editor, Ms. Tiffany Lu. Without a doubt, her thoughts, suggestions, and advice surely made this book a much better product than I could ever imagine. You are a pro, Tiffany, and I was fortunate to have you as my editor.

The Lloyd A. Jacobs Interprofessional Immersive Simulation Center (IISC) at the University of Toledo requires a special acknowledgment. A major part of my "second life" as an educator has been spent at the "Sim Center" developing and executing scenarios, devising drills, and teaching enhanced skills. Many of my photographs in this book illustrating the benefits of simulation medicine were taken there. So, I extend my gratitude to IISC's faculty and staff for working with me in developing an exciting pedagogy in disaster medicine.

Introduction

The 20th century saw its share of death and destruction, including two world wars, a couple of pandemics, and an assortment of natural, technological, intentional, and accidental disasters. Now, we are one-fifth of the way into the 21st century and have already witnessed international terrorism, emerging infectious disease outbreaks, global conflicts, population migrations, and a pandemic the likes of which may even surpass the Great Pandemic of 1917–1918. And in the background lurks the ominous specter of climate change—a potentially cataclysmic event that could logarithmically wreak devastation upon humankind in a matter of decades and last for centuries.

So, how can we assimilate, comprehend, prepare for, and respond to these inevitable wars, diseases, tsunamis, cyclones, floods, droughts, technological mishaps, and acts of terror? This, indeed, can be a daunting prospect for any emergency physician. To appreciate the nuances and intricacies of the term "disaster," it would be useful to examine select case histories of mass casualty incidents (MCIs).

FOUR CASE HISTORIES

Case report #1

On January 9, 2013, the Seastreak Wall Street ferry was transporting 331 passengers and crew from New Jersey to Pier 11 near Wall Street in Lower Manhattan. For one reason or another, the ferry failed to slow down sufficiently in the process of docking and instead smashed into the dock. Many of the passengers were up and about getting ready to exit when the accident occurred, so they were extremely vulnerable to propulsive forces. There were 74 passengers injured as a result. Most of the injuries could be classified as minor. EMS rapidly triaged and stabilized them and transported them to nearby hospitals. One victim, however, sustained serious head and facial trauma and required transportation 6 miles away to New York-Presbyterian Hospital on the Upper East Side. With Bellevue Hospital only partially functional in the aftermath of Hurricane Sandy and with St. Vincent's Hospital closed down in 2010, New York-Presbyterian was the closest Level 1 Trauma Center. Experts, at that time, agreed that Lower Manhattan was extremely vulnerable to managing an MCI due to the extent to which its emergency healthcare infrastructure was crippled by Hurricane Sandy.

Case report #2

On August 29, 2005, Hurricane Katrina made landfall along the Louisiana–Missouri border. At that point, it was a Category 3 tropical cyclone with sustained wind speeds of 125 mph. That cyclonic event killed more than 1,800 people, demolished or made uninhabitable almost 300,000 homes, disrupted the physical and mental well-being of millions of individuals, and came with an early price tag estimated to be $151 billion. This disaster extended over a geographic area of more than tens of thousands of square miles and required a national response that was beyond the scope of the official "groupthink." Even 10 years after Katrina, the New Orleans metropolitan area had not reached its pre-Katrina baseline in terms of population, housing units, and businesses. The region and its people have still not fully returned to the pre-Katrina era.

Case report #3

At the time it occurred (June 11, 2016), the Pulse Nightclub shooting was the deadliest mass shooting event in U.S. history, only to be supplanted by the Las Vegas massacre 1 year later. At about 2 a.m. Omar Mateen entered the nightclub and began a cascade of shooting and hostage-taking that lasted for 3 hours before he was "neutralized." Of the more than 300 revelers, 49 were killed and 53 more were wounded. Orlando Regional Medical Center was not only the area's major trauma center but was also very close to the attack. Within minutes and with no advance warning, the victims were being dropped off at Orlando Regional one after the other. The emergency department and trauma bays were described by staff as a "war scene." A total of 44 victims arrived at the trauma center that horrific morning. Nine died during that time.

Case report #4

The influenza pandemic of 1918 is the pandemic by which all others are judged. It is estimated that around the world more than 50 million people perished. In the United States, 675,000 people died; if extrapolated to the year 2020, that number would be equivalent to 2 million deaths. Medical students were being graduated early and took responsibility for patient care, communities were hijacking railroad cars for their coffin shipments, and local civilians came together to care for their neighbors when the normal infrastructure failed. In terms of morbidity and mortality, the COVID-19 pandemic, arguably, pales in comparison.

HOW DO WE PREPARE FOR DISASTERS?

So, how does an emergency physician process these events, these disasters? Each one is unique, and yet there is a method that can identify the fundamentals of virtually any disaster. Otherwise, the magnitude of the disaster or its individual components can overwhelm the neophyte physician at a time when the expertise associated with the breadth and depth of emergency medicine is most needed.

Leaving the science and art of disaster medicine to nurses or administrators or other specialties is an abrogation of one's responsibility as an emergency physician. This is a critical concept to appreciate. No matter the disaster, emergency physicians by their very nature and their unique skillset are the perfect specialists to take charge of a chaotic situation and regain normalcy for the emergency department, the hospital, and the community, even if it becomes the "new" normal. In any case, whether you come to this book willingly or unwillingly, you will be in the thick of the disaster. Acquiring core fundamentals will serve you well.

The point of this book is to teach you the basic concepts that will serve as a safeguard for you, your family, your hospital, and your community. It is a matter of focusing on the essentials and maintaining a proper perspective as you negotiate the byzantine byways and alleyways of disasters and other MCIs. As you access the on-ramp leading to the highway of disaster medical competency, consider these initial concepts.

All disasters are local

Keeping that in the back of your mind forces you and your community to rely on yourselves to manage the incident, at least initially. "Initially" is an open-ended term: It could mean a matter of hours for a multiple vehicular collision or days for a tornado that levels a trailer park. During that time, your community's resources (and possibly mutual aid) may be all that's available to handle the situation. Therefore, each community needs to assess its resources and resolve any impediments. To rely on the immediate arrival of personnel and supplies from the state or the federal government is foolhardy. Those external resources will arrive at some point, but it may take days, weeks, even months for this assistance, depending on the extent of the disaster and the presence of other exigencies that may be occurring simultaneously.

Of course, we should still be aware of what is happening in the rest of the country and the rest of the world. Learning how other communities address their disasters will be of enormous assistance in helping your community prepare for its own future challenges. For right now, however, concentrate on the things that can happen in your own community and prepare for them. Conducting a hazard vulnerability-risk analysis involves appraising what disaster-related risks may occur in your community and assessing how well disposed your community is in meeting the challenge.

Three magnitudes of severity

Disasters can be simple, complex, or catastrophic. This delineation will help you appreciate what needs to be done immediately, in the short term, and over the long haul.

Simple disasters

Most of the disasters or MCIs you will face are *simple disasters*, meaning that they are rather straightforward and transparent. They are classically limited in time, space, damage, injuries, and mortality. Examples include a tornado ripping through a mobile home park, a chain-reaction crash along the turnpike, or a ferry crashing into a dock in lower Manhattan. They typically involve a finite number of victims and are usually resolved in a matter of hours, possibly days. Injuries are typically traumatic and/or respiratory in nature. While the response system will be taxed and stressed, the community's infrastructure is intact and both pre-hospital and hospital resources are available to overcome the event. Long-term complexities are negligible.

Complex disasters

Type 1 complex disasters cripple the community's infrastructure for a limitless period of time. EMS, fire, law enforcement, and the healthcare system will not be able to respond to the immediate needs of the community because those agencies themselves are negatively impacted by the disaster. The acute and long-term impacts on a community's social order, economy, environment, and population are clouded.

Hurricane Andrew (1992), at one time, was considered one of the most devastating Category 5 hurricanes in U.S. history. I was honored to serve as medical commander with my OH-1 Disaster Medical Assistance Team (National Disaster Medical System) (Figure I.1). It was part of the federal response effort to that disaster. While it resulted in fewer than 100 deaths, it destroyed over 60,000 homes, damaged another 124,000, and incurred an economic loss of more than $23 billion. To illustrate the impact that Andrew had on the infrastructure, there was the anecdote of a homeowner who called the local fire department because her house was on fire.

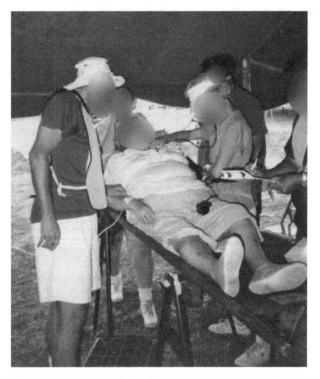

FIGURE I.1   Patient care during Hurricane Andrew.

Figure credit: OH-1 DMAT.

Instead of responding immediately with lights and sirens, the department admitted that they were unable to assist and advised that she and any family members simply get out of the house. In another instance, I recall my case of an elderly lady who arrived at our OH-1 tent and collapsed. She was quickly resuscitated and stabilized. Before she departed by air ambulance to a functional Miami hospital, she talked about how she was scheduled to have a cardiac intervention at a local hospital. Unfortunately, the day of her scheduled procedure was the day that Andrew made landfall. Needless to say, her intervention was canceled; also, her home was destroyed. She had been spending the intervening days walking from shelter to shelter for food, water, and sundries before she collapsed at our doorstep. Hurricane Andrew's complexities paled in comparison with the events that occurred during and after Hurricane Katrina made landfall in 2005.

In *type 2 complex disasters*, although the community's infrastructure is intact and the community's geographic footprint remains untouched, special resources and expertise are required relatively quickly to meet the unusual challenges. One example would be the Paris terrorist attacks of November 13, 2015. The terrorists divided themselves into three groups and attacked six sites in and around Paris with bombs and weaponry. The deaths numbered 130, and 416 more innocent victims were wounded, about a quarter of them gravely. Paris remained intact. Its infrastructure remained intact. However, due to the size, scope, and prognosis of the event, the Orsan (*organisation de la réponse du système de santé en situations sanitaires exceptionnelles*) plan was activated. This was not merely a Parisian disaster plan, but a national disaster plan that immediately coordinated responses among healthcare, law enforcement, EMS, and more.

A foodborne botulism outbreak in central Ohio in 2015 is another example of a type 2 complex disaster. Due to improperly prepared potato salad at a church picnic, over 20 people were stricken with botulism. One died. Besides the immediate management of the patients, a number of actions were required, including notification of Centers for Disease Control and Prevention (CDC) for release of the botulinum antitoxin, triage and transport of certain victims to regional medical centers, just-in-time training on the administration of the antitoxin, and the involvement of local public health agencies in the immediate epidemiologic investigation.

Catastrophic disasters

Catastrophic disasters should be rare phenomena in many industrialized nations. However, as most of us have learned, one cannot rule out the possibility even among the industrialized nations should there be a global disaster like a pandemic or a nuclear cataclysm. What makes these events catastrophic is that a stricken nation may not be able to respond to the specific event locally, regionally, or even nationally. Whatever response is potentially available may have to come from other nations' resources and manpower, and that response may be limited, late, or never. Whatever community infrastructure is viable will be altered temporarily or permanently. This could even be more unfathomable should there ever be a global nuclear war.

Mental impact of disasters

One key aspect that must not be forgotten in disaster response is mental health—not only for the victims and their families, who may be incapacitated for weeks, months, or years, but also for the community, both the typical townsperson and emergency responders and caregivers. While much of the focus of a disaster response deals with the physical impact of an event on an individual, the mental impact also needs to be addressed. The mental health of a community must be addressed both in the short term and long-term. This is relevant across all types of disasters but is particularly critical in complex and catastrophic disasters.

For example, Hurricane Irma in 2017 wreaked considerable havoc as it crossed the Caribbean and struck the Florida Keys as a Category 4 tropical cyclone. In the Keys, 65% of the homes were damaged, 40 people were injured, and 17 others lost their lives. That represented the physical impact of the storm. Twenty months after the event, 17% of the residents of the Florida Keys reported increased anxiety, 11.3% reported depression, and 17% expressed a need for mental health services. In 2018 the suicide rate in that region increased to 34.9/100,000 from a 2013–2017 average of 25.2/100,000.

IMPACT OF CLIMATE CHANGE

Right now, the unturned card in Earth's futuristic poker deck is climate change. How will global warming, worsening droughts, ever-increasing wildfires, and overwhelming flooding augment the "routine" exigencies of nature and human frailty and establish a world where complex and catastrophic disasters become the norm and not the exception?

We have seen glimpses into future disasters by studying events of the recent past. On September 20, 2017, when Category 4 hurricane Maria swept through Puerto Rico, the aftermath was horrific. Of the 3.5 million total population, 44% lost access to clean water. Cellphone towers were down and internet connectivity was lost. The entire island lost power. Out of the 69 hospitals on the island, only one remained operational. With all this destruction, a major consideration that cannot be ignored in any disaster is the baseline health of the affected community. Compared to the average U.S. population, the average Puerto Rican resident is entrenched in poverty and unlikely to improve their situation. In addition to that, the incidence of heart disease, cancer, and diabetes mellitus is higher on this island that in the rest of the United States. How well these people managed on a day-to-day basis was logarithmically worsened by a catastrophic disaster such as Maria. Two weeks after landfall, a federal medical shelter, manned by personnel from the U.S. Department of Health and Human Services and the National Disaster Medical System, was treating approximately 188 people per day for diverse problems such as infections and musculoskeletal injuries. A key finding was that almost 12% of these patients presented because of exacerbations of their chronic medical conditions. This needs to be emphasized when managing the healthcare needs of a population pummeled with a complex or catastrophic event. With a sudden dearth of pharmacies, hospitals, clinics, and native healthcare providers, it stands to reason that people's preexisting health conditions will deteriorate.

ABOUT THIS BOOK

However, if you prepare for the typical simple disaster, the lessons you learn from these situations will stand you in good stead should an aberrant MCI occur. The purpose of this book is to evaluate these disasters in their various iterations and search for and articulate a commonality that will assist emergency physicians in managing, at least initially, any MCI that should befall them, their hospital, and their community. In short, I hope to provide you with the basics of disaster medicine and management.

This will be done in a sequential narrative format. It starts with an MCI that an emergency physician happens upon while driving to work; continues with the more common types of disasters that may be encountered while practicing emergency medicine, including both internal and external events; and finishes up with disasters that require greater flexibility of response and a honed sense of crisis leadership.

Unique characteristics of certain types of disasters will receive special attention in this book. One chapter deals with the acute, subacute, and long-term consequences of a botulism MCI. Another chapter is devoted to the unique characteristics a hydrofluoric MCI. These two cases are highlighted because triage parameters, tactical issues, and strategic planning will be different than the usual day-to-day biologic or hazardous materials (HAZMAT) event.

Staff, residents, students, and medical personnel need to be trained on the key aspects of disaster medicine, so I have included a section that provides didactic education coupled with tabletop scenarios, drills, functional exercises, and full-scale exercises. I have also provided scripts for disaster cases, scenarios, and drills that can be used to help train your colleagues, staff, and students. One of the most difficult aspects of providing this education is finding the time to create and write these types of educational platforms. I have developed and honed them through 11 years of educating healthcare students, residents, EMS, and university faculty. Hopefully, this endeavor will take some of the burden off your shoulders in preparing your training exercises; they might even inspire you to create better ones.

Remember, you already know how to manage multiple patients simultaneously. That is part of your discipline and your skillset in emergency medicine. The goal of this book is to take that expertise and expand it in order to provide you with both tactics and strategies of disaster management, so that you and your team can manage a unique disaster situation competently and safely.

Further reading

Centers for Disease Control and Prevention. 1918 Pandemic (H1N1 virus) | Pandemic Influenza (Flu) | CDC.

Flegenheimer M, Moynihan C. Several dozen are injured in ferry crash in Lower Manhattan. *New York Times*, January 9, 2013.

Ghosh AK, Mecklenburg M, Ibrahim S, Daniel P. Health care needs in the aftermath of Hurricane Maria in Puerto Rico: A perspective from Federal Medical Shelter Manatí. *Prehosp Disaster Med*. 2021;36(3):260–264.

Grossman A. City trauma showing signs of strain. *Wall Street Journal*, January 11, 2013. doi:10.1017/S1049023X21000339

McCarty CL, Angelo K, Beer KD, Cibulskas-White K, Quinn K, de Fijter S, Bokanyi R, St Germain E, Baransi K, Barlow K, Shafer G, Hanna L, Spindler K, Walz E, DiOrio M, Jackson BR, Luquez C, Mahon BE, Basler C, Curran K, et al. Large outbreak of botulism associated with a church potluck meal—Ohio, 2015. *MMWR Morb Mortal Wkly Rep*. 2015;64(29):802–803.

Torres-Mendoza Y, Kerr A, Schnall AH, Blackmore C, Hartley SD. Community assessment for mental and physical health effects after Hurricane Irma—Florida Keys, May 2019. *MMWR Morb Mortal Wkly Rep*. 2021;70:937–941.

U.S. Census Bureau. Facts for Features: Hurricane Katrina 10th Anniversary: Aug. 29, 2015. July 29, 2015 (release number: CB15-FF.16).

1 Pile-up on the pike: First in

You are running late and you sure don't want to stick your colleague with that posterior epistaxis patient at 0705; you will never hear the end of it! Therefore, you take the highway. It is early morning and the ground fog is a bit heavier than usual. As you round the top of the hill heading into the valley, screeching tires and crunching metal assault your eardrums ahead of you. Some gray smoke starts to billow in the air. What is playing out is a chain-reaction multiple vehicular accident about a mile downwind of your position.

This is a classic example of a "simple" disaster. It is an event limited in time, space, and victims, and the local infrastructure, with or without mutual aid, has the resources to respond efficaciously. Figures 1.1, 1.2, and 1.3 show photos from a multiple vehicular accident field exercise.

What do I do now?

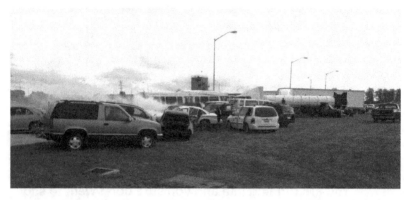

FIGURE 1.1 The planners of this September 25, 2013, field exercise inserted a couple of issues that the responders needed to address, such as the presence of smoke and a tanker car.

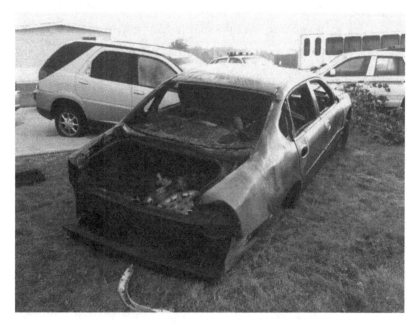

FIGURE 1.2 A burned-out car at the multiple vehicular accident field exercise.

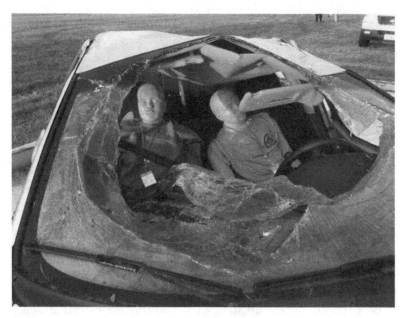

FIGURE 1.3 Dummies, with their injuries listed on lanyards, are used to simulate crash victims in the field exercise.

Pull over to the side of the road, activate your hazard lights, and stop at a position that is both safe from the accident and safe from vehicles approaching behind you. One axiom that really has not changed over the years is that if you can cover the scene of a disaster with your thumb, you won't be significantly impacted by its effects. Another adage, by the way, is "uphill, upwind, upstream." These are a series of commands that are helpful in avoiding a HAZMAT (hazardous material) incident. More about HAZMAT issues a little bit later.

All of this boils down to one question you should always consider when involved in a disaster situation: Is the scene safe?

Assuming you and your vehicle are in the safest place possible and the vehicles behind you have slowed down to a stop and are avoiding being sucked into the situation down below, make your 911 call. Tell the police as succinctly as possible:

1. Who you are: "I am Dr. So-and-So. I'm an ER doc. I want to report a multiple-vehicle accident." I find that if I am at a scene

and I give report to EMS or law enforcement, they seem to listen more attentively.

2. What happened: Do not postulate. Just the facts. What you are seeing.

3. Location: It can help responders with ingress to and egress from the site. Look for mile markers, signage, closest exit, direction of travel, etc.

4. The approximate number of vehicles involved: cars, buses, trucks, semis (potential for transporting hazardous materials). The types of vehicles can serve as a clue to the possible number of victims.

5. Any obvious ongoing or potential hazards: smoke, color of the smoke, leaking fluids, fires, explosions, stability of the ground, downed power lines, unusual odors.

6. Weather/road conditions at the site: rainy, foggy, oil slicks, etc.

Let's also consider a situation similar to this except that it is happening during a major hurricane. On August 25, 2017, Hurricane Harvey made landfall near Corpus Christi, Texas. Over a 5-day period, Texas and Louisiana were inundated by 51 inches of rain. During this time, over 330,000 residents were without power. This and other factors forced the evacuation of approximately 150,000 residents. In the process of that evacuation, flooding stranded tens of thousands on roads and highways. Road accidents were inevitable. In fact, 30,000 water rescues were documented. Your initial actions could be lifesaving, but they are also complicated by several factors: (1) While you may not be part of the chain-reaction collision, you are still victimized by hurricane's intemperate aftermath and (2) response times by EMS, firefighters, and law enforcement will be prolonged. Your talents as a leader in a crisis will be tested to the extreme.

KEY POINTS TO REMEMBER

· Always ask yourself: Is the scene safe?
· Contact 911 and provide concise and pertinent information about the event.

Further reading

Kaiser R, Karaye IM, Olokeinlade T, Hammond TM, Goldberg DW, Horney JA. Hemodialysis clinics in flood zones: A case study of Hurricane Harvey. *Prehosp Disaster Med.* 2021;36(2):135–140.

Rega P. Emergency medical services in disasters. In: Suresh D, ed. *Textbook of Emergency Medicine* (Vol. 1 & 2). Wolters Kluwer; 2011:1319–1325.

2 Triage and Napoleon Bonaparte

You are making your call to 911. You are trying to convey the most important information in the shortest time possible. Adapting journalism's "5 Ws and 1H" may be helpful in providing the necessary information as succinctly as possible (Table 2.1). This information will assist first responders' arrival at the scene of the disaster in terms of equipment, personnel, and specialized needs.

Fire, emergency medical services (EMS) personnel, and law enforcement agencies are on the way. It may take a while due to fog, distance, and road conditions. You look over the scene before you and decide that the scene is safe, and you are going in to assist the injured.

What do I do now?

TABLE 2.1 **Information to provide to the 911 operator**

WHO	"My name is _____. I am an emergency physician. I'm reporting a mass casualty incident."
WHAT	Declare: multiple vehicular accident.
	Estimate number of vehicles.
	Estimate number of special vehicles: trucks, semis, trains.
	Estimate number of victims.
WHERE	Street/cross-street
	Highway mile marker number
	Closest ingress
	Closest egress
	GPS coordinates
WEATHER	Conditions: clear, fog, rain, wind, snow, etc.
	Temperature: hot, temperate, cold, wind chill, heat index
WHY	Natural
	Technological
	Na-Tech (Natural + technological)
	Accidental
	Intentional
	Suspicious
HAZARDS	Sounds: explosions
	Smoke: atypical colors
	Spills
	Smells
	Fire

efore you go into the lion's den, prepare yourself as best as possible. Do not forget your first aid kit. What, you don't have one? That would be an action item for you this week. Meanwhile, for the immediate exigency, take along some essentials like volunteers (healthcare and/or military would be the best and the safest), pens or markers, water for hydration purposes, any pocket food for energy (e.g., candy bars), strips of cloth (bandages/tourniquets), and any head, ear, and eye protection. Keep in mind that you may be walking on ground that could have sharp objects scattered about. If you have boots, change into them. If you do not, be careful where you walk and exhort your cadre of volunteers to do likewise. Remember, the situation calls for crisis leadership, and you have been elected.

Now, you are at the scene and are confronted with sights and sounds that you hopefully will never hear again. What comes next?

The answer emanates from Dominique Jean Larrey, the surgeon-general of Napoleon's army. As background, before Napoleon, great armies would clash on vast battlefields and leave their wounded, dying, and dead on the field until the battle was over. Wounded soldiers subsequently died of exsanguination, thirst, and/or adverse climatic conditions (e.g., hypothermia/hyperthermia). It was Dr. Larrey who proposed to Napoleon the idea of an *ambulance volant*—a brigade of emergency responders who, with horses and carriages, would ride into the field of battle, extricate the wounded, and transport them to the rear so they could be cared for in order of the severity of their wounds, regardless of rank, friend or foe. As such, Dr. Larrey is often called the father of EMS, the father of triage, the father of pre-hospital care.

So, that's your mission: triage, from the French word meaning "to sort." You will be sorting the urgent from the non-urgent and providing the most rudimentary medical care that you can. The adage is: "The greatest good for the greatest number." With resources stretched to the limit, you can only identify and save those who can be saved until reinforcements arrive.

ADULTS AND START TRIAGE

Arguably, the most popular triage technique is START triage (Simple Triage and Rapid Treatment). It is used on a global level, but keep in mind that while it may be the most popular, it is, like the rest, not validated for disasters. We will use it in this scenario because it is quick, simple, and well known (Table 2.2).

TABLE 2.2 START triage

Category	Description	Actions
Red	In danger of immediate death or loss of limb without an intervention	Clear airway; stop hemorrhage; evacuate
Yellow	Death is not imminent; they are severely injured but have an expectation of living as long as medical care is delivered in an expeditious fashion	Maintain airway; stop hemorrhage; evacuate after Red victims
Green	No danger of immediate death or loss of limb	Evacuate after Red and Yellow victims
Black	No pulse, respiration, consciousness	None; any means of resuscitation would take away precious resources from others more salvageable. Await coroner

Figure 2.1 outlines the algorithm used for the START process. (This is for adults; kids have their own Jump-START triage system, described in the next section in the chapter.)

Tactically, START begins with separating the Green victims from the Red, Yellow, and Black ones. The process begins with your calling out in as loud a voice as possible, "Anybody who can hear me, get up and move over to the side of the road by that sign" (or whatever landmark is convenient). The concept is that those who can obey that command more than likely do not have life-threatening injuries. Send over a couple of your volunteers to assess them. Triage is not a static process; it is a continual process. Admittedly, this is a crude, insensitive process. After all, your voice may not carry very far with all the confusion, but it's a beginning. Theoretically, those remaining on the ground and in the vehicles are the Red, Yellow, and Black victims.

Now, as we come upon the remaining victims, keep in mind that with START only two medical interventions are permitted: (1) clearing the airway and (2) stopping any life-threatening hemorrhage. As you go from victim to victim, the key to separating the Reds from the Yellows

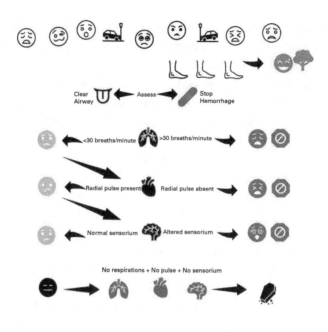

Algorithm

Step 1: Those who can walk ![] are tagged GREEN and move away from the site.

Step 2: The rest are RED ![], YELLOW ![], or BLACK ![] victims. Physiologic parameters will determine the appropriate color.

Step 3: RED patients are identified by respirations/minute over 30 (or under 8) ![], absence of a radial pulse ![], and/or an altered sensorium ![]. Tag: ![]

Step 4: YELLOW patients are identified by respirations/minute under 30, presence of a radial pulse, and a normal sensorium. Tag: ![]

Step 5: BLACK patients have catastrophic injuries with absent vital signs. Tag: ![]

FIGURE 2.1 The algorithm used for the START triage process.

is by assessing specific physiologic parameters, summarized by the mnemonic R-P-M (reminders for the assessment of breathing [R], pulse [P], and mentation [M]. The 30-2-Can Do triage aid represents the cut-off for number of respirations per minute [R], the cut-off for the number of seconds required for capillary refill in the nailbeds [P], and a reminder to ascertain whether the victim can obey commands/instructions [Can Do]. Remember, this is disaster medicine. You are trying to provide the greatest good for the greatest number.

You come upon your first victim and your initial assessment is for breathing. The respiratory rate is over 30. The person is tagged Red. Just make sure that the airway is cleared of debris. Some experts also prefer tagging Red those with a respiratory rate of 8 or below. In any case, once you have tagged a person Red and breathing and bleeding issues have been assessed, you should move on to the next victim. There is nothing more you can or should do for the initial victim. No need to assess pulse or mentation because you have already established that the person is indeed critical, you have corrected what can be corrected expeditiously, and you have communicated that to those responders coming in after you.

So, how do you communicate? You probably will not have triage tags or colored ribbons. Hopefully, you'll have a pen or marker and you can spell out the color on the person's forehead or palm. All this should not take you longer than 30 seconds. That is purposeful since it forces you to manage the most important aspects of lifesaving and still allow you time to move on to the other victims.

Now, you come upon your next victim. The respiratory rate is less than 30 and greater than 8. So far, so good. Now check circulation. A radial pulse check reveals no pulse and, as per START, that signifies shock. Another way to assess blood pressure is by checking capillary refill. Pinch the nailbed with your finger. Count "1-Mississippi, 2-Mississippi." If the capillary refill is less than 2 seconds, blood pressure is adequate. If it is greater than 2 seconds, that signifies hypotension. However, this assessment technique is limited. For example, a nailbed examination in the dark is useless. Additionally, false positives will occur while performing nailbed examinations in a cold environment. If there are no signs of any external bleeding that would require pressure, bandages, or tourniquets, tag the victim Red and move on.

The third victim's respiratory rate is greater than 8 and less than 30. Her radial pulse is nicely palpable. You have assessed, in short order, the R and P in the R-P-M mnemonic. Now you must assess her mentation. If she does not answer your simple question, if she answers illogically, or if she's simply articulating gibberish, she has failed the mentation test and has become a Red patient.

Any patient should be considered Yellow until they fail a specific physiologic parameter, in which case they become Red. The one exception is the victim who is without respirations, without pulse, and without any evidence of neurologic function, who should be tagged Black. Once you have tagged a victim Black, that person should receive no further interventions, resources, or care. To do so would waste precious resources and take away time from identifying and caring for another victim down the line who is more salvageable. Victims tagged Black should never be moved except in two circumstances: (1) when the coroner declares the bodies can be moved and (2) when responders must move lifeless bodies to rescue a living victim trapped beneath them.

CHILDREN AND JUMP-START TRIAGE

With children, my preference is to simply tag them Red regardless of how minor their injuries seem. Their physiologic parameters, especially blood pressure, can deceptively maintain themselves for a longer time than adults'—and then they can suddenly decompensate. So, tagging them Red right away eliminates discussion, delay, and deceptive vital signs and enhances their innate salvageability. This may especially be the case when those performing triage have only the barest of fundamentals regarding emergency pediatric care. Table 2.3 outlines triage considerations for various categories of victims in a mass casualty incident.

TABLE 2.3 **Triage considerations in a mass casualty incident**

Victim categories	Tagging	Rationale
Children	Red	More salvageable if managed expeditiously; deceptive vital signs
Children	Black	No signs of life after basic airway techniques
Adults	Red, Yellow, Green, Black	Based on basic START skills
Pregnant (gravid uterus at level of umbilicus)	Red	Minor trauma to mother may still increase of fetal demise.
First responders	Red	Morale

If multiple children are involved (e.g., a school shooting), a pediatric version of START called Jump-START can be employed (Figure 2.2). It follows START's general algorithm with one notable exception: If a child is not breathing, giving five quick breaths might "jump-start" the child, in which case the child is tagged Red. Otherwise, with no response after the five breaths, the child is tagged Black. If the rescue breaths are successful, then assessment of blood pressure and mentation follows. Mentation is based on the AVPU technique (A = alert, V = responsive to verbal stimuli, P = responsive to painful stimuli, and U = unresponsive to any stimuli).

Another consideration that is not really addressed with START is the obviously pregnant female. In this situation, you are dealing with more than one potentially viable victim. However, the triage responder can only adequately assess one victim, and it is well accepted that even seemingly trivial injuries may predispose the future mother to abruptio placentae and

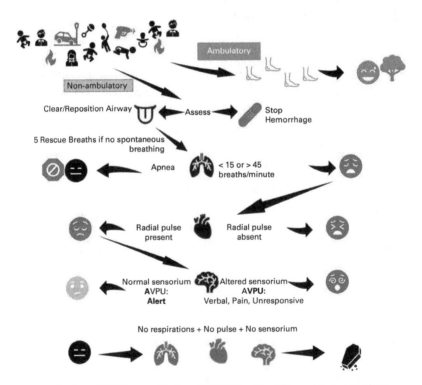

FIGURE 2.2 Jump-START is a modification of START triage for children under 8 years of age.

therefore place the unborn in jeopardy. So, regardless of how minor Mom's injuries may be, it makes medical sense to tag her Red so that she and her future offspring can be cared for as expeditiously as possible. This was how these victims were triaged at the first World Trade Center bombing in 1993.

Finally, we come to the first responders who suddenly become ill or injured while at the scene. Arguments can be made for and against prioritizing their care above other victims. It can be decided on a case-by-case basis, but keep in mind the following factors:

- First responders like many healthcare personnel will work until they drop.
- Many first responders may be older, voluntary workers with chronic medical conditions.
- Removing a stricken first responder immediately from the scene may improve the morale of other associates at the scene who appreciate that one of their own has not been sidestepped.

While START is a generally accepted triage tool around the world, it is not perfect. Like a number of other similar tools, none has been validated in a randomized, double-blind, case-controlled disaster situation study. Table 2.4 lists a selection of the diverse triage tools that have been developed, proposed, and employed around the world. The diversity underscores the conundrum that there is no triage tool that has been studied in a true disaster using a randomized, case-control methodology.

However, START is based on sound physiologic principles, and it is accessible to the most basic rescuer-responder. It is also the foundation of many subsequent triage tools that have been circulated globally. Nevertheless, it should not replace your medical knowledge, expertise, and experience as you evaluate multiple victims virtually simultaneously. If your gut tells you that a patient should be triaged higher than START's algorithm, go with your gut. For example, using the multiple vehicular accident as an example, you, as physician, come upon a 21-year-old victim complaining of abdominal pain. He is awake and alert with a palpable radial pulse and a respiratory rate of 25, so it would be understandable to classify him as Yellow based on the START criteria. However, your clinical acumen also detects significant bruising along his left upper quadrant. Now, you classify him as

TABLE 2.4 **Triage tools used around the world**

Triage tools	Key aspects	Reference
Reverse	Those with minor injuries receive priority. Useful in wartime.	*Eur J Emerg Med.* 2016;23(4):240–247.
Military	Identify and treat those who are most likely to survive to return to the frontlines.	Triage priorities and military physicians. In: *Physicians at War.* Springer; 2008:215–236.
MASS (Move, Assess, Sort, Send)	Similarities to both START and SALT	Koenig KL, Schultz CH. *Koenig and Schultz's Disaster Medicine: Comprehensive Principles and Practices.* Cambridge University Press; 2010.
Sieve	Similar to START. Used in areas of Europe and Australia.	UK triage–an improved tool for an evolving threat. *Injury.* 2013;44(1):23–28.
CESIRA	Similar to START. Three classes of triage.	Mass casualty triage: An evaluation of the data and development of a proposed national guideline. *Disaster Med Public Health Prep.* 2008;2(S1):S25–S34.
Homebush	Based on START and SAVE triage systems. Five classes of triage. Employed in Australia.	Australian disaster triage: A colour maze in the Tower of Babel. *Austr N Z J Surg.* 1999;69(8):598–602.
Careflight	Ability to obey commands receives higher priority than pulses and respirations.	Mass-casualty triage: Time for an evidence-based approach. *Prehospital Disaster Med.* 2008;23(1):3–8.
STM (Sacco Triage Method)	Mathematical model based on patient condition, resource availability, and facilities.	Precise formulation and evidence-based application of resource-constrained triage. *Acad Emerg Med.* 2005;12(8):759–770.

TABLE 2.4 **Continued**

Triage tools	Key aspects	Reference
META	Stabilization triage and evacuation triage.	The development and features of the Spanish prehospital advanced triage method (META) for mass casualty incidents. *Scand J Trauma Resusc Emerg Med.* 2016;24(1):63.
MASS Gathering	An Australian triage tool. Four triage categories: resuscitation, urgent, minor, self-help.	Development of a mass-gathering triage tool: An Australian perspective. *Prehospital Disaster Med.* 2017;32(1):101–105.
SWiFT	Triage tool for older adults: Senior Without Families Team.	SWiFT: A rapid triage tool for vulnerable older adults in disaster situations. *Disaster Med Public Health Prep.* 2008;2(S1):S45–S50.
Medical	Similar to START	*Integrated Emergency Management for Mass Casualty Emergencies.* 2013:101.
TEWS (Triage Early Warning Score)	For injured people over 12 years of age and 150 cm in height. Uses five triage colors.	An evaluation of the Triage Early Warning Score in an urban accident and emergency department in KwaZulu-Natal. *S Afr Fam Pract.* 2014;56(1):69–73.
MPTT (Modified Physiological Triage Tool)	Similar to START.	Major incident triage: Derivation and comparative analysis of the Modified Physiological Triage Tool (MPTT). *Injury.* 2017;48(5):992–999.

Continued

TABLE 2.4 **Continued**

Triage tools	Key aspects	Reference
ASAV (Amberg-Schwandorf Algorithm for Primary Triage)	Similar to START.	Evaluation of a novel algorithm for primary mass casualty triage by paramedics in a physician manned EMS system: A dummy-based trial. *Scand J Trauma Resusc Emerg Med*. 2014;22(1):50.
Smart	Similar to START.	Comparison of the SALT and Smart triage systems using a virtual reality simulator with paramedic students. *Eur J Emerg Med*. 2011;13(6):314–321.
Tactical	Similar to START	*Tactical Emergency Care: Military and Operational Out-of-Hospital Medicine*. Prentice Hall; 1999.
SAVE (Secondary Assessment Victim Endpoint)	Secondary triage tool to identify victims requiring extensive resources for survival.	*Koenig and Schultz's Disaster Medicine: Comprehensive Principles and Practices*. Cambridge University Press; 2010.
SORT	Secondary triage tool. Victims tagged based on scoring system.	Triage in mass casualty situations. *Contin Med Ed*. 2012;30(11):413–415.
CRAMS (Circulation, Respiration, Abdominal and Thorax Exam, Motor Response, Speech)	Employed in some American and European countries. Triage category based upon number score.	A comparison of EMT judgment and prehospital trauma triage instruments. *J Trauma*. 1991;31(10):1369–1375.
Emergency Severity Index (ESI) Triage	Victim triage coupled with facilities and resources required for each victim.	The Emergency Severity Index triage algorithm version 2 is reliable and valid. *Acad Emerg Med*. 2003;10(10):1070–1080.

Red, suspecting that he may have a rupturing spleen and that his vitals may be deceptively stable.

Whatever you decide, you won't be wrong. You're only wrong if you take too much time to deliberate. Wasting time is wasting time. Triage should take 15 seconds per person unless an immediate medical intervention is required based on the START criteria.

SALT TRIAGE

For the sake of completeness, while START is the principal triage tool in many locations, nationally and internationally, we should also consider SALT triage (Figure 2.3). SALT (Sort—Assess—Life-saving interventions—Treatment/transport) has been endorsed by the American College of Emergency Physicians, American College of Surgeons Committee on Trauma, American Trauma Society, National Association of EMS Physicians, National Disaster Life Support Education Consortium, and State and Territorial Injury Prevention Directors Association.

How this developed was that experts at various levels of local, state, and federal agencies plus other stakeholders felt that the current state of triage was deficient. There are multiple triage systems around the world, arguably START being the most popular, that were not sensitive and specific enough to manage mass numbers of casualties. There was concern for over-triaging victims and overwhelming trauma hospitals with minimally injured individuals. There was also a matter of under-triaging victims and preventing their access to competent trauma care. So, experts were identified and asked to provide their collective opinion as to which triage system was the best. Because they found each of these systems lacking in one way or the other, they developed their own. That is how SALT was born in 2008.

The SALT steps are as follows:

1. Separate Green victims (those who can follow simple commands such as walking to a nearby location or by waving).
2. For those remaining, determine who may require one or more of four life-saving interventions.

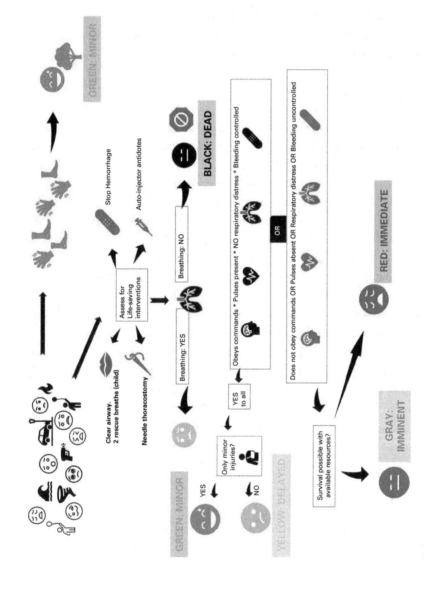

GREEN: MINOR

Stop Hemorrhage

Auto-injector antidotes

BLACK: DEAD

Breathing: NO

Assess for Life-saving interventions

Clear airway.
2 rescue breaths (child)

Needle thoracostomy

Breathing: YES

Obeys commands * Pulses present * NO respiratory distress * Bleeding controlled

OR

Does not obey commands OR Pulses absent OR Respiratory distress OR Bleeding uncontrolled

RED: IMMEDIATE

YES
to all

Only minor injuries?

YES

GREEN: MINOR

NO

YELLOW: DELAYED

Survival possible with available resources?

GRAY: IMMINENT

FIGURE 2.3   SALT triage.

3. Determine who is Red, Yellow, and Green based upon mental awareness, radial pulses, and bleeding severity.
4. Identify as Gray those victims who are still alive but for whom survival is improbable based on existing resources.

In SALT, the initial sorting is based on who can and cannot follow simple verbal commands (e.g., waving hands or walking to safety). Those who comprehend and obey are classified as Green. Those who cannot respond to those commands fall into the Red, Yellow, Black, and Gray categories and are assessed individually based on the usual physiologic parameters (respirations, circulation, and mentation). With SALT, that assessment also includes providing emergency medical management that is more sophisticated than what START triage allows. These interventions include, besides START's hemorrhage control and airway opening, performing a needle thoracostomy to resolve a tension pneumothorax and administering auto-injector antidotal therapy (e.g., sarin attack). The SALT algorithm allows for the delivery of two rescue breaths in a pediatric respiratory arrest. That is one of the benefits of SALT triage: It involves only one algorithm for both adult and pediatric populations. START is not meant for children under 8 years of age; for that population, the Jump-START algorithm is used. SALT, on the other hand, addresses both populations with one algorithm.

In tandem with this initial victim management is the need to identify whether the victim is Red, Yellow, Gray, or Black. SALT acknowledges that some victims have such catastrophic injuries that there is virtually no hope of survival, but they still are alive in terms of maintaining some semblance of vital signs, no matter how transitory. If these victims are tagged Red, it could allow the wasting of precious resources on them when they can be used for the more salvageable. However, to tag them Black will provide them no resources, not even palliative therapy or even human companionship at the very last moments of life. The Gray category recognizes these individuals as "expectant" and makes provisions for their final care, even if it is hopeless.

SALT has been appearing in the literature for 12 years or so, but it is like Avis car rental company to START's Hertz. There have been multiple peer-reviewed studies on the merits and deficiencies of both. The problem is that these studies are not prospective, double-blind studies comparing outcomes in an actual disaster population, because that would violate the disaster ethical framework. The bottom line is that there has been no triage system that has been scientifically validated during an actual disaster.

The other problem that SALT has in becoming the triage "law of the land" is that START is entrenched in American EMS and other pre-hospital responders' education. To introduce SALT means that it must be used by virtually all the stakeholder agencies across the region. Otherwise, responders from one regional response unit will certainly be confused if they see victims tagged Gray by another community's response unit coming in as part of mutual aid. Re-education and developing new drills and exercises to demonstrate SALT in action require time and money, two elements that are in short supply in EMS.

To summarize, the major differences between START and SALT are the following:

1. SALT uses one algorithm for both children and adults.
2. Instead of the two medical interventions used in START, SALT includes four:
   a. Clearing the airway
   b. Stopping hemorrhage
   c. Needling a tension pneumothorax
   d. Administering antidotes in certain HAZMAT situations (e.g., atropine/pralidoxime Cl for organophosphate toxicity)
3. SALT involves an additional color, Gray for the "expectant" patient. Gray victims are still alive but have sustained injuries that will ultimately be fatal. If they were tagged Red (as they would be in START), they could be receiving preciously scarce resources that could have benefited a more salvageable victim. If they were tagged Black, they would receive absolutely nothing. However, victims who are tagged Gray could receive palliative care and human comfort.

Since you are the highest healthcare authority on the scene, you are not married to any specific triage system. You are still allowed to triage patients based on your knowledge of the literature and your own clinical experience. For example, if you come upon a 20-year-old with abdominal trauma and physiologic parameters that would merit a Yellow tag, you could easily upgrade him to a Red tag simply because you noticed a 5-cm-diameter bruise in the left upper quadrant.

THE CAVALRY ARRIVES

When you and your volunteers have finished the initial triage, rehydrate yourselves if possible and re-triage. As noted earlier, triage is not static; it is a continual process. A patient who is Green initially may turn Yellow or even Red in time. Also, since you may represent the highest level of medical care at the scene, check on your volunteers and make sure they have not inadvertently added themselves to the victim list.

Finally, fire, law enforcement, EMS, and additional agencies begin arriving. It may have only been 15 to 20 minutes, but it felt like hours to you! Their arrival will provide us an opportunity to summarize their traditional roles and responsibilities out in the field during a mass casualty incident (Table 2.5). Why? Much of what has been established in hospitals and on global disaster relief missions has been developed and honed by these knights of pre-hospital safety and care.

The three agencies will establish a command post. This is where inter- and intra-agency communications will be coordinated and where the designated head of each agency will be face to face to confer and interact. It should be located uphill and upwind from the disaster site and outside of the internal perimeter where the victims are located and where search-and-rescue activities will be developing. The *primus inter pares* is the local fire chief—the incident commander. This person and the fire department are responsible for everything: site management, scene safety, operations, victim and personnel safety, hazardous material management, staging, etc. Law enforcement may serve as incident commander or as part of unified command should there be an intentional mass casualty incident or an ongoing crime scene such as a hostage situation. Law enforcement establishes control of the area: ingress and egress to and from the disaster site, internal perimeter,

TABLE 2.5 **Key pre-hospital personnel at a disaster site: roles and responsibilities**

Selected senior personnel on site	Roles and responsibilities
Incident commander	Supervises all activities at the disaster site.
	Usually, the local fire chief or designee.
	May be law enforcement in an intentional incident or when the perpetrator remains at large, or in hostage situations.
Joint command	Several agencies may share command, such as fire and law enforcement.
EMS command	Responsible for all medical care at site.
	Identifies key EMS personnel: triage, treatment, transport officers.
	Works in conjunction with incident commander at command post.
	Coordinates activities with fire and law enforcement.
	Search and rescue activities with fire personnel.
Triage officer	Provides oversight of triage activities within the disaster site.
	Maintains safety of personnel.
	Determines triage parameters.
	Assigns appropriate personnel.
Treatment officer	Oversees activities at field hospital.
	Assigns appropriate personnel for advanced medical procedures.
	Acquires the necessary resources for medical care.
	Prioritizes victims for transport.
	Coordinates activities with transport officer for evacuation prioritization.

TABLE 2.5 **Continued**

Selected senior personnel on site	Roles and responsibilities
Law enforcement	May assume incident command function in the event of perpetrator-at-large or hostage situations.
	Demarcates internal and external perimeters of disaster site.
	Controls access to disaster site.
	Preserves site for forensic investigation.
	Protection of victims and personnel.
Transport officer	Determines hospital capabilities in managing influx of disaster victims.
	Coordinates victim disposition activities with treatment officer.
	Coordinates with staging officer.
	Assigns appropriate conveyance for each victim.
Safety officer	Evaluates environmental, structural, and climatic conditions to determine ongoing safety of personnel and victims at disaster site.
Staging officer	Oversees site(s) for the arrival and disposition of incoming personnel, vehicles, and other resources.
	Logs all resources and provides information to senior command officials.

external perimeter, crowd control, etc. Figure 2.4 shows a map of the scene, including:

1. Command post: One location for the command officers from fire, EMS, law enforcement.
2. Staging: Specific sites are delineated to stage and log in additional personnel, response vehicles, and other resources that may be needed. Requires a staging officer. An additional helicopter landing zone may require development.

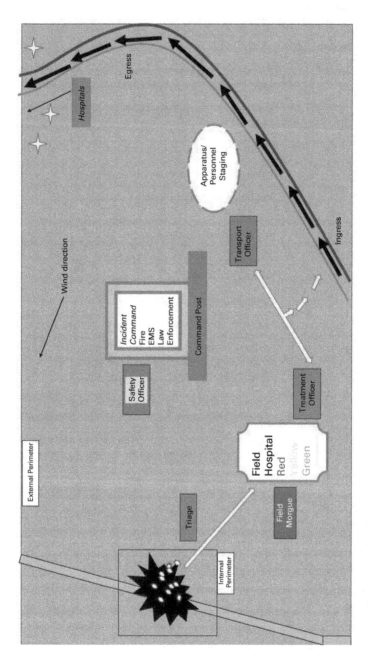

FIGURE 2.4 Diagram of pre-hospital management.

3. Field hospital: Location where the victims receive more sophisticated care.
4. Field morgue: Location where the dead at the field hospital are relocated.
5. Ingress: One-way entry of permitted personnel, vehicles, and other resources.
6. Egress: One-way exit of permitted personnel, vehicles, and casualties.
7. Internal perimeter: Boundary of the actual disaster site and its victims. Personnel may be limited to suitably trained and donned EMS, fire, and search-and-rescue personnel. The first triaging of victims occurs within this perimeter. May be controlled by law enforcement.
8. External perimeter: Boundary between the site where all response efforts for the disaster are occurring and the surrounding uninvolved locations.

EMS activities consist of victim extrication (shared with fire, viz. search and rescue), triage, basic and advanced medical care in the field (from the disaster site to the field hospital), and transport to the hospitals for definitive care. Ideally, your most basic EMTs would be the preferred responders to triage victims at the disaster site. Their basic training should allow them to triage, stop hemorrhage, clear airways, and translocate victims competently. More advanced EMTs or EMT-paramedics (EMT-Ps) should be assigned to the field hospital. Here, more advanced stabilization measures may be required, such as emergency medications, chest thoracostomy, airway intubations, intraosseous infusions, spine stabilization, etc.

In the current situation, once incident command determines that the scene is safe, EMS and fire personnel will begin the process of search and rescue, extrication, and triaging and re-triaging the victims. You have already performed your initial triage of the victims, and that should be satisfactory. However, as we have emphasized, triage is a dynamic process; it is never static. It should occur at multiple locations and at different times at the scene. It will also continue at the hospital and in the hospital. For example, a diabetic victim with an ankle sprain may have given herself insulin that morning but never had time to consume her regular diet. It is not inconceivable that although she was once tagged Green, she may gradually become disoriented or worse. By keeping the concept of dynamic triage in mind, this change in status will be more quickly identified and she would be upgraded to Red for immediate evacuation to the adjacent field hospital or treatment area for more advanced care by EMT-paramedics. After you have identified yourself as a medical professional (especially if you are an emergency physician) and given report, expect to be asked to serve at the field hospital or treatment area to assist with the more advanced patient care.

At the field hospital (Figure 2.5), once a victim has been as stabilized as best as possible, the field hospital officer, in conjunction with the

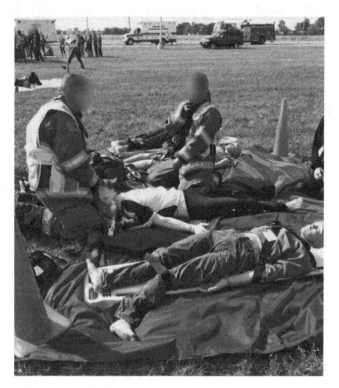

FIGURE 2.5 Part of the field hospital during a community mass casualty incident functional exercise. The red tarpaulin represents the Red zone, where more aggressive and invasive patient care skills occur, such as preoxygenation prior to intubation. EMT-Ps represent a significant part of the care team at this site. Emergency healthcare volunteers may be assigned here also. While tarpaulins are used in drills, bear in mind that they may become slippery with inclement weather or exsanguinating victims.

transport officer, will determine what is the best way for them to reach the hospital (e.g., what type of conveyance, what types of medical personnel transporting, to what type of hospital). Sometimes that can be quite problematic when dealing with a family of different ages and levels of injury; try to keep families together if at all possible.

Should the scene become unsafe or potentially unsafe (inclement weather, unrecognized hazard situation), the incident commander, upon counsel from the safety officer, may shift to a "load-and-go" strategy and order the victims to be loaded into ambulances immediately and transported to the hospitals as the EMT-Ps attempt to stabilize them in route.

Classically, the Red victims are evacuated first, then the Yellows, and finally the Greens. All the Black-tagged victims should remain at the scene and will be processed by the local coroner. These bodies do not leave the area until the coroner orders it. Once Black or dead victims are pronounced dead at the scene, they are not to be touched by anyone for whatever reason without approval of the coroner. The only exception would be to rescue a survivor who may be trapped underneath the body.

For victims who die in the field hospital, for the sake of propriety and out of consideration for the living victims, it is reasonable to move the bodies to an adjacent site out of the view of others. Respect for the bodies must always be maintained.

While our discussion in this chapter has focused on START and SALT triage, keep in mind that these tools appear to work best with the traditional mass casualty incident. There is no consensus of opinion that these tools will be suitable for non-classical events like a biological or radiation incident.

KEY POINTS TO REMEMBER

- Scene safety comes first.
- START triage = 30-2-Can Do.
- START triage's medical interventions are clearing the airway and stopping hemorrhage.
- SALT triage adds needle thoracostomy and antidotal therapy as medical interventions during triage.

Further reading

Bazyar J, Farrokhi M, Khankeh H. Triage systems in mass casualty incidents and disasters: A review study with a worldwide approach. *Open Access Maced J Med Sci*. 2019;7(3):482–494.

Bhalla MC, Frey J, Rider C, Nord M, Hegerhorst M. Simple triage algorithm and rapid treatment and sort, assess, lifesaving, interventions, treatment, and transportation mass casualty triage methods for sensitivity, specificity, and predictive values. *Am J Emerg Med*. 2015;33(11):1687–1691.

Christian MD. Triage. *Crit Care Clin*. 2019;35(4):575–589

Fink BN, Rega PP, Sexton ME, Wishner C. START versus SALT triage: Which is preferred by the 21st-century health care student? *Prehosp Disaster Med*. 2018;33(4):381–386.

Iserson KV, Moskop JC. Triage in medicine, part I: Concept, history, and types. *Ann Emerg Med*. 2007;49(3):275–281.

Lerner EB, Schwartz RB, Coule PL, Weinstein ES, Cone DC, Hunt RC, Sasser SM, Liu JM, Nudell NG, Wedmore IS, Hammond J, Bulger EM, Salomone JP, Sanddal TL, Markenson D, O'Connor RE. Mass casualty triage: An evaluation of the data and development of a proposed national guideline. *Disaster Med Public Health Prep*. 2008;2(Suppl 1):S25–S34.

Moskop JC, Iserson KV. Triage in medicine, part II: Underlying values and principles. *Ann Emerg Med*. 2007;49(3):282–287.

Nakao H, Ukai I, Kotani J. A review of the history of the origin of triage from a disaster medicine perspective. *Acute Med Surg*. 2017;4(4):379–384.

Pepper M, Archer F, Moloney J. Triage in complex, coordinated terrorist attacks. *Prehosp Disaster Med*. 2019;34(4):442–448.

3   The hospital disaster committee: A challenge, a curse, or both?

A spot on the hospital's disaster committee has opened up. You have been asked to "volunteer." The committee typically is populated with middle-management types who have more pressing concerns on their front burners. Your role is to provide an emergency medicine perspective on mass casualties. Hopefully, a disaster medical care perspective will be shared by representatives from surgery, anesthesia, and critical care disciplines.

What do I do now?

Above all, be thankful. You and by extension your ED now have the opportunity to influence all aspects of the disaster cycle instead of merely being a departmental "puppet" manipulated by hospital bureaucratic "strings." But you need to get up to speed as quickly as possible. One never knows when and how the next mass casualty incident will occur. So, in no particular order, the following actions are your immediate priorities.

THE DISASTER RESPONSE AND RECOVERY CYCLE

Disaster response and recovery does not begin when the disaster strikes. Rather, it is a continuing cycle that includes in equal measure preparedness and mitigation strategies (in some quarters, the term "spiral" is substituted for "cycle"). The point is that after recovery from an event, there will be a community debriefing that will address the successes and the challenges that developed in the response to the latest disaster. Then it is hoped that mitigation and preparedness strategies will improve for the next disaster. Hence, the term "spiral" as opposed to "cycle"—it is meant to indicate that your plans will keep improving. This also is an inducement to attend these hospital disaster meetings even though a disaster situation may not appear imminent in your own mind. It is during these quiescent periods that serious discussions can be had about training, resources, and other mitigation and preparedness issues.

Figure 3.1 shows the disaster cycle. Many events will have a warning phase ("disaster warning") to allow time to cogitate, consult, and act. Others, like an earthquake or an active shooter event, will have no warning. In these situations, prior planning and drills will have to suffice. The "disaster recovery" phase represents a time for an unbiased assessment about what actions worked and what challenges need to be addressed for the future. The "mitigation" phase involves identifying and using measures that will prevent the effects of a disaster from impacting something or someone (e.g., moving a house away from a flood zone). The "preparedness" phase addresses actions that need to be employed to blunt the effects of a disaster when it cannot be prevented (e.g., potable water caches). Both the mitigation and preparedness phases constitute the planning process, which, to a large extent, will dictate the success or failure of the next disaster response.

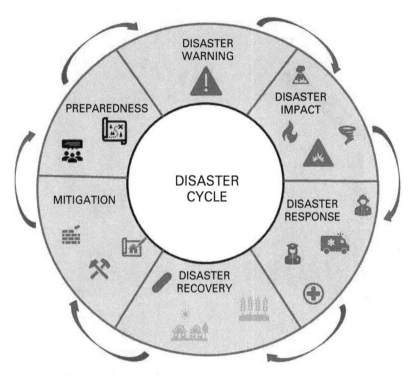

FIGURE 3.1 The disaster cycle.

HOSPITAL DISASTER MANUAL

Read the hospital disaster manual. There is no need to devour the entire tome. Concentrate on the hospital incident command system (HICS); the geographic locations and controllers of the Red, Yellow, and Green zones; the location of the incident command post and the staging area; the incident commander; and the roles and responsibilities of the ED personnel (Figure 3.2).

The disaster plan outlines locations for the Red, Yellow, and Green zones; the roles and responsibilities of all the hospital disaster responders; and the chain of command relative to the HICS. Once the hospital disaster code has been activated, many aspects of the plan should be working concurrently. The HICS command post becomes operational with its personnel and its diverse communication channels open. It should be near but not part of any patient care areas. Similarly, an area

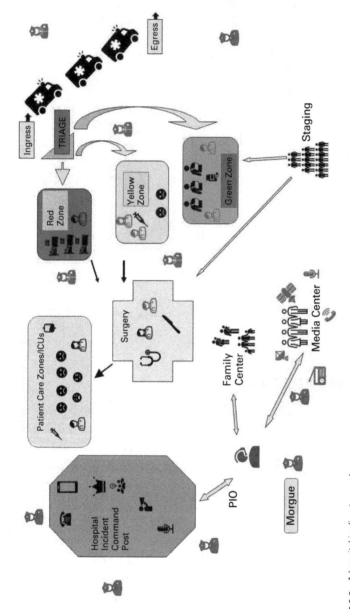

FIGURE 3.2 A hospital in disaster mode.

should be designated for family and friends of the victims (family center or family reunification center) where they can receive information from the hospital's public information officer (PIO). The mental, medical, and physical needs of the families/friends should be managed here, so computers, phones, food, and medical and psychological teams should be readily available in this zone. Another area should be reserved for the media, and it should be equipped with all the journalistic tools required by the print and electronic media. Members of the media may also benefit from nourishment, enhanced communication channels, and medical/psychological assistance. Neither the family center nor the media center should be within geographic proximity of the patient care areas. Likewise, there should be no communication between the media center and the family center. Information to everyone must flow from the PIO in order to minimize misinformation.

The staging area is a key location for a hospital's surge capacity. Individuals, including physicians, who are not immediately needed for the crisis may stage here for impending and future assignments. Names, titles, capabilities, and contact information would be collected here for future use. Security is omnipresent and lockdown has been activated, especially in the more sensitive areas of the hospital.

INCIDENT MANAGEMENT SYSTEMS

Learn about the incident command system (ICS). This is relatively easy to accomplish by simply taking the FEMA Emergency Management Institute (EMI)'s independent study courses (https://training.fema.gov/is/). There are hundreds of them, but the one course to get you started is IS-100.C: Introduction to the Incident Command System, ICS 100. The course provides an overview on the organizational structure (Figure 3.3), the importance of communications, and its command-and-control essentials (e.g., "Who reports to me and to whom do I report?"). The course is free and once you finish the 2-hour session, a test is available (you will first be required to apply for a FEMA student identification number). If you complete the online final exam successfully, a certificate is issued. Keep it for future documentation and verification.

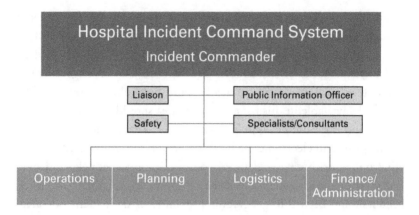

FIGURE 3.3 The top-level command officers in the HICS.

The principles behind the ICS are the same whether it is being employed in the field or in the hospital:

- Common terminology
- Modular organization
- Integrated communications
- Organized and unified command structure
- Coordinated action plan
- Manageable span of control
- Organized and comprehensive resource management

Once you have learned the basics of ICS, then take FEMA EMI's IS-700.B: Introduction to the National Incident Management System (NIMS). NIMS goes beyond ICS (Figure 3.4). It provides an overview of how local, state, tribal, federal, private, and public governmental and non-governmental stakeholders come together to prepare for and respond to a critical incident—any incident, from local to national. It involves command and control of incidents, resource management, and information management. NIMS is a system that organizes a preparedness and response strategy; coordinates communications; provides a unified, consistent voice for information management and dissemination; and manages current and future resource needs. While NIMS may be used for any event, it is imperative that it be activated during a complex or catastrophic disaster when many stakeholders near and far come together to provide timely assistance.

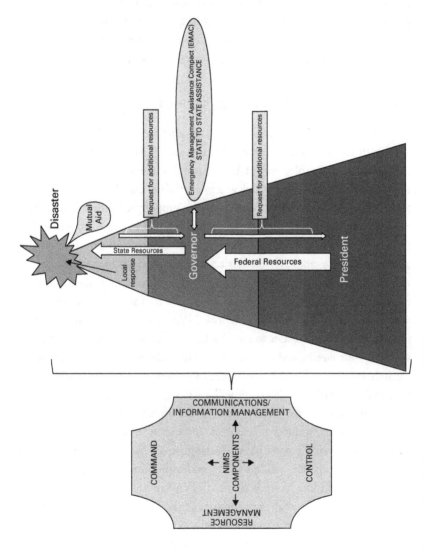

FIGURE 3.4 The National Incident Management System (NIMS).

Granted that this additional knowledge may not be necessary in the typical mass casualty incident, but remember that the diverse natural and technological stressors that were evident in the 20th century will likely be compounded and fracture societal underpinnings in the 21st century. The NIMS course is about 3.5 hours long and has an online final exam (again, you will need a FEMA student identification number). Once you've passed it, you are issued a certificate. Save this document too.

HAZARDS VULNERABILITY ANALYSIS (HVA)

Review the hospital's HVA. This is the hospital's attempt to enumerate the specific threats that may occur in the community. They can be natural, technological, or a combination of both natural and technological, and accidental or intentional. A thorough analysis estimates each hazard's probability and its potential impact (human, business, property), historical frequency, and impact. Factors that should be considered include an historical review of the types of emergencies and disasters that have struck the hospital and/or community, geographic characteristics (fault zone, coastline, etc.), community characteristics/demographics (mean age, diversity, language challenges, etc.), distance from transportation routes, cities, industries, or military bases, and climatic changes. A comprehensive HVA procures and evaluates these multifactorial data in order to identify factors that may be serious threats to yourself, your family, and your hospital. This vulnerability assessment is intimately intertwined with the community's efforts to recognize each threat's potential for death and destruction. This recognition serves to mitigate the threat entirely or to prepare for its eventual impact. This is done through planning sessions, caching of resources, and extensive training.

There are multiple ways of conducting the HVA in terms of numbers, percentages, or merely qualitative adjectives (i.e., low, medium, or high). What you would like to see is that the HVA is evaluated at least annually, that it is the product of all the members of the disaster team, and that it is shared with the rest of the community.

Figure 3.5 shows examples of HVAs for two fictitious communities in the United States. Your hospital's or your community's risk is the sum of the likelihood of a particular event and its potential impact minus all the preparedness strategies to mitigate that impact. These assessments are typically

EVENT (natural, human accident, human, intentional, technological)	How likely will a particular event occur? (Score: 0 = not likely–5 = very likely)	Potential impact on people, property, and infrastructure (Score: 0 = no impact–5 = very significant impact)			How prepared is the hospital/community in planning for and responding to the event? Training, resources, etc. Score: 0 = unprepared–5 = fully prepared)			RISK level (Scoring: Potential + Impact – Preparedness = Risk Level)
		Human	Property	Infrastructure	Training	Resources	Mutual Aid	
Wildfires	4	4	5	5	5	3	4	18–12 = 6
Earthquakes (>7M)	2	4	5	4	4	3	0	15–7 = 8

HVA for the fictitious community of Opalonka, California

EVENT (natural, human accident, human, intentional, technological)	How likely will a particular event occur? (Score: 0 = not likely–5 = very likely)	Potential impact on people, property, and infrastructure (Score: 0 = no impact–5 = very significant impact)			How prepared is the hospital/community in planning for and responding to the event? Training, resources, etc. Score: 0 = unprepared–5 = fully prepared)			RISK level (Scoring: Potential + Impact – Preparedness = Risk Level)
		Human	Property	Infrastructure	Training	Resources	Mutual Aid	
Terrorism	1	2	1	0	3	2	4	4–9 = 5
Flooding	4	3	5	4	4	3	5	16–12 = 4

HVA for the fictitious coastal community of Toolip, Long Island, N.Y.

FIGURE 3.5 Examples of HVAs for two fictitious U.S. communities.

subjective on the part of the committee members, and the final document should represent a consensus of those members.

Let's consider some examples. A tsunami in Iowa is an impossibility. Therefore, the risk is 0 or not likely at all, and the HVA for that event has a risk of 0. Nothing further needs to be analyzed. On the other hand, a rural community may deem that a terrorist attack is worth a "1" on the threat level. However, should it occur, it could create a significant negative impact on the population, the businesses, and the infrastructure due to lack of precedent, interest, resources, and training. Then it is up to the hospital/community to decide how to proceed after that evaluation.

Meanwhile, the hospitals in Washington, D.C., should consider terrorism events. The risk there is high in terms of morbidity, mortality and infrastructural compromise, and the HVA scoring of its impact should reflect that possibility. On the other hand, the resources and training of governmental and non-governmental stakeholders may be such that the final risk assessment may actually be at the medium level in the aggregate. However, a city like Washington, D.C., or New York City would go deeper into generic terrorism events to gauge the risk for the multiple types of intentional acts like a "dirty bomb," a sarin attack, or even armed insurrection.

While institutional HVAs tend to be somewhat static (meaning that they get dusted off once or twice a year), you should not be locked into that same mindset. If an event is occurring that may involve large crowds (e.g., charity drives, marathons, and festivals) or may have some controversial activities associated with it (e.g., protests, political conferences), it would not be unreasonable to alert your ED personnel about the possibility and prepare accordingly. In fact, mass gathering medicine is a subspecialty within disaster medicine. Anytime there is an event that will involve significant numbers of participants and/or attendees, it behooves the hospital disaster committee to convene outside of the usual meeting schedule and simply touch base about the event and any preparedness issues (Box 3.1).

Finally, consider developing an HVA for you, your family, and your home. It will help in developing your own disaster plan.

BOX 3.1 **Mass gathering considerations**

WHO
– Participants: demographics, numbers, ages, event stressors
– Spectators: demographics, numbers, ages, likely medical conditions

WHAT
– Historical overview of the event

WHERE
– Geography
– Climate
– Indoors vs. outdoors: hazards
– Mobile: main route, secondary routes, ingress, egress
– Fixed: Ingress, egress

WHEN
– Gates opening/closing
– Event start time
– Event closing time
–Total hours
–Total days: hours/day
–Total weeks: days/week

WHY
– Religious event
– Sporting event
– Political event

HOW
– Medical preparedness and response
– Manpower numbers
– Medical disciplines
–Work hours
– Personal preparedness/gear: routine
– Personal preparedness/gear: unusual
– Medical equipment: routine
– Medical equipment: extraordinary

KEY POINTS TO REMEMBER

· Review the hospital's disaster manual.
· Understand the hospital's HICS.
· Understand the implications of the NIMS.

- Perform your own HVA and risk assessment.
- Know where you fit in to the hospital's HICS (role and responsibilities).

Further reading

FEMA. Hazard Identification and Risk Assessment. https://www.fema.gov/hazard-identification-and-risk-assessment

FEMA. *National Incident Management System* (3rd ed.). FEMA; 2017.

Mclsaac J, Gentz BA. Preparing for mass casualty events. *Anesthesiol Clin.* 2020;38:821–837.

4 When even the birds die

That highway scene filled with mangled trucks
and cars just does not look right. There are
trauma victims, coughing and vomiting. Birds
and squirrels near the scene are lying still along
the road. A sickly yellow-green smoke is issuing
from one of the semis and is hovering over the
trauma field.

What do I do now?

top exactly where you are. The scene is not safe. Alert any potential rescuers arriving at the MCI. All of you should consider yourselves as potential victims, not potential rescuers. Keep in mind the adage "Uphill, upwind, upstream":

- Uphill because those chemicals that are heavier than air will increase your exposure time
- Upwind because downstream air currents will carry the toxic cloud away from the emission site
- Upstream because the toxins in the waters will flow with the current, not against the current

Additionally, what is the traditional distance at which you may consider yourself secure? The rule of thumb is the rule of thumb, meaning that if you can cover the disaster site with your raised thumb, then you should be safe from its impact.

INCIDENCE OF HAZMAT EVENTS

A mass casualty HAZMAT event is not common. In fact, it is quite rare in the United States. A recent review of more than 17 million EMS activations indicated that a little more than 2,500 were HAZMAT related. Out of that sub-group, just 5.6% were coded as an MCI.

Since these situations are so infrequent, a scene response may be prone to errors. In 2019 in Illinois, a farm tractor's mechanical failure resulted in the release of approximately 500 gallons of anhydrous ammonia. Drivers, passengers, and responders who were exposed to the plume of white gas were overcome with coughing, choking, and difficulty breathing. Among the 35 patients who required EMS transport to local EDs, 13 were first responders who smelled the acrid gas and entered the plume without donning proper PPE. One of them required intubation and mechanical ventilation in the ICU.

IF YOU SUSPECT A HAZMAT EVENT

Should you suspect a HAZMAT incident, go no farther yourself, and direct any potential rescuers to go no farther as well. Call 911 and alert the dispatcher of your suspicions. Double-check your current location to ensure that it is safe from potential HAZMAT spread. Usually that would mean that you are at an altitude higher than the disaster site's, the wind is at your back, and you can cover the disaster site with your outstretched thumb.

Clues that a disaster site may involve or has the potential to involve hazardous materials include the following:

1. Crunched trucks, semis, and railroad cars. Legal and illegal hazardous materials travel the highways, byways, and railways of this country. Vehicles and railcars that transport hazardous materials are required by the U.S. Department of Transportation (DOT) to carry specific documents and to post what they are carrying on the outside of their containers. The symbols on the placards would alert responders and the public about the exact contents. Having the DOT's emergency response guidebook or at least the DOT Chart 16 in your vehicle for a quick reference demonstrates both initiative and foresight on your part. In fact, the DOT Chart 16 is a free downloadable app to your smartphone. Of course, since you will be at a safe distance from the site, having either excellent eyesight or binoculars would be a blessing. However, just relaying to 911 that you are seeing a diamond-shaped placard on a container and little else is still important information to deliver.

2. Dead or dying animals. Creatures of the wild may not be part of the event, but they are still exposed to the noxious chemicals issuing from the conveyances and they can easily be symptomatic.

3. Multicolored smoke. Smoke arising from fires is typically degrees of white and black. Green, yellow, or any other color that blends in with the smoke suggests hazardous material. Chlorine, for example, can create a yellow-green smoke. In the Illinois anhydrous ammonia case, the plume was described as "white," which may have created a false sense of security among the initial responders.

4. Unusual odors. If you are smelling anything emanating from the scene, you are too close and downwind; clear out! Again, regarding the Illinois accidental ammonia release, that particular chemical has a distinct, easily recognizable odor and should have been enough of

a warning to the responders that it was a HAZMAT situation and they should don appropriate gear.

5. Liquid spills. Anything on the ground could simply be water from ruptured radiators, but it could be gasoline or worse. Do not consider gasoline as benign: It can generate fires and lead to chain-reaction explosions.

6. Seizing victims. Seizures may indicate head injuries and hypoxia, but they could also signify exposure to a noxious agent, such as an organophosphate or carbamate leak.

Contaminated victims might be heading in your direction for assistance. By doing so they are expanding the HAZMAT "hot zone" and incorporating you into it. To minimize the potential for your exposure, encourage them to stop away from you, remove their outer clothes, and have them douse themselves with whatever liquids may be in your possession. Removing their outer garments should remove up to 90% of their contaminants.

EMS RESPONSE

When the first responders come on scene and confirm the possibility of a HAZMAT situation, their response will be more structured and deliberate. The incident commander, typically the local fire chief, will have multiple objectives that need to be addressed immediately (Box 4.1). The actions in this case, as with any disaster response, will be more concurrent than sequential. Simply stated, the role and responsibility of the incident

---

BOX 4.1 **Responsibilities of the incident commander when coming upon a possible HAZMAT event**

- Confirm a HAZMAT incident.
- Identify the agent and its associated repercussions.
- Stop or control the release of the agent.
- Ensure rescuer safety.
- Provide victim care.
- Protect against contamination of potential victims in the vicinity.
- Protect environment.
- Consider an intentional release and alert proper authorities.

commander is to serve and protect the responders, save and protect the victims, guard against the contamination of additional victims in the path of the release, and protect the environment.

THREE ZONES

Depending on the agent's characteristics and risk potential, the disaster site will be divided into three sectors: hot, warm, and cold (Figure 4.1).

The hot zone is the contamination zone. It contains the non-ambulatory victims and the source of the hazardous material. The perimeter of that zone can stay stable or expand depending on various factors such as volatility of the agent, the severity of the wind and its direction, and other environmental factors (e.g., natural water sources). It is in this zone that the local HAZMAT team in their Level A PPE operate. They are there for search and rescue as well as gross decontamination of the victims (Figure 4.2). Medical management of the victims will be problematic due to the constraints of the Level A PPE and the amount of time the HAZMAT team can work in them. The other principal objective is to stop ongoing hazards and quell the spread of the hazardous materials to virgin territory.

At some point, the victims will be transferred to the warm zone, where more sophisticated decontamination equipment will be positioned. Here, more medical interventions can begin, such as antidote administration. The responders in this zone could be wearing Level B PPE. Theoretically, by this time the victims, with their outer clothes removed, are free of about 90% to 95% of any surface contamination and present little to no contamination threat to their rescuers.

With the conclusion of the decontamination process, they are allowed entry into the cold zone, where further triage, stabilization, and sophisticated medical interventions are under way.

It is important to consider two potential complications:

1. There will be contaminated ambulatory victims who have no idea about HAZMAT zones. They are looking for help, but in the process of doing so, they are at risk for contaminating others. Mini-teams may need to be developed on the spot to corral

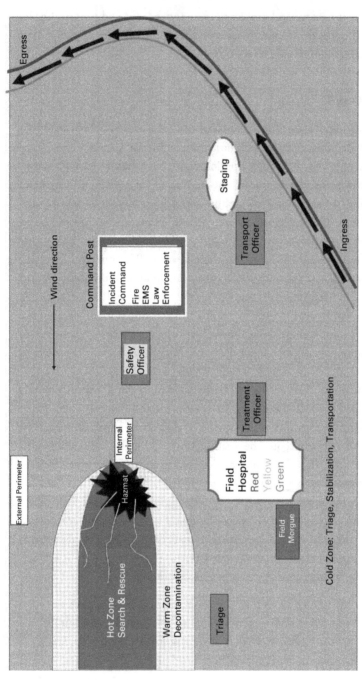

FIGURE 4.1 HAZMAT scene response. The key to a proper response to a HAZMAT incident is to identify, mark off, and control the three zones of response. The hot zone, where the HAZMAT release has occurred, is also the site where non-ambulatory and/or trapped contaminated victims are located. The warm zone is the site for initial management and decontamination of the victims. The cold zone is the HAZMAT-free site, where normal operations are occurring. Note that the cold zone operations are upwind from the release site.

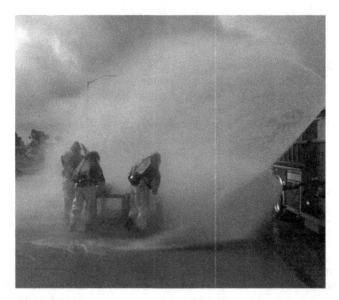

FIGURE 4.2 An example of HAZMAT decontamination in the field. Note that in this exercise, the responders are in Level B PPE. While in this drill the "victim" is non-ambulatory, the set-up could easily function as an expeditious modality to decontaminate a large number of ambulatory victims. During this process, attention must be given to infants and children, who can easily become hypothermic before, during, and after the process. Similarly, the geriatric population must receive careful attention; due to possible mental and physical infirmities, they may become confused, agitated, and injured.

these individuals in order to protect them from further harm to themselves and to others.

2. A HAZMAT scene is a dynamic situation and therefore more unpredictable than a routine MCI. Sudden wind shifts can dramatically alter the geographic demarcations of the three operational zones and create a situation where the responders become additional victims. There may be no other options than to relocate the operational areas of the cold zone and declare that further patient care, after decontamination, will follow "load-and-go" procedures.

LEVELS OF PPE

PPE is essential. There are four basic types: Level A, B, C, and D. Table 4.1 summarizes Levels C and D PPE commonly employed in hospitals.

TABLE 4.1 **Levels C and D PPE**

Gear	Purpose	Usage
Level C PPE		
Chemical-resistant suit, gloves, boots (seams)	Threat of severe ocular and skin damage is low.	Pre-hospital cold zone
Air-purifying respirators (APRs) and powered air-purifying respirators (PAPRs)	Respiratory threat is possible, but not likely to be severe.	Hospital personnel
Level D PPE		
Street clothes, work clothes, scrub suits	No dermatologic hazard. Minimize nuisance contamination.	Pre-hospital cold zone personnel and hospital personnel
Surgical masks Face/eye shields	Respiratory threat is possible, but not likely to be severe. Infectious disease prevention.	Pre-hospital cold zone personnel and hospital personnel

KEY POINTS TO REMEMBER

- Upload the DOT's Emergency Response Guidebook to your smartphone.
- Before entering the scene, look for indications of a HAZMAT release.
- Stay uphill, upwind, and upstream from a possible HAZMAT release.
- Removing a victim's external clothes will remove the majority of their contamination.

Further reading

Martin AJ, Lohse CM, Sztajnkrycer MD. A descriptive analysis of prehospital response to hazardous materials events. *Prehosp Disaster Med.* 2015;30(5):466–471.

Rispens JR, Jones SA, Clemmons NS, Ahmed S, Harduar-Morano L, Johnson MD, Edge C 3rd, Vyas A, Bourgikos E, Orr MF. Anhydrous ammonia chemical release—Lake County, Illinois, April 2019. *MMWR Morb Mortal Wkly Rep.* 2020;69(4):109–113.

U.S. Department of Transportation. DOT Chart 16: Hazardous Materials Markings, Labeling, and Placarding Guide. https://www.phmsa.dot.gov/sites/phmsa.dot.gov/files/2020-07/USDOT%20Chart%2016%20PHH50%200162%201117%20WEB.pdf [also available as a free mobile app]

U.S. Department of Transportation. Emergency Response Guidebook 2020. https://www.phmsa.dot.gov/hazmat/erg/emergency-response-guidebook-erg

5 The Bat-Phone rings: The tornado and the trailer park

It is 3:46 p.m. on a Sunday afternoon that, according to the local meteorologists, will shortly be inundated by a threatening weather system. The ER is moderately busy with the usual assortment of chest pains, ankle sprains, earaches, and fender-benders. The weather people were a little behind in their predictions as the beeps, clicks, and rings of the ER compete with the thunder outside the ambulance bay. A call from EMS grabs the attention of the nurse who answered it. She quickly calls you, saying there is a disaster. Your physical and mental posture shifts from casual to resolute. You are ready for report while waving your charge nurse to your side, "Go ahead, Squad 10." She says, "It looks like a tornado hit the trailer park on Central and West. We are thinking about a couple of hundred people were there at the time. There are bodies all over the place. Search and rescue are going through the debris right now. The weather still sucks, so we might load and go with whoever is alive. You are the closest hospital. That's it." The phone goes dead. The nurse and you look at each other, enveloped by the cacophony of the ER.

What do I do now?

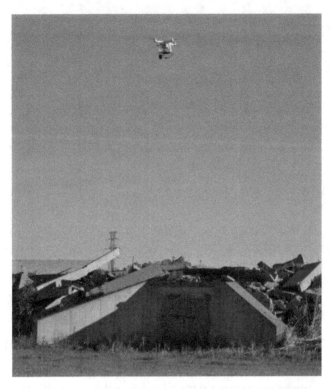

FIGURE 5.1   An unmanned aerial vehicle (UAV) hovering over the disaster site. This was an exercise demonstrating the value of a drone in viewing and televising a disaster site from a bird's-eye viewpoint. Properly equipped UAVs or drones can be quite useful in identifying living and dead victims and any ongoing threats.

GETTING READY

In the old days, the emergency physician, after getting report, would instruct the operator to announce a "Code: Disaster." Disaster code activation can be somewhat more complicated once the hospital hierarchy is alerted, but it does improve overall communications within the hospital. More than likely the nursing administrator on call will have to be notified with the particulars and then will activate the "Code: Disaster." Regardless of how the announcement is made, your role is straightforward:

1. Notify the administration.
2. Alert ED staff.

3. Designate ED disaster leadership.
4. Assign specific roles and responsibilities to specific individuals on the ED team.
5. Don disaster vests.
6. Emergency task management.

Once the administration has been notified, convene the ED staff and for a couple of minutes tell everyone what you know, who is in charge, and what needs to happen (Figure 5.2). Staff members need to ready themselves both physically and mentally, and as quickly as possible. As they are absorbing the shock of the upcoming disaster response, you are going to need to go into overdrive yourself. Why this sense of urgency? Let's review a couple of historical examples:

- On March 11, 2004, Madrid exploded with multiple terrorist bombings within the rail system. These explosions killed 177 people immediately and sent more than 2,000 wounded to hospitals. Gregorio Marañón University General Hospital (GMUGH) received 312 casualties; 272 of them arrived through its ED doors between 8 and 10:30 a.m.

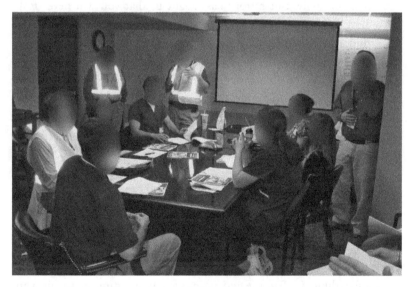

FIGURE 5.2 Hospital incident command drill. Note that certain key personnel have donned identifying vests.

- On June 27, 1995, Tokyo's subway system was the target of the multiple nerve-agent attacks around 7:55 a.m.—rush hour. St. Luke's Hospital received its first call from EMS at 8:16 a.m. Within the first half-hour, the hospital's first sarin victim arrived on foot, complaining of visual difficulties. Within the first hour, St. Luke's received about 500 victims because the hospital was within 2 miles of the subway stations where the sarin releases occurred.

The point is that you, your ED, and your hospital must get ready quickly because the victims may begin arriving within minutes. There may not be a delay during which they are rescued, triaged, and stabilized by EMS before being transported to your facility. After the Las Vegas-MGM mass shooting on October 1, 2017, even before EMS arrived, many of the wounded drove themselves to the nearby hospitals using mapping apps on their smartphones or were driven to the closest EDs by the heroic efforts of those at the scene. Those heroes included law enforcement personnel who believed they could get the victims to the ED faster than waiting for an ambulance.

If you have practiced your table-top exercises and your drills, pretty much everyone should comprehend the significance of what is happening and act accordingly. But history has taught us that you will never really know how many victims are coming, how quickly they are coming, and what kind of dangers they may present to you and your staff.

The bottom line here is: Hope for the best but prepare for the worst. Do it quickly, calmly, and efficiently. A team huddle is important since, as the emergency physician, you are the incident commander of the ED in conjunction with your charge nurse. Let everyone know what is coming and what to expect. This is crisis leadership at its most pristine. Remind them that this is the reason you have been training.

COMMUNICATIONS

Notice that the underlying theme in the first few moments of this new event is communications. In improperly managed MCIs, the first element to fail is communications. Communication channels should be open, constant, and redundant. Because one means of communications can fail at any moment, it is critical to have diverse means of communications, including face to face; runners, notepads, and pencils; bullhorns; hospital phones; personal cellphones; text messaging; hand-held radios; the hospital public address system; social media; the internet; and ham radios. What you stock and what you will use as first-, second-, and third-line means of communications should have already been discussed, procured, taught, and drilled. Naturally, the resources and guidance from your information technology and legal departments are important. When "disaster communications" is on the agenda of the disaster committee, lay out the framework as to how certain people need to speak to other people. Everyone needs to understand that one system may be compromised, accidentally or intentionally, and that another system must come online immediately while a backup is being prepared.

To underscore the importance of redundancy in communications, there is no way to minimize the importance of ham radio operators. Because of their established networks and expertise, they can communicate short distances, long distances, and very long distances when no one else can. During Hurricane Marilyn, we were able to communicate from St. Thomas in the Virgin Islands to Toledo, Ohio, by way of ham radio operators when our team could not do so using satellite phones. Therefore, in your plans and drills, invite these communications experts to participate and be part of your team.

Donning ED disaster vests is another important aspect of communications. Knowing at a glance who is "triage" or "ED command" or "chaplain" based on their vest informs everyone without needless chatter.

FIRST WAVE AND SECOND WAVE

If you are the closest hospital to the disaster site, your hospital is going to get hit first and significantly so. Regardless of how much fire, EMS, and law enforcement personnel train and teach about distributing victims as evenly as possible to all the hospitals in the community, a disproportionate number will arrive at the closest hospital. This can be even more nettlesome if that hospital is also a Level 1 Trauma institution. This is the "First Wave Phenomenon": The hospital nearest the disaster will be receiving the initial onslaught of victims. These victims may have evacuated themselves, in which case they are more than likely Green patients. On the other hand, expect that even Red or Yellow patients may be arriving at your ED, having been transported by Good Samaritans whose only goal is to reach the closest hospital as quickly as possible. These victims, therefore, will not have not been triaged or stabilized by EMS; in fact, EMS may not even have arrived prior to their evacuation. Therefore, this first wave will consist of victims at all levels of severity, from the "walking wounded," to the "moribund," to the dead.

The "second wave" of victims will be the more traditional ones who have been rescued, triaged, and transported. The degree of medical stabilization will be determined by the decision of the EMS personnel to "stay and play" or "load and go."

Of course, hospitals farther away from the disaster site will also be involved to some extent. Consider that in a major MCI, field operations personnel at the scene may have decided to transport the Green patients by bus to more distant hospitals in order to alleviate the patient load on the nearest hospitals. This is what occurred on November 21, 1980, at the MGM Grand fire in Las Vegas, Nevada. Apart from the 84 deaths, EMS had to triage about 3,000 people at the scene. Incident command drafted school buses to transport the Green victims. If non-medical transportation (e.g., a commercial bus) is being employed to move Green victims from one place to another, it would be prudent to insert a medic on the bus in case of any emergency and to have an ambulance following along for an emergency transportation.

What happens when there are few hospitals? The ED team of the closest hospital may elect to triage the incoming victims by managing the Red and Yellow victims themselves while triaging the Green ones to outlying hospitals. This tactic should be discussed and vetted at regional disaster meetings so that no one is surprised.

DISPOSITION OF CURRENT ED PATIENTS

Efforts must be made to clear the ED of the current patients expeditiously but safely. It seems simple to discharge to home the patients who appear non-acute, but beware! Is that 39-year-old patient with heartburn waiting impatiently in the waiting room really a case of acid indigestion, or a myocardial infarction in evolution? How about the 18-year-old with the chief complaint of "foreign body, right eye" who is waiting for a slit-lamp examination? Might it not be a penetrating injury to the globe? Discharging patients with conditions that appear innocuous may be detrimental to the patient as well as to you and the hospital. What are some safer alternatives?

One way of handling these cases is to triage all these patients to the most appropriate disaster zones that are being activated within the hospital: Red, Yellow, and Green zones. Yes, the Red zone can still be the ED itself, with its critical care nurses and physicians at the ready, but at least your Green and Yellow patients can be transported to other areas of the hospital where they will be assessed by others. Plan to have their ED records easily accessible by the caregivers in those zones.

The best way of handling the current ED patients may be to use a "disaster admit team," developed as part of the hospital's disaster plan. When the disaster code is activated, the ED team no longer takes primary responsibility for the patients currently in the department. The admit team receives patient transfer from the ED team and expeditiously evaluates and decides on a disposition for them. This allows the ED team to concentrate on the arriving disaster victims.

This is a strategy that has been employed in Israel as hospitals received bombing victims. It was also used during the Boston Marathon bombing, which occurred at 2:49 p.m. April 15, 2013. This was especially relevant in Boston, given the fact that the bombing site was cleared of serious victims within 22 minutes. While these examples were intentional incidents, there is no reason why this strategy cannot be applied to any type of MCI.

While the most severe patients will be herded into the ED, consider establishing a "Redder" microsite within the ED. Patients with the most life-threatening conditions would be filtered to that area, where the staff and physicians with the greatest expertise would be located. Airway carts, chest tube trays, and intraosseous drills would be out and ready to use. This may not be needed in an area where physicians and physician extenders are plentiful, but if only one or two ED physicians are readily available, concentrate your expertise.

Is there a role for a surgeon to take over ED command? Definitely not! The ED physician knows the ED and the ED staff and can perform all the life-saving techniques as well as anyone. What specialty can handle the A, B, Cs in a chaotic environment better than an ED physician? Surgery and anesthesia personnel are useful adjuncts to the emergency physician, but ultimately their expertise is best suited for the surgical suites.

TRIAGE

When discussing disaster triage at an ED, three issues should be discussed during the planning stage:

- Who will conduct triage as the victims begin arriving?
- What triage tool will be employed?
- What resources will be needed at triage?

Who will conduct triage? Who will be the triage officer? Triage comes from the French word *trier*, "to sort." Sorting patients based on severity is well within the wheelhouse of experienced ED nurses. They perform this skill every day, and practice makes perfect. Emergency physicians, while they are equipped to perform triage duties, should be prepared to receive victims and render expert medical care. This guidance would also hold true for other physicians regardless of specialty. Physician resources are limited compared to nursing; therefore, physicians' skills would be needed at the bedside. Generally speaking, this would also hold true for physician assistants and nurse practitioners. Within the ED, the victims' surgical, imaging, and ancillary requirements will be prioritized by the appropriate physician specialty available. That will be part of the internal triage process.

What triage tool should be used? It can be a continuation of the triage tool being used in the pre-hospital environment (e.g., START or SALT) or it can be an extension or modification of the ED's everyday Emergency Severity Index (ESI) triage algorithm. International studies have proposed alternative tools and now there is ongoing research dealing with machine learning and ED triage. Whatever tool has been decided upon internally must also be drilled at regular intervals.

What triage resources should accompany the triage officer at the triage station? The simple answer is "as little as possible." The triage officer who has been selected based upon experience, training, stamina, and steadiness will have the benefit of four of their five senses (touch, sight, hearing, and smell) to make rapid triage decisions. Monitors and blood pressure equipment take too much time and delay definitive care. At most, a portable pulse oximeter may be useful. However, the triage officer will need the following additional manpower to expedite the triage process:

- A registrar to enter the victim into the hospital's in-patient tracking and tracing system (e.g., a barcode registration system). This function may have already been initiated in the field.
- A photographer to photograph the victim's face and any easily available alternative means of identification (e.g., tattoos, scars). With the assistance of the information technology and legal departments, these photographs may be added to a secure website to assist families in locating and identifying their loved ones in large-scale disasters.
- A scribe to document and attach the triage officer's assessment of each patient as well as the patient's assignment to one of the patient care zones.
- Transporters
- A clean-up crew

IMAGING

If the disaster occurs any afternoon from Monday to Friday, imaging resources both in terms of personnel and equipment may be plentiful. Nevertheless, while you can hope for the best, always prepare for the worst. Use the radiology department judiciously. Work with them to develop a disaster imaging guidance. Not everyone from an MCI merits a "Pan-Scan." Here are several guidelines that can alleviate the pressures on the radiology personnel and still maintain good patient care:

- No patients in the Green zone should receive an X-ray, except under extraordinary conditions. And if the situation is extraordinary, then it is more than likely the patient was mis-triaged and should have been sent to the Yellow or even the Red zone. Extremity trauma, for example, require splinting and non-weightbearing. Imaging can be deferred at a later date once it has been determined that no vascular or neurologic problem is present. To order and obtain an ankle film on a Green patient would needlessly occupy the time of both the equipment and the personnel that could be used more efficaciously in the Yellow or Red zones.

· In Red and Yellow zones, bedside imaging should be confined to the torso. Therefore, C-spine, AP CXR, pelvis, and extended FAST exams are reasonable. On the other hand, extremity X-rays serve no immediate purpose. The judicious use of routine point-of-care radiologic imaging will allow the radiology department to concentrate on those cases that indeed do require CT scans and MRIs.

· Consider having a radiologist immediately available, at least in the ED, as part of the ED team. They will be of great assistance in triaging victims into the radiologic suites and will be of enormous assistance in synchronous imaging interpretation.

· The Green and Yellow zones may not be in normal patient care areas of the hospital. If feasible, dispatching portable X-ray equipment to those sites could save time and needless communications.

LABORATORY SERVICES

Treat laboratory services the same way you are treating radiology. Again, not every victim requires a Chem Profile or toxicology panels. The emergency physician needs to avoid the easy knee-jerk reflex and concentrate on ordering only the tests that are needed now. When the dust settles, then more elaborate testing would be appropriate.

Therefore, you can obtain enough blood and urine for myriad testing down the line, but you may want to consider developing a guidance or advisory stating which tests are permissible in the immediate aftermath of an MCI. Here are some examples of appropriate lab studies in the immediate aftermath of a disaster:

· Hemoglobin/hematocrit
· Type and screen or type and crossmatch
· Fingerstick glucose
· Urine dipstick
· UCG (pregnancy test)

This minimalist approach could free up laboratory equipment and personnel when the ED must evaluate and resuscitate a series of Red victims such as a 60-year-old male bombing victim with a BP of 80 mmHg and a Glasgow Coma Scale (GCS) score of 9 who is wearing medical alert bracelets for diabetes and blood thinners.

BLOOD PRODUCTS AND SERVICES

Since the majority of simple disasters deal with trauma, the resources of your blood bank must be addressed. How can one predict how much blood is required in an MCI? One study from Israel looked at nearly 1,000 victims from 18 terrorist attacks in Tel Aviv. A total of 332 units of packed red blood cells (PRBCs) were transfused. Half of the units were administered to less than 5% of the patients and within the first couple of hours of presentation. The researchers concluded that 1 to 2 units of blood per victim should be considered for planning purposes. This conclusion was validated by another study emanating from Operation Iraqi Freedom. Over 770 evacuees required blood transfusions (4.2% required mass transfusions), with a mean number of PRBCs + whole blood of 1.4 units per patient. The qualifier, to ensure that everyone is on the same page, is the "packed cells per patient index" (PPI).

IN THE AFTERMATH

Eventually, your ED has received its allotment of victims and your team has provided the best in disaster medical care. In keeping with the concept of a "simple" disaster (i.e., an MCI at which the infrastructure remains intact to resolve the crisis), it only took a matter of hours. Your ED is now settling down to providing care for the usual assortment of routine patients: the MIs, the belly pains, the ocular foreign body. With good planning by the planning and logistics arms of the hospital incident command system, those individuals who arduously rendered care in extreme circumstances will be relieved of their duties by relief personnel. That is an important aspect of surge capacity. The hospital meanwhile will continue in disaster mode as there will be an ongoing management of trauma patients in the operating suites and the ICU. The hospital incident command system will be constantly assessing the situation for days, if not weeks. Their activities will include issuing press releases, possible patient transfers to specialty centers, attention to the needs of the victims' families, etc.

To illustrate the intricacies of a "simple" disaster, it would be worthwhile to examine in greater detail what occurred at San Francisco General Hospital (SFGH) when Asiana Airlines Flight 214 crashed at San Francisco International Airport on Saturday, July 6, 2013. At that time, SFGH was the only Level 1 Trauma Center in the city and county. The crash occurred in the late morning. Of the more than 300 passengers and crew, 192 victims were injured, 49 seriously. The hospital received 63 victims, including 10 deemed to be in critical condition.

In anticipation of mass casualties, the hospital erected triage tents outside of the ED, transferred non-critical ICU patients to the floor, and expedited the discharge of in-house patients. The first victims arrived by ambulances within 45 minutes of the crash, and several of the critical cases were transferred to the operating suites within minutes of arrival. On hand to meet these victims and expedite care was a team of five ED attendings and three trauma surgeons. Four attending radiologists were drafted to expedite imaging interpretations. This was critical because due to the type of blunt-force impact, there was a liberal use of CT scans (50.8% of the cases) as well as eFAST (Extended Focused Assessment with Sonography for Trauma) exams. The senior trauma surgeon determined which victims received a CT and in what order.

Blood resources were also a critical logistical issue (as in any MCI). Within the first 2 days, the victims at SFGH received 52 units of PRBCs, 53 units of plasma, 8 pooled units of platelets, and 4 units of cryoprecipitate. Needless to say, communication with the blood bank from the very beginning of the incident is compulsory.

This report came from a major hospital with a Level 1 Trauma Center. How these logistical matters are handled in non-academic, non-trauma suburban hospitals is rather nebulous due to lack of peer-reviewed literature.

All of the hospitals involved with the Air Asiana incident had to deal with the press, the National Transportation Safety Board, the Federal Aviation Administration, and South Korean embassy officials. In addition, many of the passengers only spoke Korean. The last factor may not be an issue in cosmopolitan San Francisco, but what if the crash had occurred in DuBois, Pennsylvania? The issue of language barriers is not a minimal one, and the repercussions go well beyond disaster medicine and into everyday emergency medicine. In a study published in 2004 in *American Surgeon*, the authors performed a nine-year retrospective review of trauma patients who were intubated at a trauma center. Forty-nine percent of Spanish-speaking patients were intubated for less than 48 hours compared to 38% of the English-speaking patients. There was no statistical difference between the two cohorts in terms of mechanisms of injury, injury severity scores, drug or alcohol use, hypotension levels, or payer source. The major statistical difference between them was that the Glasgow Coma Scale (GCS) score was 14 in the Spanish-speaking group and 12 in the English-speaking group; nevertheless, more intubations occurred in the Spanish-speaking group. The authors concluded that the language barrier between patient and physician was the sole reason these patients were intubated. Consider this issue in your normal response during the daily mechanics of emergency medicine. It could pay off huge dividends during a disaster response.

MENTAL HEALTH

While the ED is resuming normal operations, don't let your guard down. There may be consequences related to an F5 tornado, and those consequences may find themselves knocking on the ED entrance. Obviously, mental health issues will be of concern as survivors deal with losses of varying magnitude. Since you are on the disaster committee, you should have the occasion to determine what mental health capabilities exist in your hospital and your community and see how they can be streamlined to provide the most benefit in the shortest amount of time. Mental health services should not be limited to the victims; they should be made available to all those who labored in the hospital during the incident. This need should be addressed immediately after the incident and at some point in the near future. This includes offering this assistance to physicians who may be hesitant or resistant to debriefings and stress management.

- In a "simple" disaster, the infrastructure is intact and will respond appropriately. Mutual aid resources may assist. Traumatic injuries dominate.
- Identify proper utilization of the diverse services that may be employed (e.g., radiology, lab, blood services).
- Redundancy of communications is essential.
- Identify the triage system to be employed.
- Identify the role, responsibilities, and resources of the triage system.

Further reading

Austin CL, Finley PJ, Mikkelson DR, Tibbs B. Mucormycosis: A rare fungal infection in tornado victims. *J Burn Care Res*. 2014;35(3):e164–e171.

Bard MR, Goettler CE, Schenarts PJ, Collins BA, Toschlog EA, Sagraves SG, Rotondo MF. Language barrier leads to the unnecessary intubation of trauma patients. *Am Surg*. 2004;70(9):783–786.

Beekley AC, Martin MJ, Spinella PC, Telian SP, Holcomb JB. Predicting resource needs for multiple and mass casualty events in combat: Lessons learned from combat support hospital experience in Operation Iraqi Freedom. *J Trauma*. 2009;66(4 Suppl):S129–S137.

Campion EM, Juillard C, Knudson MM, Dicker R, Cohen MJ, Mackersie R, Campbell AR, Callcut RA. Reconsidering the resources needed for multiple casualty events: Lessons learned from the crash of Asiana Airlines Flight 214. *JAMA Surg*. 2016;151(6):512–517.

Gutierrez de Ceballos JP, Turégano Fuentes F, Perez Diaz D, Sanz Sanchez M, Martin Llorente C, Guerrero Sanz JE. Casualties treated at the closest hospital in the Madrid, March 11, terrorist bombings. *Crit Care Med*. 2005;33(1 Suppl):S107–S112.

Haverkort JJM, Bouman JH, Wind JDD, Leenen LPH. Continuous development of a major incident in-hospital victim tracking and tracing system, withstanding the challenges of time. *Disaster Med Public Health Prep*. 2017;11(2):244–250.

Kikta KJ. 45 seconds: Memoirs of an ER physician. When the deadly EF-5 tornado struck Joplin, May 22, 2011. *Mo Med*. 2011;108(3):150–154.

Lake C. *A Day Like No Other: A Case Study of the Las Vegas Mass Shooting*. Nevada Hospital Association; 2018. https://nvha.net/a-day-like-no-other-case-study-of-the-las-vegas-mass-shooting/

Leonard HB, Cole CM, Howitt AM, Heyman PB. *Why Was Boston Strong? Lessons from the Boston Marathon Bombing*. Harvard Kennedy School; 2014.

https://www.hks.harvard.edu/sites/default/files/centers/research-initiatives/
crisisleadership/files/WhyWasBostonStrong.pdf

Neblett Fanfair R, Benedict K, Bos J, Bennett SD, Lo YC, Adebanjo T, Etienne K, Deak
E, Derado G, Shieh WJ, Drew C, Zaki S, Sugerman D, Gade L, Thompson EH,
Sutton DA, Engelthaler DM, Schupp JM, Brandt ME, et al. Necrotizing cutaneous
mucormycosis after a tornado in Joplin, Missouri, in 2011. *N Engl J Med.*
2012;367 (23):2214–2225.

Soffer D, Klausner J, Bar-Zohar D, Szold O, Schulman CI, Halpern P, Shimonov
A, Hareuveni M, Ben-Tal O. Usage of blood products in multiple-casualty
incidents: The experience of a level I trauma center in Israel. *Arch Surg.* 2008
Oct;143(10):983–989.

Yancey CC, O'Rourke MC. Emergency department triage. 2020. StatPearls. https://
pubmed.ncbi.nlm.nih.gov/32491515/

6 The Bat-Phone rings again: A basketball game, a yellow-green cloud, and seizing victims

The tones from the Bat-Phone sound more ominous than usual. Maybe you are overreacting to the FBI notice about credible threats from homegrown terror cells. In any case, your worst fears have been realized: During the community's championship basketball game between East Overshoe High and Buckle Down Prep, an ominous cloud rose from under the stands, causing scores of spectators to cough, wheeze, and seize. For the other spectators who were not directly involved, it was a race off the stands and toward the exits. "Race" is too mild a term. It was more like a stampede—a fight for fresh air. In addition to the HAZMAT victims, you will also be receiving additional casualties as a result of blunt-force trauma in the rush to the exits.

The responders have established hot, warm, and cold zones at the scene to rescue and decontaminate the victims as safely as possible. HAZMAT teams have donned their Level A suits to perform search and rescue and begin the decontamination process. Gross decontamination procedures are being operationalized and EMS is telling you to expect up to 100 cases after decontamination and stabilization. In the back of your head, you are concerned that with the "first-wave phenomenon," victims may be arriving who could not wait to be decontaminated.

What do I do now?

When dealing with a HAZMAT event, be it accidental or intentional, there are two principal objectives:

1. Prevent contamination of and injury to the healthcare providers.
2. Provide appropriate care to the victims.

To paraphrase John Donne, "No person is an island"—and that is never truer than when dealing with a HAZMAT situation. This particular situation is even more complicated because of three additional factors that are guaranteed to make your life more difficult unless you prepared yourself and your team for any eventuality:

1. This was evidently an intentional event. Once you accept that possibility, you will need to accept other possibilities—including the likelihood that one of the victims coming to you is the perpetrator of the gaseous release. That person, feigning injury, could be seeking entry to the ED to create greater havoc or could actually be injured from a self-induced mishap. Either way, that person may be concealing additional weaponry on their person. Fortunately, the removal of clothes from these victims will help prevent that from happening. Having security at the decontamination area will be essential.

2. The victims coming to you may or may not have experienced some level of decontamination. Some may have received little to no decontamination because they navigated themselves to the ED for care or were transported by well-meaning, non-medical Good Samaritans. Therefore, these victims are potential threats to the ED personnel due to off-gassing. This is exactly what occurred during the 1995 sarin attack in Tokyo. Many of these victims arrived at the hospitals without being decontaminated at the scene. Many of the hospital responders who were caring for them did not don proper PPE and they became symptomatic too. The caregivers who were exposed and became symptomatic ranged from clerks to physicians, and the sites of their exposures ranged from the ED to the hospital chapel, as these were the hospital sites where the victims received care. Fortunately, for the nearly 500 hospital personnel who were exposed, their complaints were not

life-threatening (e.g., headaches, visual disturbances, nausea, and dyspnea). However, it did add to their mental and emotional stress.

3. These patients are not strictly HAZMAT patients; rather, they are "HAZMAT plus." The "plus" signifies the trauma they received while attempting to escape from the gas. Most of the injuries will inevitably be blunt trauma, from head to toe. Therefore, these victims will require not only decontamination and possible antidotal therapy but also trauma management (primary and secondary trauma surveys). In reviewing case histories in many closed space disasters (e.g. fires, earthquakes, explosions, etc.), many of the victims perished from crush injuries in the general stampede.

STAMPEDE

In any MCI involving hazardous materials, we need to be on guard for a stampede. Any sudden event that is perceived by a vulnerable population as being dangerous or even lethal will induce that population to escape in any manner possible. The very visceral act of escaping can cause injury to those trying to escape as well as those who get between the runners and safety. Rational decision-making is in short supply.

One of the most extreme examples of a stampede is what occurs period- ically during the Hajj, the annual Islamic pilgrimage to Mecca and Mina in Saudi Arabia. Over the course of 5 days, millions of Muslim worshippers come from around the world to profess their faith and fulfill their ritual obligations. For instance, in September 2015, a stampede killed 717 wor- shippers and injured another 900. It developed when two massive groups of people on two different paths converged on their way to the "Stoning of the Devil" in Mina. It is hypothesized that the encounter created a panic situation, and the crush began. Safety-valve exits were said to be closed, which contributed to the crush and the panic. According to one eyewitness, "It's literally a pile of bodies of people who . . . pushed, they shoved, they panicked, they screamed . . . It was hot, someone fell, others trampled and they got stampeded."

The stampede that occurred in Sheffield, England, on April 15, 1989, was not related to religion but to football (or, as it is termed in "The

Colonies," soccer). At Hillsborough Stadium, Liverpool was set to battle with Nottingham Forest in the FA Cup semifinal match. In one area of the stadium, one of the pens that had been created to keep the fans enclosed became overcrowded as those seeking to gain entrance stampeded forward over the earlier arrivals to view the match. No crowd control, no police vigilance, and the lack of an expeditious EMS response were key factors that led to the deaths of 96 men, women, and children. The oldest was 67 years old; the youngest was only 10 years old. Hundreds more were injured, 20 seriously.

Studies indicate that there are two basic types of trauma seen with stampedes. One is related to trampling or crushing of multiple people over another. The other is traumatic asphyxia related to the crush. The inability of the thorax to expand will lead to suffocation, and this injury is said to be the most common cause of death in a stampede. In this case we are discussing in this chapter, the stampede victims may not even have any manifestations related to HAZMAT; rather, they may have crush injuries, fractures, crush syndrome, massive brain injury, hemopneumothorax, hepato-spleno-renal hemorrhage, cervico-facial plethora, cyanosis, facial/conjunctival petechiae, coma, and cardiac arrest.

So, with these confounders in mind, consider the following actions:

1. Activate your version of "Code Disaster-HAZMAT." That should get the incident command system up and running right away.
2. Activate the hospital HAZMAT team to deploy the decontamination tent or similar structure.
3. Instruct the appropriate individuals in the ED to don the requisite PPE. This can be a Level B or C suit with appropriate respiratory protection mentioned earlier. There is an unwritten tenet of emergency HAZMAT management that if a contaminated victim arrives alive to the ED, their contamination is not severe enough to cause significant morbidity to hospital personnel. That was evident with the Tokyo sarin incident in 1995. Nevertheless, donning Level B or C PPE is appropriate, especially for individuals conducting triage and working in the decontamination area (Figure 6.1).

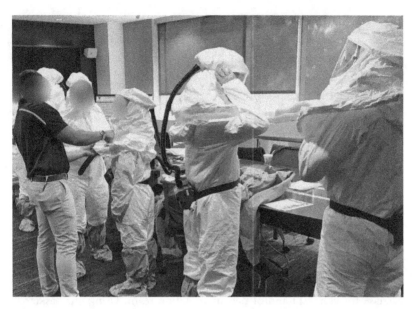

FIGURE 6.1 Emergency Medicine PGY-1 residents are receiving an introduction in donning and doffing Level B PPE.

4. Triage the existing ED patients away from the center of action. Having a triage team or disposition team from the other parts of the hospital will allow you and your team time to prepare for the incoming victims in a safe and efficacious manner. In some EDs, part of the ED staff is used to establish the decontamination process.

5. When victims arrive by EMS or private vehicle, check out the responders and the Good Samaritans and see if they have been accidentally contaminated by their patients. Then take the appropriate action, which means decontaminating them and isolating their vehicles.

As the victims arrive, they are theoretically carrying the hot zone with them. If ambulatory, they will be divesting themselves of their clothes and undergoing decontamination procedures before they are ultimately allowed to enter the cold zone (i.e., ED central; see Figure 3.2 in Chapter 3). These individuals may feel more secure if they are given a waterproof bag or container for their clothes and other personal and valuable items and carry it with them. The other option is to collect all personal items and bag and tag them until they can be returned to their owners. Caution must be taken with whatever strategy is being employed because of the possibility of off-gassing from the victims' clothes.

DECONTAMINATING NON-AMBULATORY INDIVIDUALS

Another issue that must be considered in the decontamination process is that some individuals will be unable to traverse the decontamination area independently and must be placed on a backboard or some other conveyance to undergo decontamination by the team. These patients may be tagged Yellow or Red and in normal situations would require IVs and basic and/or advanced airway management.

Let's take one victim as an example and perhaps use it as a table-top exercise for your ED and/or decontamination team. Using our basketball game scenario, an ambulance comes to your decontamination area carrying a middle-aged female in a cervical collar and on a backboard. She is awake, eyes open, and mumbling incoherently. She is extremely diaphoretic, and her breaths are fast and noisy. She is bruised on the face and legs, and there is blood visible from one ear. Her outer garments were removed at the scene, but she is still wearing her blouse and skirt. Because you are wearing a double set of gloves, you cannot appreciate a radial pulse. Medics state on the hand-off that she was trampled by others as she tried to escape down a long flight of stairs. If this were not a HAZMAT incident, you would know exactly what needs to be done for this patient. However, the complication of contamination forces you to consider safely log-rolling her in order to decontaminate her back as well as the backboard. This can only be done by specially trained medical personnel. In any case, simple but efficacious decontamination may be all that you would want to do for this patient. However, consider that certain medical procedures may be performed while decontamination is proceeding apace.

Starting IVs, administering antidotes and medications, and performing endotracheal intubations during decontamination would indeed be problematic. In this type of patient, consider intraosseous infusions (IOs) and a bag-valve mask. The IO would be helpful to treat seizures or to provide

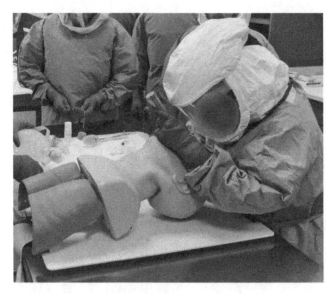

FIGURE 6.2 PGY-1 Emergency Medicine residents are receiving training in advanced airway management while wearing Level B PPE.

antidotes in a timely fashion. Obviously, this requires an ED medical team sufficiently trained to insert IOs and to handle basic airway management while suited up in Level B PPE (Figure 6.2).

In the past, decontamination took place in a room off the ED that was set up to decontaminate one or two patients. With increasing concerns that a chemical attack can occur anytime, anyplace, and anywhere, there have been initiatives to rethink hospital decontamination strategies. What is currently in place is the development of a decontamination area that can be set up quickly and that permits the decontamination of multiple victims in as short a time as possible (Figures 6.3, 6.4, 6.5, 6.6, and 6.7). The decontamination area is divided into three zones:

- The red zone is the area that the victims enter prior to decontamination. It is considered the red zone because until the victims are decontaminated, they are "hot" (i.e., have hazardous materials deposited on their clothing and therefore represent a hazard to hospital personnel). Here the stable victims receive a decontamination kit that contains nonabrasive cleaning material,

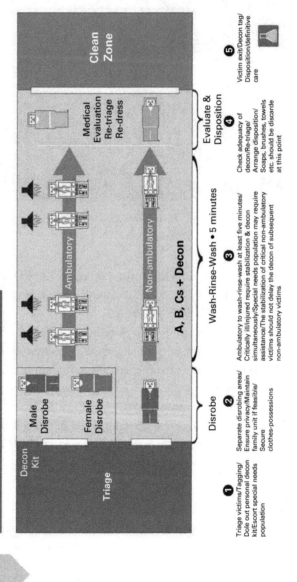

DECONTAMINATION PROCESS

Decon Kit

Triage

Male Disrobe

Female Disrobe

Ambulatory

Non-ambulatory

A, B, Cs + Decon

Medical Evaluation Re-triage Re-dress

Clean Zone

❶ Triage

Triage victims/Tagging/
Dole out personal decon
kit/Escort special needs
population

❷ Disrobe

Separate disrobing areas/
Ensure privacy/Maintain
family unit if feasible/
Secure
clothes-possessions

❸ Wash-Rinse-Wash • 5 minutes

Ambulatory to wash-rinse-wash at least five minutes/
Critically ill/injured require stabilization & decon
simultaneously/Special needs population may require
assistance/The stabilization of critical non-ambulatory
victims should not delay the decon of subsequent
non-ambulatory victims

❹ Evaluate & Disposition

Check adequacy of
decon/Re-triage/
Arrange disposition/
Soaps, brushes, towels
etc. should be discarde
at this point

❺

Victim exit/Decon tag/
Disposition/definitive
care

FIGURE 6.3 The decontamination process.

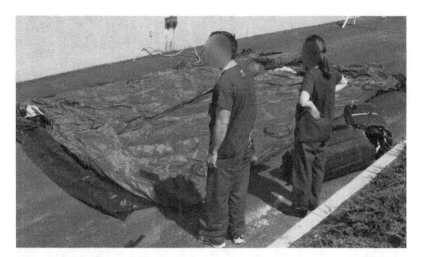

FIGURE 6.4 In a decontamination exercise, the decontamination tent is unfolded and ready to be inflated.

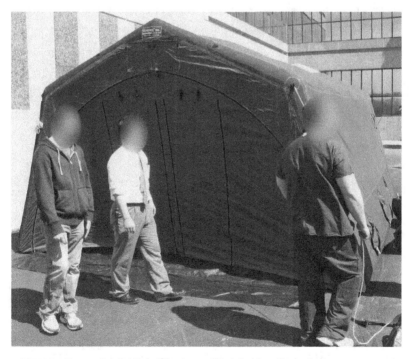

FIGURE 6.5 The tent is fully inflated. The time to fully inflate is a matter of minutes.

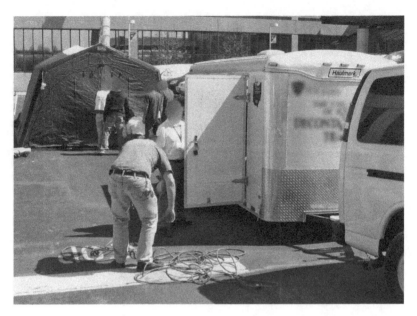

FIGURE 6.6 The tent is being readied to be deflated and stored in the decontamination vehicle.

waterproof bags to contain personal valuables, and clothing to don after the decontamination process is concluded.

- In the yellow or "warm" zone, the ambulatory victims are given privacy to remove their clothes and then go through the decontamination process, where they will wash, rinse, wash, rinse. Once through the "warm" zone, the decontamination and medical personnel will reevaluate each victim's status.
- In the green or "cold" zone, normal patient care operations begin. Patients enter this zone once they have been decontaminated sufficiently that they no longer pose a threat to themselves or anyone else.

This discussion about hazardous materials exposure sounds basic and not worthy of over-analysis. However, it was only in April 2019 that an Illinois transportation accident involving an anhydrous ammonia release resulted in the secondary contamination of five ICU staff members. Why? Simple: The initial patients at the scene of the release were not decontaminated either in the field or when they first presented at one hospital. They were

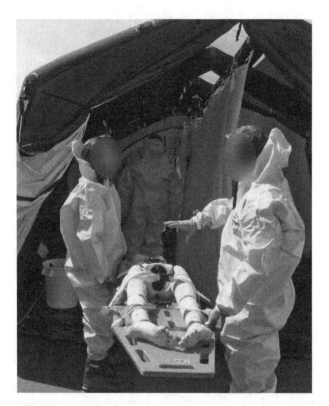

FIGURE 6.7 Inside the decontamination tent there is a separation. One side can be used for the ambulatory victims and the other for the non-ambulatory victims. A roller system helps move a victim on a backboard down the line.

finally decontaminated when five ICU staff members became symptomatic as a result of off-gassing from the victims' clothing.

DECONTAMINATING PEDIATRIC PATIENTS

Infants, babies, and children are an extremely vulnerable population no matter the type of disaster, but these vulnerabilities are particularly important in a HAZMAT incident (Figure 6.8). It is important to scan the triage decontamination line for children and babies and escort them and their caregivers right to the front so they can be decontaminated as rapidly as possible. This is especially the case if the decontamination line is outdoors and the weather is

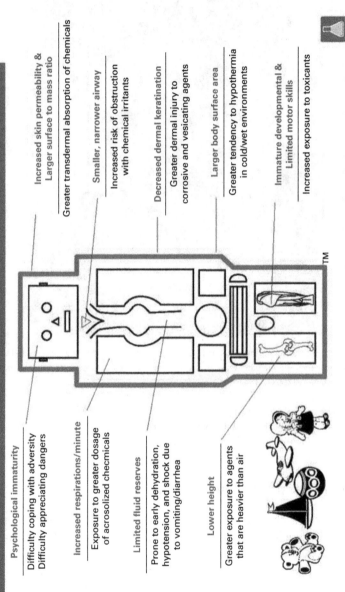

PEDIATRIC ISSUES IN THE FACE OF CHEMICAL TERRORISM

Psychological immaturity
Difficulty coping with adversity
Difficulty appreciating dangers

Increased respirations/minute
Exposure to greater dosage
of acrosolized checmicals

Limited fluid reserves
Prone to early dehydration,
hypotension, and shock due
to vomiting/diarrhea

Lower height
Greater exposure to agents
that are heavier than air

Increased skin permeability &
Larger surface to mass ratio

Greater transdermal absorption of chemicals

Smaller, narrower airway

Increased risk of obstruction
with chemical irritants

Decreased dermal keratination
Greater dermal injury to
corrosive and vesicating agents

Larger body surface area

Greater tendency to hypothermia
in cold/wet environments

Immature developmental &
Limited motor skills

Increased exposure to toxicants

TM

FIGURE 6.8 Pediatric vulnerabilities in a HAZMAT incident.

intemperate. The children's caregivers may need assistance to decontaminate themselves as well as their kids. This is another reason why experienced medical oversight in needed in the decontamination area.

DECONTAMINATING SPECIAL POPULATIONS

Consider the unique vulnerabilities of special populations like the functionally or mentally compromised, the elderly, and those who may require interpreters, and manage them on a case-by-case basis. For example, how would you decontaminate a person with a $7,000 motorized wheelchair? Both the person and the wheelchair need decontamination, but will the process ruin the wheelchair? Remember that these devices, as well as assistance animals, are valuable lifelines for these individuals. Strategies are needed to manage them and keep the mental well-being of the victim in the forefront of operations.

KEY POINTS TO REMEMBER

- A HAZMAT incident threatens initial victims, rescuers, responders, and the community.
- When dealing with a HAZMAT situation, evaluate for blunt and penetrating trauma secondary to a stampede.
- If the incident may be intentional, remember that your patient may actually be the perpetrator. Take proper precautions.
- Develop decontamination strategies that will benefit the vulnerable populations.

Further reading

de Almeida MM, von Schreeb J. Human stampedes: An updated review of current literature. *Prehosp Disaster Med.* 2019;34(1):82–88.

Rispens JR, Jones SA, Clemmons NS, Ahmed S, Harduar-Morano L, Johnson MD, Edge III C, Vyas A, Bourgikos E, Orr MF. Anhydrous ammonia chemical release—Lake County, Illinois, April 2019. *MMWR Morb Mortal Wkly Rep.* 2020;69(4):109–113.

Steindl D, Boehmerle W, Körner R, Praeger D, Haug M, Nee J, Schreiber A, Scheibe F, Demin K, Jacoby P, Tauber R, Hartwig S, Endres M, Eckardt K-U. Novichok nerve agent poisoning. *Lancet.* 2021;397(10270):249–252.

7 The case of the pesticide and the melancholy farmer

You are receiving a stat page to the waiting room. You are greeted by some surprised and anxious people who are distancing themselves from a coughing, gagging individual. He is being supported by a friend. The friend, let's call him Horatio, quickly explains that Josiah tried to harm himself a short while ago. Josiah was commiserating with Horatio in the garage after he received word that he lost custody of his children. Impulsively, Josiah grabbed a bottle of pesticide from the shelf and took a large gulp. His friend grabbed the bottle, saw the poison warning on the label, and drove him to the closest ER . . . your ER. Fortunately, Horatio brought the bottle with him. It is an organophosphate pesticide. During the 20-minute trip to the ED, Josiah became diaphoretic, dyspneic, and somewhat confused. Horatio is asymptomatic.

What do I do now?

This is more than a depressed, possibly suicidal, patient in your waiting room; this is a HAZMAT situation. Your patient is not just *in* the hot zone; he *is* the hot zone. While, according to Horatio, Josiah did not spill the contents of the bottle on himself, and therefore it is likely there is no external hazard, consider what could happen should he abruptly vomit. The key action is to ensure the safety of the potential victims while, secondarily, expediting the care of the patient.

An indication as to how you might act may be found in an article published in the Centers for Disease Control and Prevention's *Morbidity and Mortality Weekly Report*. It was a case of attempted suicide in which the patient drank 100 grams of an organophosphate insecticide. He was coughing and vomiting as he was being cared for by three ED personnel. Personnel attended to the patient without considering that this was a HAZMAT situation and they were in the hot zone. The donning of PPE and decontamination of the patient were not considered early in the course of management. As a result, those who were providing direct care to the patient were contaminated by the aerosolization of secretions and emesis. One 45-year-old nursing assistant developed respiratory distress due to bronchial spasms and secretions, diaphoresis, and vomiting. She required antidote and endotracheal intubation. A young ED nurse had no direct tactile contact with the patient, but they shared the same environment. That nurse developed confusion, respiratory distress, and weakness. The administration of 10 mg of atropine and pralidoxime over 12 hours saved her from intubation. The final case, a 56-year-old RN, also had no tactile contact with the patient, but because they shared the same breathing space, the nurse developed confusion and dyspnea. Atropine and overnight observation were required.

This episode crystallizes what needs to be done when encountering a HAZMAT event in your own ED. The patient needs to be isolated and decontaminated and stabilized, but priority must go to the people, patients, and staff in the ED to avoid secondary contamination.

Since Horatio is asymptomatic, the pesticide remains within Josiah, and there may be time to load him up on a gurney and transport him to the decontamination area while his care team dons suitable PPE. It is unlikely you will have Level A suits available, but Level B protection for respiratory and skin precautions may be the best you can provide yourselves in this emergency. Treating him in the decontamination room will keep the ED safe, and you should be able to manage him medically until you have assured yourself that he is externally decontaminated.

If you decide to stabilize the patient in the waiting room, evacuate unnecessary personnel and prospective patients. Have the entourage led to a safe area for further evaluation of possible contamination and their other medical needs.

Wherever Josiah is being managed (i.e., the waiting room or the decontamination zone), the team should be in appropriate PPE and begin administering supportive therapy. This will include obtaining vascular access and may even include aggressive airway control. You may feel your technical skills will be hampered by the bulky PPE with decreased tactile sense and poor visibility (see Figure 6.2 in Chapter 6).

While IV access is optimum it may be next to impossible. However, vascular access can still be accomplished by IO infusion and, through it, the administration of atropine and 2-pralidoxime chloride. As far as intubations are concerned, with practice, an airway can be successfully accomplished by traditional means or through a videoscope mechanism. If that fails, simply rely on the Ambu bag to oxygenate and ventilate. There may be a great deal of resistance at first due to the bronchorrhea, but with aggressive administration of atropine that will subside.

Management consists of atropine, 2-pralidoxime chloride, and diazepam (seizure prophylaxis in severe poisonings) in conjunction with the usual supportive measures (Figure 7.1). Dosing amounts and scheduling vary depending on current peer-reviewed research and expert opinion. As a guide for planning purposes, the severe cases in the Tokyo sarin attack required doses of atropine that varied from 1.5 to 9 mg (IM, IV, IO). Meanwhile, for organophosphate pesticide poisoning, the mean initial atropine dose was 23 mg. Cannibalization of atropine from the pharmacy department, from crash carts all over the hospital, and even from other hospitals or EMS units may be required. The biomarker for successful "atropinization" is lessening of the bronchorrhea and improvement in ventilatory mechanics. Frequency of dosing is usually at 5-minute intervals.

Emergency physicians are comfortable with general adult and pediatric dosing guidelines for atropine and the benzodiazepines, but that may not be the case for administering pralidoxime chloride. A weight-based infusion

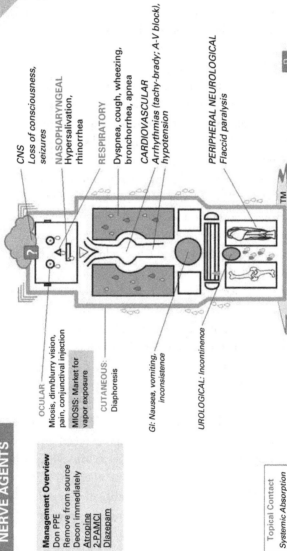

NERVE AGENTS

Management Overview
Don PPE
Remove from source
Decon immediately
Atropine
2-PAMCl
Diazepam

OCULAR
Miosis, dim/blurry vision, pain, conjunctival injection
MIOSIS: Market for vapor exposure

CUTANEOUS:
Diaphoresis

GI: Nausea, vomiting, inconsistence

UROLOGICAL: Incontinence

CNS
Loss of consciousness, seizures

NASOPHARYNGEAL
Hypersalivation, rhinorrhea

RESPIRATORY
Dyspnea, cough, wheezing, bronchorrhea, apnea

CARDIOVASCULAR
Arrhythmias (tachy-brady; A-V block), hypotension

PERIPHERAL NEUROLOGICAL
Flaccid paralysis

TM

Topical Contact
Systemic Absorption
Major Affected Areas

FIGURE 7.1 Nerve agents.

of 25 mg/kg for both adults and children can serve as a safe dosing regimen until expert consultation is available. Nevertheless, while both atropine and pralidoxime work synergistically, atropine is key.

All bodily fluids must be kept isolated and secure to avoid secondary contamination. Whatever means you choose, if you choose any at all to decontaminate the GI tract, remember that those fluids are contaminated. It may be days before the patient is considered not to be a hazard to anyone else, and until that day comes, PPE for the care team is essential.

While this conversation has centered on the suicidal or unintentional (e.g., infants and children) ingestion of the well-known organophosphates, it has only been in this 21st century that a newer class of organophosphate agent, Novichok, has been used, arguably as an assassin's weapon. Five individuals have been poisoned with it; one died. One of the first peer-reviewed articles dealing with the effects of Novichok on a Russian dissident revealed that clinical findings, although consistent with muscarinic actions, may be misinterpreted and that the key to good resuscitation remains aggressive management of the ABCs as well as aggressive administration of atropine, even if it is delayed. Oximes such as pralidoxime or obidoxime may not have the impact previously thought for this particular agent.

KEY POINTS TO REMEMBER

· Consider appropriate PPE when managing a patient who may have ingested a hazardous agent.
· Evaluate all individuals who transported the HAZMAT victim to determine their need for decontamination and treatment.
· Aggressive administration of antidotes, especially atropine, is important in an organophosphate exposure.

Further reading

Centers for Disease Control and Prevention (CDC). Nosocomial poisoning associated with emergency department treatment of organophosphate toxicity—Georgia, 2000. *MMWR Morb Mortal Wkly Rep.* 2001;49(51–52):1156–1158.

Geller RJ, Singleton KL, Tarantino ML, Drenzek CL, Toomey KE. Nosocomial poisoning associated with emergency department treatment of organophosphate toxicity—Georgia, 2000. *J Toxicol Clin Toxicol.* 2001;39(1):109–111.

Hulse EJ, Haslam JD, Emmett SR, Woolley T. Organophosphorus nerve agent poisoning: Managing the poisoned patient. *Br J Anaesth*. 2019;123(4):457–463.

Stacey R, Morfey D, Payne S. Secondary contamination in organophosphate poisoning: Analysis of an incident. *QJM*. 2004;97(2):75–80.

Steindl D, Boehmerle W, Körner R, Praeger D, Haug M, Nee J, Schreiber A, Scheibe F, Demin K, Jacoby P, Tauber R, Hartwig S, Endres M, Eckardt KU. Novichok nerve agent poisoning. *Lancet*. 2021;397(10270):249–252.

8 Hydrofluoric acid: One of the worst HAZMAT agents you never heard of

EMS is calling in. The voice on the other end of the line sounds out of breath. The medic does not want to give report to the nurse; she wants the doctor—now! You get on the line and indicate to your charge nurse to stay close.

"It's HAZMAT, Doc," says the medic. "Multiple victims at a glass factory. A coworker just sprayed a lunchroom of workers with hydrofluoric acid. We don't know much about it, but five of the victims are getting deconned right now. But two just died and one is getting chest compressions. No chance for vital signs on the survivors right now, but they're in a lot of pain and we sure could use some advice. By the way, you're the closest. They're all coming to you."

What do I do now?

With your hand over the speaker, tell your nurse to alert administration, the HAZMAT/decontamination team, and the initial consultants from the pharmacy, nephrology, and respiratory departments. After that, you can turn your attention to the medic. These victims obviously require decontamination, but this is a unique event and a number of response actions are not necessarily within the ken of many emergency healthcare providers. It is a matter of the primary survey: A, B, C, D, and E. With HAZMAT, the "D" represents "decontamination." However, with particular reference to hydrofluoric acid (HFA), the letter "D" also represents "drugs"—and with HFA, those drugs include calcium and magnesium. Victims of HFA die early because they have absorbed enough of the chemical that they develop life-threatening hypocalcemia, not to mention hyperkalemia. So, your immediate counsel can go along one of two paths: (1) Either have the medics monitor QT prolongation and peaked T waves and treat with the antidotes, if necessary, or (2) empirically administer calcium chloride or gluconate when resources are scarce, monitoring capabilities are nonexistent, and victims are too many. Keep in mind that calcium chloride ($CaCl_2$) has more elemental calcium than calcium gluconate ($C_{12}H_{22}CaO_{14}$).

Now the initial steps are progressing, and while you are awaiting the call-backs, it is time to tell your people what it is all about and what they need to do. This means donning appropriate PPE. After all, you never knows if someone will be arriving who escaped detection by law enforcement and EMS at the scene of the incident.

With just-in-time training, you can cover the main points of HFA, caregiver safety, and care for the victims. HFA acts as both a weak acid and an alkali. Therefore, its effects on human tissue are consistent with coagulation necrosis and liquefactive necrosis. The severity of HFA's actions is related to three factors:

1. The concentration of HFA. Since the incident occurred at a glass factory and since the living patients were in severe pain, one can intuit that the concentration was high.
2. The percentage of total body surface area (TBSA) contaminated
3. The duration of exposure

Once HFA attacks the eyes, skin, and/or mucosa, the process of tissue destruction begins, and that process can extend beyond epidermis and

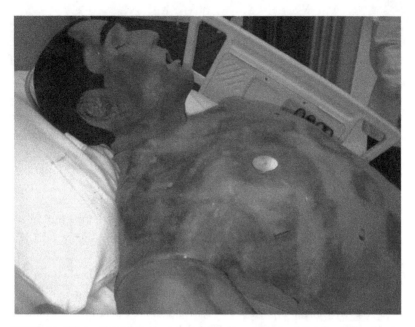

FIGURE 8.1 This is a high-fidelity simulator moulaged to represent a victim of an HFA accident at a glass manufacturer. In the control center, the victim is scripted to yell in pain, and on the video monitor the EKG shows prolonged QT intervals and peaked T waves. The emergency medicine residents, after a brief didactic session, are now challenged to manage the "patient's" hyperkalemia, hypocalcemia, and pain.

dermis and destroy fascia and muscles, down to bone (Figure 8.1). HFA will disassociate into H^+ and F^-. Simultaneously, the fluoride ion will then combine with the body's calcium to form CaF_2. The more the body's calcium is inactivated by its attachment to fluoride, the greater the risk of symptomatic hypocalcemia. The fluoride ion can also attach to the body's magnesium (MgF_2), and while hypomagnesemia does not have the clinical import of low serum calcium, frequent magnesium levels should be ordered. Another complication is the excess hydrogen ion entering cells and the concomitant movement of intracellular potassium into the systemic circulation. Therefore, frequent serum levels and cardiac monitoring are needed to avoid hyperkalemia, hypocalcemia, and hypomagnesemia.

However, when dealing with an MCI in the ED, the simpler course would be to prophylactically administer an appropriate dose of calcium gluconate as soon as these victims present, whether it is in the decontamination area or in the ED. Incidentally, even if a victim presents in cardiac arrest, it would be worth continuing ACLS measures and add a couple of doses of calcium.

Once the patients are in the cold zone, it is a matter of conducting continual primary surveys (A, B, C, D2, and E), intervene as needed, and go on to the secondary survey. With specific attention to an HFA exposure, the following should be considered, either under your own authority or in conjunction with your consultants:

1. Pain control: Pain is a sign that the patient was exposed to a significant concentration of HFA. If it continues despite topical administration of the antidotes and analgesia, pain suggests that therapy is not working.
2. Monitoring: Lab studies should be obtained immediately upon arrival and repeated every half-hour to hour depending on the severity of the exposure. The critical labs are calcium, potassium, and magnesium. If point-of-care lab testing is not immediately available, then cardiac monitoring is vital. A baseline rhythm strip will indicate QT prolongation and peaked T waves. This should be evaluated at regular intervals, especially if there is a delay in obtaining the serum values.
3. Antidotes: Treatment of hyperkalemia, while critical, is already within the scope of practice for emergency physicians. However, there are a number of ways to manage the burns associated with an HFA exposure and to reverse hypocalcemia.
   a. Topical: This involves massaging a calcium slurry with a water-soluble lubricant into the burn area.
   b. Subcutaneous/intradermal injections of $C_{12}H_{22}CaO_{14}$ into large burn areas or when the pain is refractory to topical applications
   c. Intravenous: This can be given as an infusion, both for calcium and magnesium.
   d. Intra-arterial: This should be done only in consultation with interventional radiology and other specialists. This technique could be particularly useful in significant extremity burns.

e. Nebulization: An aerosol nebulizer that contains an appropriate amount of calcium can be helpful in acute airway injuries as topical therapy, but calcium's systemic absorption by this means can be a reasonable temporizing measure as the victims begin arriving at your back door.

f. Hemodialysis: There have been reports that hemodialysis can reduce fluoride levels and lessen the risk of hypocalcemia as well as hyperkalemia.

g. Consultations: These will be numerous as you get deeper into the incident and as you get a better handle on the situation. However, even before the patients start arriving, it would be reasonable to consult nephrology, pulmonary, respiratory therapy, anesthesia, and pharmacy. In time, there will be calls made to surgery, orthopedics, plastic surgery, psychiatry, medicine, etc. Among the first calls, pharmacy will, arguably, be the most important in terms of not only assisting with the dosing of the medicines but also obtaining the antidotes from within the hospital complex and maybe even from other hospitals.

KEY POINTS TO REMEMBER

- Acute management of an HFA exposure consists of airway, breathing, circulation, decontamination, antidotes, and pain control.
- With an HFA exposure, consider the effects of an acid (coagulation necrosis) and alkali (liquefactive necrosis) exposure.
- When HFA dissociates, its fluoride ion binds to the body's calcium stores.
- A drop in serum calcium could be significant enough to cause sudden death.
- Additional electrolyte imbalances include hypomagnesemia and hyperkalemia.
- In the absence of immediate serum calcium levels, look for the prolonged QT intervals indicative of severe hypocalcemia.

- In the absence of immediate serum potassium levels, look for the peakedT waves as an early indication of hyperkalemia.
- In your hazard vulnerability analysis, look specifically for those companies or storehouses that have HFA.
- Conduct readiness and response exercises for those companies, as well as EMS and hospital personnel.

Further reading

Bajraktarova-Valjakova E, Korunoska-Stevkovska V, Georgieva S, Ivanovski K, Bajraktarova-Misevska C, Mijoska A, Grozdanov A. Hydrofluoric acid: Burns and systemic toxicity, protective measures, immediate and hospital medical treatment. *Open Access Maced J Med Sci.* 2018;6(11):2257–2269.

Rega PP. Hydrofluoric acid mass casualty incident. In: Ciottone GR, editor-in-chief. *Ciottone's Disaster Medicine* (2nd ed.). Elsevier; 2015:680–684.

ZhangY, Wang X, Sharma K, Mao X, Qiu X, Ni L, Han C. Injuries following a serious hydrofluoric acid leak: First aid and lessons. *Burns.* 2015;41(7):1593–1598.

Fever, rash, and one helluva cough: One approach to a biological incident, etiology unknown

It has been a slow morning. The ED is quiet and here is your chance to run over to the coffee kiosk and grab a mocha double latte and a bagel. At the cashier, you receive a text message on your phone: "Get back. Stat. Room 13."

You throw down a 10-spot on the counter and canter the 50 yards to the ED.

You open the door to 13 and you see the patient care nurse tending to the patient who was just brought in by ambulance. The patient looks "sick." He looks about 60 and his skin has the mottled appearance of one who is in extremis. You notice petechiae, purpura, and purplish pustular lesions on his face, hands, and feet. He is coughing incessantly. The nurse applies the monitor leads on the patient as well as nasal oxygen. His vital signs are worse than you expected: temp 103.6° F; pulse 124/minute; sinus tachycardia; respirations 28 with retractions; BP 80/54. The GCS as best as you can tell hovers around 10 to 11. You call to him and all he can do is mumble.

Your head swirls as you try to recall the litany of neglected tropical diseases and Category A bioterror agents. You cannot decide if this may be the index case of some exotic disease or even a bioterrorism attack.

What do I do now?

Whether this presentation is the result of an intentional attack or a severe manifestation of some neglected tropical disease is irrelevant. What you realize, however, is that this patient may be an infectious disease threat, not only to you and your nurse, but also to your ED, your hospital, and your community.

You have multiple obligations, and they have to be accomplished virtually simultaneously. Call out to your charge nurse and have the team clear a path to the room with a negative-pressure environment. This will take time. In the meantime, have someone get you and your nurse the proper PPE: cap, gown, double gloving, eye protection, and at least N95 respirators.

Provide the minimum amount of care to the patient in order to keep them alive enough to make the short journey to the negative-pressure environment. You really want to avoid the spread of infectious disease contamination associated with definitive airway control and increase the risk of aerosolization. If it is feasible, shut down HVAC to your ED to confine the infectious disease spread. Have someone notify EMS, and alert them to place the team that brought the patient to you in quarantine. Until further notice, it would also be prudent to divert EMS traffic. Patients in the waiting room, as long as they are stable, can be shuttled to other areas of the hospital for further evaluation. For this to happen smoothly, the chief medical or nursing officer of the hospital needs to be contacted. You have in a short period of time taken the necessary steps to protect yourselves, your staff, your patients, your ED, and your hospital. Now with hospital administration on board, they may be able to activate a specific "code" to alert everyone that a biological incident is taking place. This, hopefully, should precipitate a series of actions that have been developed and drilled in prior discussions and exercises. These actions will have to include, apart from the infectious disease department, local public health authorities. While your point of view is focused on your patient and the patient's threat to the immediate venue, local public health, through its community outreach and its local, regional, state, and national connections, will determine whether this is an isolated incident, the index case of an epidemic, or the presage of an intentional incident.

With the negative-pressure room ready and prepared and with you and your nurse in proper PPE, cover the patient in one or two sheets or a thermal blanket, mask them to prevent droplet exposure to the ED, and convey them to the room. Once there, the team can begin the process of definitive resuscitation, meaning IOs, nebulizers, BVM, intubation, etc. Any equipment that you require, such as EKG machines and portable x-ray machines, should remain in that room. Had asymptomatic family or friends accompanied your patient to the ED, the safe course would be to keep them together in the patient's first ED room. In a sense, following good infectious disease practice, you are isolating the person who is symptomatic and quarantining those who were exposed but asymptomatic. They will remain there until evaluated for final disposition by your in-house or public health experts.

With the transportation of the patient from one room to the other, there has been an extension of the "hot zone," and that entire area should be cordoned off except to those individuals in proper PPE who will serve to support the patient care team.

Now, over the course of the next one-half to 1 hour, your patient has stabilized. Airway and breathing have been secured through endotracheal intubation. Circulation has been improved by means of intraosseous infusions, followed by two large-bore IVs with fluids wide open and a pressor agent. With the emergency secured, standard ED management of a critical patient continues. Recognizing a septic patient etiology unknown, you may have even ordered cultures and empirical antibiotic and antiviral therapy.

Repeat vitals now indicate temp 101.3°F; pulse 104; sinus tachycardia; respirations 18 (ventilator); BP 96/64. Meanwhile, a search through the patient's personal effects reveal that he is a journalist from a local newspaper and his passport indicates that he has just returned from touring Southeast Asia, the Middle East, and Western Africa.

With the judicious use of pharmaceuticals and ophthalmological ultrasonography to rule out increased intracranial pressure, the patient undergoes a lumbar puncture. Blood and spinal fluid, under infectious disease precautions, have been sent to the lab for analysis. Tests for traditional and atypical diseases, as well as the "zebras," have also been ordered in phone consultation with infectious disease and pathology specialists. With all the cultures from all sources obtained (blood, CSF, urine, lesions, etc.), you start your patient on broad-spectrum antimicrobials, if you have not already done so. It is also likely that with appropriate consultation, you could be broadening your selection of antimicrobial agents to include specific antiviral, antifungal, and antiparasitic agents.

Somewhere along the way, your charge nurse has contacted one of your emergency medicine colleagues to cover the department, to allow you and your team to concentrate on the index patients without possibly contaminating anyone else.

At this point, with no external information coming in, the differential diagnosis of this patient's condition is long and complex. After all, a key historical fact is the patient's travels throughout the ever-shrinking global environment. While it is likely that a more mundane diagnosis will be made, nevertheless, farther down the differential diagnostic list, there remains the possibility of an intentional biological attack. Your patient may have been the inadvertent human bioweapon. In the meantime, regardless of the etiology, you have taken the necessary steps to protect your people, care for your patient, shield your hospital, and alert your community.

An intentional biological assault is difficult to diagnose. One reason is that the incubation period will vary from victim to victim: Clinical manifestations can begin anywhere from hours to weeks from the initial assault. Additionally, it is likely that the victims may be going to various healthcare agencies for evaluation and care. Therefore, no one clinician will have the situational awareness that an unusual incident has struck the community. Local public health is, therefore, essential in evaluating community vulnerabilities based on the surveillance mechanisms. In the meantime, it is never inappropriate to reacquaint your people about certain clues suggesting a biological attack (Box 9.1). They should also be empowered to bring their concerns to your attention.

BOX 9.1 **Covert assault clues**

- Severe disease manifestations in previously healthy people
- Higher-than-normal number of patients with fever and respiratory/ GI complaints
- Multiple people with similar complaints from a common location
- An endemic disease appearing during an unusual time of year
- Unusual number of rapidly fatal cases
- Greater number of ill/dead animals
- Rapidly rising and falling epidemic curve
- Greater numbers of patients with severe pneumonia, sepsis, sepsis with coagulopathy, fever with rash, diplopia with progressive weakness

---

- It does not matter initially whether the patient is a victim of bioterrorism or of nature.
- Initial management, regardless of etiology, is basically the same.
- Protect yourselves with appropriate PPE.
- Protect your environment with isolation of patient, quarantine of entourage, negative-pressure treatment room, and shutting down HVAC.

Further reading

Dembek ZF, Kortepeter MG, Pavlin JA. Discernment between deliberate and natural infectious disease outbreaks. Epidemiol Infect. 2007;135(3):353–371. [Erratum in: Epidemiol Infect. 2007 Aug;135(6):1055.]

Koch L, Lopes AA, Maiguy A, Guillier S, Guillier L, Tournier JN, Biot F. Natural outbreaks and bioterrorism: How to deal with the two sides of the same coin? J Glob Health. 2020;10(2):020317.

10 A pruno party gone awry

You labor in a small ED in rural America. As you attend the occasional asthmatic patient or thresher mishap, you receive a call from an unusual source: the nurse practitioner at the state prison 10 miles away. She tells you that for the past day, she has been caring for a number of prisoners who have come down with an assortment of weird complaints: nausea, vomiting, blurred vision, and difficulty speaking. A couple of them have worsened and manifested droopy eyelids and really slurred speech, and now several have developed shortness of breath. She discovered that the common thread among this group of 10 is that two nights earlier, they celebrated their crony's birthday with illicit pruno. She began to put two and two together and came up with a dangerous interim diagnosis: "Doctor, I think they all have botulism! I can't do much here and you're the closest ER in a 50-mile radius, so I'm sending them to you with armed guards. They're coming by the prison bus, and it's leaving now. Their vital signs are OK. Thank you."

What do I do now?

efore she hangs up, have the nurse practitioner send along all the medical records the prisoners might have collected while "in stir."

Activate your disaster plan now. An ED team huddle is clearly warranted. Botulism is not a disease entity that is well known by many in the healthcare profession, so just-in-time training is appropriate. What needs to be conveyed to your team is the following:

· Botulism is not infectious. However, standard PPE is appropriate, including mask and eye protection as well as double gloving, which would offer added protection against any chronic comorbidities the prisoners might have.

· Botulism can cause death acutely from two complications: (1) aspiration due to a dysfunctional swallowing mechanism and (2) respiratory failure due to paresis and paralysis of the intercostal muscles and diaphragm.

Figure 10.1 shows the manifestations of botulism. The lack of a fever in an awake and alert patient can be deceptive in terms of the gravity of the situation.

As the patients arrive, have the triage team shuttle those who are in obvious respiratory distress or who have altered mental status (possibly related to hypercarbia) to the "reddest" of the red zone in the ED. Here, you and your "airway cohort" (consisting of nurses and respiratory therapists) are preparing yourselves for emergency airway intervention.

Once these patients are safely ensconced in their appropriate areas, they are automatically NPO (to prevent aspiration). They also receive an IV and are assessed for signs of respiratory compromise using any of a number of methodologies that would measure any impairment in the mechanics of breathing, such as ABGs, capnography, negative inspiratory force (NIF), and vital capacity (VC) measurements, and single breath counts. Discuss this with your respiratory therapist ahead of time.

Once you have addressed and resolved any respiratory issues, the next step is to contact local and/or state health departments and, if necessary, the CDC (24/7 at 770-488-7100). The principal reason for making this contact as quickly as possible is to obtain the release of botulism antitoxin heptavalent (A, B, C, D, E, F, G)—(equine), also known as BAT (botulinum antitoxin). The faster this antitoxin is administered, the less the circulating

Botulinum Toxin (Clostridium botulinum)

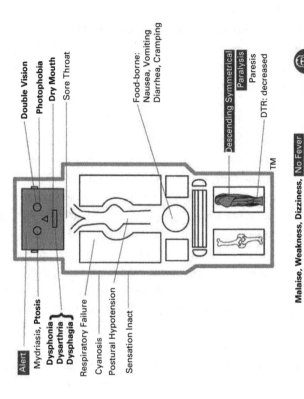

Syndromes
NEUROLOGICAL

Alert

Double Vision
Photophobia
Dry Mouth
Sore Throat

Mydriasis, Ptosis
Dysphonia
Dysarthria
Dysphagia

Respiratory Failure
Cyanosis
Postural Hypotension
Sensation Inact

Food-borne:
Nausea, Vomiting
Diarrhea, Cramping

Descending Symmetrical
Paralysis
Paresis
DTR: decreased

TM

Malaise, Weakness, Dizziness, No Fever

Early Symptoms
Delayed Symptoms
Classic Symptoms

FIGURE 10.1 Manifestations of botulism.

botulinum neurotoxin (BoNT) can be internalized by specific nerve cells at neuromuscular junctions. Studies have indicated that early administration of the antitoxin translates into fewer days on a ventilator, days in ICU, and days of hospitalization.

A number of years ago, there was a botulism MCI in central Ohio as a result of improperly stored potato salad at a church picnic. Once the correct diagnosis was considered, CDC was called and BAT was released. From the call to the administration, it took a total of 12 hours. Therefore, a call to CDC should be made expeditiously. Even if you have public health or your own hospital consult handle that task, make sure they understand that this is not a "back-burner" item. Trust them to do their job, but always verify. Additionally, it is critical for local public health to be notified early so that its personnel can perform an expeditious epidemiological evaluation. Many times it is not simple to isolate the cause of a botulism outbreak and even the suspicion of one case in a community is a public health emergency.

Once all the patients have been stabilized to your satisfaction, then the next consideration is which, if any, require transfer to another healthcare institution. The safest patients to transfer would be those whose airway has been secured by intubation and ventilation. If you transfer those who have evidence of respiratory insufficiency but whose airway has not been aggressively stabilized, you run the risk of respiratory deterioration in the ambulance or life flight.

Box 10.1 outlines CDC's classification of biological agents into Categories A, B, and C. Botulism is a Category A agent.

KEY POINTS TO REMEMBER

- Patients die acutely from aspiration and respiratory paralysis.
- The diagnosis of botulism is clinical. Do not wait for a confirmatory test result.
- Notify local public health to consider initiating a community-wide epidemiologic survey.
- Contact CDC expeditiously for the immediate release of botulism antitoxin heptavalent (A, B, C, D, E, F, G)—(equine).

CDC categories of biological agents

Why does CDC make certain biological agents **Category A agents**?
Easily dispersible and/or
Easily transmissible and/or
Easily produce significant morbidity and mortality and/or
Creators of panic and/or
Facilitate societal fragmentation and/or
Require special resources to resolve the crisis.

Category A Agents/Diseases
Anthrax: non-transmissible; organism: *Bacillus anthracis*
Botulism: non-transmissible; organism: *Clostridium botulinum* + toxins
Plague: transmissible; organism: *Yersinia pestis*
Smallpox: transmissible; organism: *Variola major virus*
Tularemia: non-transmissible; organism: *Francisella tularensis*
VHF: transmissible; organisms: *Filoviruses, Arenaviruses*
Why does CDC make certain biological agents **Category B agents**?
Dissemination potential: moderate
Morbidity potential: moderate
Mortality potential: low
CDC diagnostic and surveillance capabilities: required

Select Category B Agents/Diseases
Brucellosis (*Brucella*)
Clostridium perfringens (epsilon toxin)
Salmonella, Shigella, and *Escherichia coli* O157:H7: food vulnerabilities
Glanders (*Burkholderia mallei*)
Melioidosis (*Burkholderia pseudomallei*)
Ricin toxin (*Ricinus communis* [castor beans])
Staphylococcal enterotoxin B
Viral encephalitides (e.g., alphaviruses such as eastern equine encephalitis)
Potable water vulnerabilities: *Vibrio cholerae* and *Cryptosporidium parvum*
Why does CDC make certain biological agents **Category C** agents?
Third highest priority
Easily available
Easily produced
Easily disseminated
Ability to create significant morbidity and mortality

Select Category C Agents/Diseases
Nipah virus
Hantavirus

Further reading

Centers for Disease Control and Prevention. Bioterrorism agents/diseases by categories. https://emergency.cdc.gov/agent/agentlist-category.asp

Ni SA, Brady MF. Botulism antitoxin. StatPearls. 2021. https://www.ncbi.nlm.nih.gov/books/NBK534807/

Rao AK, Walters M, Hall J, Guymon C, Garden R, Sturdy P, Thurston D, Smith L, Dimond M, Vitek D, Bogdanow L, Hill M, Lin NH, Luquez C, Griffin PM. Outbreak of botulism due to illicit prison-brewed alcohol: Public health response to a serious and recurrent problem. *Clin Infect Dis*. 2017;66(suppl 1):S85–S91.

Rega PP. A 53-year-old social media worker with dysphonia and paresis. Medscape. 2021. https://reference.medscape.com/viewarticle/954850_1

Rega PP, Bork CE, Burkholder-Allen K, Bisesi MS, Gold JP. Single-breath-count test: An important adjunct in the triaging of patients in a mass-casualty incident due to botulism. *Prehosp Disaster Med*. 2010;25(3):219–222.

Rega P, Burkholder-Allen K, Bork C. An algorithm for the evaluation and management of red, yellow, and green zone patients during a botulism mass casualty incident. *Am J Disaster Med*. 2009;4(4):192–198.

Walters MS, Sreenivasan N, Person B, Shew M, Wheeler D, Hall J, Bogdanow L, Leniek K, Rao A. A qualitative inquiry about pruno, an illicit alcoholic beverage linked to botulism outbreaks in United States prisons. *Am J Public Health*. 2015;105(11):2256–2261.

11 "Is that a car backfiring?": The active assailant

It is a rather quiet Saturday in the ED. You are walking leisurely instead of rushing into Room 13 to see a 42-year-old tennis player who wrenched her knee jumping over the net after beating her adversary in two straight sets. She is in pain as an ice pack caresses her impressively swollen left knee. Her ACL is most likely shredded. Her vital signs are unremarkable. As you begin the process of improving your Press Ganey scores by introducing yourself and offering her both consolation and analgesia, you both hear that staccato rat-a-tat sound that once was thought to be a car backfiring but nowadays could only be an assault weapon.

What do I do now?

Whatever you do, it's never wrong because it's always right. Every active shooter situation is unique. In fact, today the term "active shooter" has become a misnomer. It may not even be a shooter; it may be an assailant with a knife or several grenades. It may not even be one assailant; there may be multiple. You may be at your computer away from your patient or directly in a care room with your patient doing what you do best. That patient may be a completely ambulatory earache and can run the 100-yard dash faster than you or it can be a patient in septic shock on three drips and a vent. The room you are currently occupying may be just off the ambulance bay or the farthest distance from the closest exit. Bottom line: Whatever action you take is the correct one (Figure 11.1).

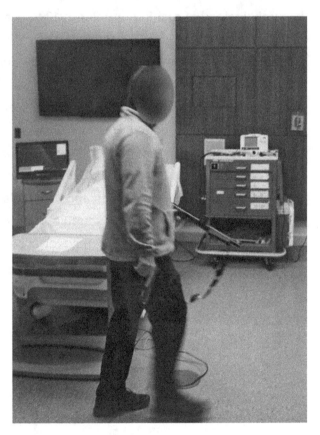

FIGURE 11.1 Active shooter in an active shooter drill.

For most individuals with diverse occupations at various locations, the standard course of action is "run, hide, fight." Many public and private stakeholders have tweaked the basic concept a bit to make it their own, but essentially, it's (1) run from the perpetrator if you can, (2) hide and barricade when you can't, and (3) fight as if your life depends on it—because it does. Encourage those nearby to follow your lead, but your primary responsibility is to yourself. Delay = Death.

This strategy can work in most places within the hospital. However, in patient care environments, especially in areas where the patients can't fend for themselves due to physical or cognitive vulnerabilities (e.g., ICU, ED, surgery), you may be facing a dual conflict: duty to yourself and duty to your patient. Healthcare professionals have a duty to care for their patients and to assume some level of personal risk in doing so. But what is the extent of that obligation to the patient? What level of risk should the healthcare practitioner assume? Recent studies indicate that healthcare students as well as ED patients believe that the healthcare professional's duty to preserve a patient's life is paramount. Nevertheless, each healthcare practitioner can easily appreciate that personal obligations to oneself and to one's family will be in direct conflict with one's obligations to one's patient.

Recently, the *New England Journal of Medicine* published an article written by a distinguished panel of healthcare practitioners and experts that proposed a counterpoint to the "run, hide, fight" strategy: "secure, preserve, fight." The objective is to save your own life as well as the life of your patient who is incapable of saving their own. "Secure" means enveloping the patient care area in a cocoon of invulnerability. "Preserve" means protecting yourself while maintaining the care and safety of the patient. And "fight" means using whatever is available to defend yourself should the area be breached.

Thinking through all of this at the time of the assault is too little too late. Critical decisions must be made in seconds. As soon as you realize that an actual attack may be happening, you need to gauge the level of the immediate threat and assess your own capabilities and vulnerabilities and those of your patient.

The events of December 2, 2015, at the Inland Regional Center in San Bernardino, California, serve as a good example. The shootings began around 11 a.m. during a holiday party. In a matter of minutes, 75 rifle rounds were fired. The two perpetrators escaped. Firefighters were the first to arrive, which they did 7 minutes after the first 911 calls were sent out. Seven minutes sounds fast, and indeed it was, but nevertheless, 14 people died and another 22 were wounded.

Delay = Death. Another point to consider is that while we think in terms of one assailant, there is no reason not to believe there may be more than one idealogue bent on murder and mayhem, as occurred in San Bernardino. Therefore, never consider yourself safe until you are behind police lines—if then.

Of course, the odds are that this will never occur at your hospital. Studies indicate that hospital shooting occurrences are rare among active assailant locations, but are you willing to gamble your life on the likelihood it will never happen?

The key is not to make decisions at the time the event is happening. Take stock of your ED *now*, before the threat appears. What this requires is a situational awareness of the department. This is especially important should you be moonlighting or work as locum tenens at a place with which you are not familiar.

- Turn off all lights in the room you are occupying. The time it takes for a perpetrator to accommodate to the darkness can provide precious time for you to hide more securely or to obtain improvised weaponry.
- Keep your phone muted or off. There's no reason for the "perp" to locate your position by the *William Tell Overture* sounding on your iPhone.
- Keep low and stay out the line of fire either through the door or if the door is slightly ajar.
- Learn the key punch codes to enter secure areas like the supply room ("safe rooms").
- Find out where the patient bathrooms are located. They often lock from inside and can accommodate several people at one time.
- Determine if the doors of the "safe" areas are wide enough to accommodate stretchers.
- Learn how to manipulate a gurney, prop it against the patient's door, and brake it. If a gurney is moved and locked in place against a closed

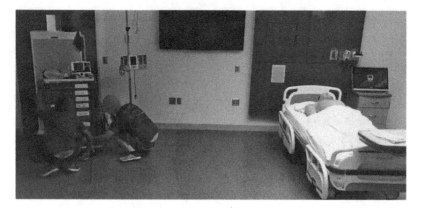

FIGURE 11.2 During an active shooter drill, medical students are barricading the entry by locking the wheels on a crash cart.

wall, this virtually ensures that no one can break in (Figure 11.2). If the gurney is occupied, consider moving the patient to the floor—IV lines, ET tube, and all—and then using the gurney as a barricade. Lives are at stake! Other equipment that can be used as barricades are the code cart, chairs, oxygen cylinders, etc. If the equipment has wheels, it is likely that you can lock it in place.

- If the entrance to your room has sliding doors, determine how best to block off the track. Many times these sliding doors are mostly glass, so you should protect yourself should it shatter for one reason or another.
- Use anyone competent in the room to assist you with barricading and with weaponry.
- Consider what you or others may have on you that can be used as improvised weapons. Shoes, pens, trauma shears, stethoscope, tuning forks, reflex hammers, etc. are easy to pick up and throw, thereby ruining the aim of the assailant.
- Figure out what "weapons" might be available in the room you're barricaded in (especially critical care rooms). Examples include IV poles, vials of medications, a sharps container, scalpels, and IO needles. Personally, I enjoy teaching my students about laryngoscopes. They're actually four weapons in one: one blade, one handle, and two batteries. There are other items—defibrillators,

chairs, stools, and oxygen tanks—but the question is whether you can lift and throw them. Find out now, not then.

- Learn how to secure an automatic door closer with surgical tape or IV tubing (Figure 11.3).

If other individuals who are with you elect to act differently from what you want to do, let them. This is not the time for rhetoric. Discussion and arguing is time-consuming. Chances are they will be looking to you for crisis leadership.

If you have decided to exit, with or without your patient, do so quickly. Keep your hands up in plain view to help law enforcement decide if you are friend or foe. This also serves as a reminder that if the perpetrator is neutralized in some fashion, kick the weapons away or place a wastepaper basket over them, but *do not* pick them up to threaten the perpetrator

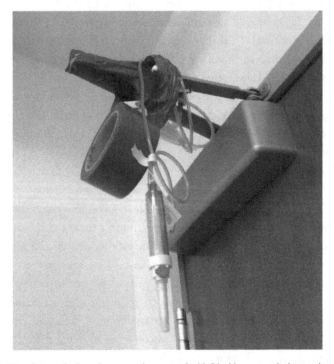

FIGURE 11.3 Automatic door closers can be secured with IV tubing or surgical tape, thereby preventing assailant access into your safe area.

or to show to your rescuers. You do not want to be confused with the assailant.

At some point, the event will be neutralized. With the permission of law enforcement, local medics and hospital personnel will be allowed to enter the hot zone and tend to the trapped patients and a whole new group of wounded ones, many of whom may be your friends and colleagues. This will not occur immediately, however, since the officers need to ensure scene safety for all concerned.

Now triage begins. The entry group can begin clearing airways, placing tourniquets on bleeds, recovery positioning those with head injuries, and determining who is tagged as Red, Yellow, Green, or Black. The next arrivals can provide advanced airway skills, place IOs, and relieve tension pneumothoraces. It's during this time that incident command and the chief surgeon should be deciding which patients should stay for surgical stabilization and which ones should be sent to other institutions. These are difficult decisions to make, given the fact that your hospital has just sustained not only a physical disaster but an emotional and a mental one.

At some point, the patients and the victims will receive the best care possible and there will be an attempt to return to a "new" normal. This is the recovery phase in the disaster cycle. The sooner it's initiated, the better. It should determine what was done correctly and what areas need improvement and should also address, in a timely fashion, the mental health needs of the professionals and staff. There should be an effort to ensure that whatever actions individuals took to save themselves or others, there should be no stigmatization. Whatever actions were taken were the best possible actions given the unique circumstances.

KEY POINTS TO REMEMBER

- In an active shooter situation, don't think; act. Analysis = paralysis = exposure = injury/death.
- Each incident is unique. Therefore, no one can predict individual behavior.
- As a healthcare provider, you have accepted a higher level of risk-taking than the average individual.

- The level of risk depends on multiple unpredictable factors coupled with your own personal duties, obligations, and infirmities. It's likely that your professional duties may conflict with your personal obligations.
- Do not try to normalize. Automobiles do not backfire. It's automatic gunfire.
- Since each person's actions will be different and may go against expectations, do not stigmatize.
- Mental health evaluation and rehabilitation should be mandatory.
- Look at the room you are in as an armory. What can be used as a potential weapon? What can be used as a barricade?

Further reading

Inaba K, Eastman AL, Jacobs LM, Mattox KL. Active-shooter response at a health care facility. *N Engl J Med*. 2018;379(6):583–586.

Kenney K, Nguyen K, Konecki E, Jones C, Kakish E, Fink E, Rega PP. What do emergency department patients and their guests expect from their health care provider in an active shooter event? *WMJ*. 2020;119(2):96–101.

Lee C, Walters E, Borger R, Clem K, Fenati G, Kiemeney M, Seng S, Yuen HW, Neeki M, Smith D. The San Bernardino, California, terror attack: Two emergency departments' response. *West J Emerg Med*. 2016;17(1):1–7.

McKenzie N, Wishner C, Sexton M, Saevig D, Fink B, Rega P. Active shooter: What would health care students do while caring for their patients? Run? Hide? Or fight? *Disaster Med Public Health Prep*. 2020;14(2):173–177.

MedPage Today Staff. Inside a massacre: What we learn from tragedy: Three physicians share the ways in which their lives were forever changed by gunmen. October 5, 2017. https://www.medpagetoday.com/emergencymedicine/emergencymedicine/68340

Ortiz E. San Bernardino shooting: Timeline of how the rampage unfolded. NBC News. https://www.nbcnews.com/storyline/san-bernardino-shooting/san-bernardino-shooting-timeline-how-rampage-unfolded-n473501

Sanchez L, Young VB, Baker M. Active shooter training in the emergency department: A safety initiative. *J Emerg Nurs*. 2018;44(6):598–604.

12 Explosions along the riverfront: A tragic accident

The sounds and vibrations from a distant explosion cause heads in your ED to turn. Almost immediately, EMS dispatch calls and directs your Level 1 Trauma Center to be prepared for the arrival of scores of victims. There has been a major explosion aboard a freighter, loaded with ammonium nitrate, anchored in your city's harbor. All signs indicate that it was an accidental event: torrential downpours, multiple lightning strikes, an uncontrolled fire on the deck of the *Marie Louise*, and, finally, a series of explosions below deck.

What do I do now?

As you get your act together, you are mindful of the event that occurred along the waterfront of Beirut, Lebanon, in 2020 (Box 12.1). Your current predicament is similar to, but hopefully not as extensive as, the ammonium nitrate maritime explosions that devastated that city's downtown.

Depending on the magnitude of the explosion, the number of victims, and the extent of the urban damage, this event may rise to the level of a complex disaster. The downtown infrastructure, including pre-hospital and hospital services, may be crippled for weeks to months. The response to that type of disaster will force the request for mutual aid, state agencies, and even federal agencies. However, these considerations are not your immediate concern. Beirut's preventable human tragedy involved nearly 3,000 tons of ammonium nitrate. The human impact consisted of 6,000 injured, at least 200 dead, and approximately 100 missing. It also caused the displacement of 300,000 inhabitants. The cost to Lebanon was approximately $10 billion USD.

BOX 12.1 **Two high-energy explosive events involving ammonium nitrate**

Vignette #1
Date: August 12, 2015
Location: Tianjin Post, Binhai New District, China
Cause: Reaction of stored hazardous chemicals
Major HAZMAT: 800 tons of ammonium nitrate (TNT equivalent: 256 tons)
Magnitude
1. Explosion #1: Equivalent to a 2.3M earthquake
2. Explosion #2: Equivalent to a 2.9M earthquake
Deaths: ~160 including first responders (~104 firefighters)
Injured: ~700

Vignette #2
Date: August 4, 2020
Location: Beirut, Lebanon
Cause: Warehouse fire/explosion
Major HAZMAT: ~2,750 tons of ammonium nitrate (TNT equivalent: 1.1 kilotons)
Magnitude: Equivalent to a 3.3M earthquake
Deaths: ~200
Injured: ~6,500

Contact hospital administration.
Activate the hospital's disaster plan.
Inform your team.
Provide just-in-time training if required.
Assume your ED disaster roles as per your plans and don vests (e.g., triage, command).
Triage your ED patient population (Yellow and Green) to alternative venues within the hospital to open up patient care rooms.

Knowing the potential impact and the likelihood of first-wave and second-wave victims, you will need to contact hospital leaders and trauma services and advise activating a Code-Disaster or its equivalent, depending on the disaster committee's previously accepted guidelines (Box 12.2). Additionally, alert the HAZMAT team and establish your decontamination zone. These victims may be covered with harmful substances that require removal (Figures 12.1 and 12.2). This may be a redundant operation since EMS and fire services at the scene may be involved in mass decontamination, but should a first-wave group of victims come to your doorway, they probably were evacuated prior to the arrival of the first responders.

Initiating communications with essential personnel and departments of the hospital should take only minutes. Now it is time to turn your attention to the ED and your team. They need to know what happened and what is expected of them. With published guidelines, procedures, and prior training, that is not an insurmountable task.

Before they get into the ED disaster mode (i.e., triaging ED patients, heightening their own PPE, and preparing rooms for the victims), it is critical to reacquaint everyone with the impact that high-energy explosives have on a human being. Even though your team members are used to trauma and all its nuances, the sudden impact of high-energy explosions can create specific trauma (i.e., blast injuries) that can rapidly become fatal if not recognized early. An explosion involves the sudden conversion of a solid or liquid to highly pressurized gases. A high-energy detonation such as what has been described in the scenario will consist of two components: the blast wave and the blast wind (Figure 12.3 and

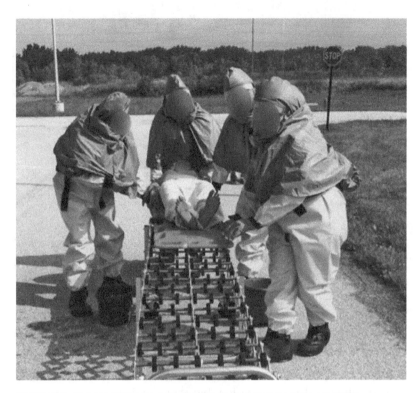

FIGURE 12.1 Part of a field decontamination drill. The responders are in Level B PPE.

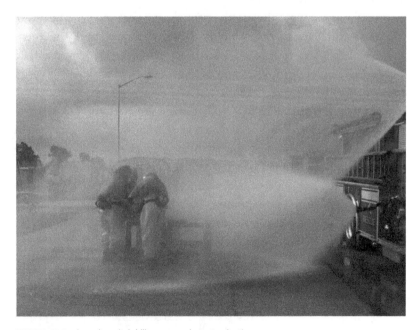

FIGURE 12.2 A pre-hospital drill on mass decontamination.

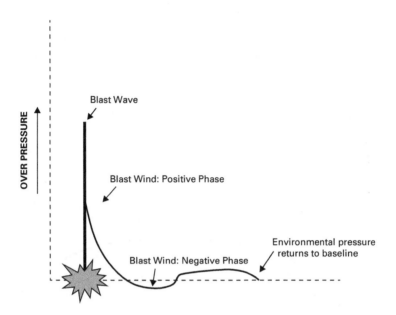

FIGURE 12.3 A schematic representation of a high-energy explosion.

TABLE 12.1 **High-energy and low-energy explosives**

Examples of high-energy explosives	Examples of low-energy explosives
Semtex/C4 (plastic)	Molotov cocktails (petroleum)
Trinitrotoluene (TNT)	Pipe bombs
Nitroglycerin/dynamite	Gunpowder
Ammonium nitrate	
Triacetone triperoxide (TAPT)	

Table 12.1). Low-velocity explosions, on the other hand, consist of the blast wind effect (Figure 12.4).

There are a number of factors that contribute to blast injuries and their level of severity:

- The type of explosive
- The sequence of events leading up to the explosion (i.e., the cause)
- Whether the victim was in a closed or open environment at the time of the explosion. The magnitude of blast mechanics is significantly greater should it be reflected by solid surfaces.

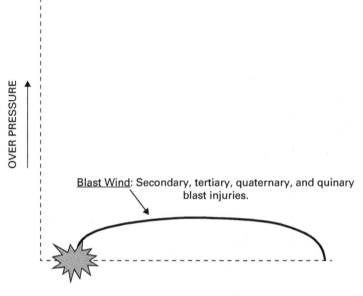

FIGURE 12.4 A schematic representation of a low-energy explosion.

- The victim's distance from the detonation site. The pressure wave drops as the cube root of the distance from the explosion. For example, a victim who is 10 feet from the detonation receives nine times the overpressure as a victim who is 20 feet away.
- The total body surface area (TBSA) that was exposed to the blast
- The presence of additional threats at the explosion site that could further injure the victim

THE BLAST WAVE

A blast wave is the sudden overpressurization and compression of the air and the environment, including anyone caught within it. The pressure wave generated by the explosion will create the compression and decompression of specific parts of the body (Figure 12.5). This mostly occurs in air-containing structures of the body, but it can also impact fluid-filled areas (e.g., brain, eyes, ears, lungs, GI tract). Much of the corporal damage is related to the physiologic stressors or forces such as shearing, implosion, and spalling. These organs will expand and contract at different frequencies, producing destabilization of that particular organ or body part. Their

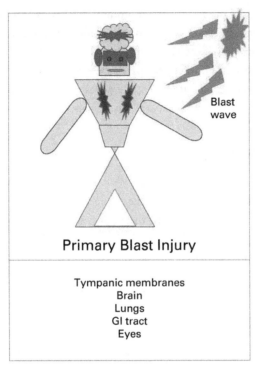

Blast wave

Primary Blast Injury

Tympanic membranes
Brain
Lungs
GI tract
Eyes

FIGURE 12.5 Primary blast injury.

ligamentous attachments can also tear apart since they will be vibrating at conflicting frequencies. The brain, encased in cerebrospinal fluid, will experience a coup–countercoup phenomenon. The middle ear's air-containing environment will expand and contract. Tympanic membranes will rupture.

The lungs and their alveoli are particularly vulnerable to the sudden changes in pressure. Alveoli will rupture, the alveoli–capillary membranes will tear, air emboli will be generated, and the lungs will easily collapse from a simple or tension pneumothorax or disintegrate completely. Many of the sudden deaths at the scene of a high-energy explosion are attributed to the significant impact on the lungs.

The GI tract will experience that same type of phenomenon, although the primary blast effect is more commonly seen with underwater explosions.

While emergency physicians and their associates are well versed in routine trauma signs and symptoms, especially working in a trauma center, their experience dealing with primary blast injury may be limited, if not nonexistent, unless they were in the military or a member of a SWAT team.

While many of the signs and symptoms will be evident upon the victim's initial presentation, there can be a delay lasting hours. Observation may be warranted, especially if the victim was in a closed-space environment when the explosion occurred. In closed spaces the effect of the blast wave is compounded; in contrast, in an open-space exposure the wave comes, impacts, and expands outward and dissipates into the environment.

THE BLAST WIND

Secondary, tertiary, and quaternary blast injuries are a result of the environmental wind generated by the explosion. Secondary blast injuries (Figure 12.6) are associated with the impact on the body of shrapnel and

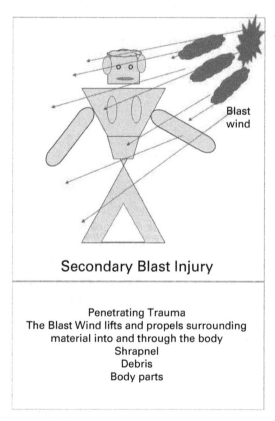

Blast wind

Secondary Blast Injury

Penetrating Trauma
The Blast Wind lifts and propels surrounding
material into and through the body
Shrapnel
Debris
Body parts

FIGURE 12.6 Secondary blast injury.

other debris, which penetrate it at velocities that can exceed 1,500 mph. Even the smallest-diameter cutaneous trauma can signal a major internal catastrophe. Anecdotally, there have been cases of peritonitis that developed weeks after tiny bits of shrapnel had penetrated the abdominal wall. The tears in the bowel wall were so small that leakage into the peritoneum was slow but inevitable.

Tertiary blast injuries (Figure 12.7) develop when the force of the explosion physically propels the victim from point A to point B. In a sense, while secondary blast injuries represent mainly penetrating trauma, consider tertiary blast injuries as representing blunt trauma. A human body that hits a solid object at a velocity of 26 feet/second has a mortality rate of 50%.

Quaternary blast injuries (Figure 12.8) are the indirect trauma that occurs in conjunction with an explosion. These types of injuries can include

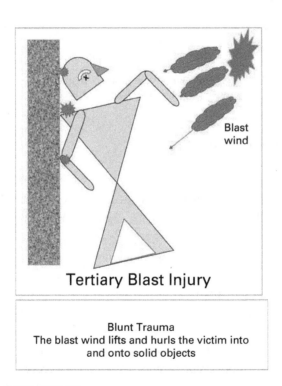

Tertiary Blast Injury

Blunt Trauma
The blast wind lifts and hurls the victim into
and onto solid objects

FIGURE 12.7 Tertiary blast injury.

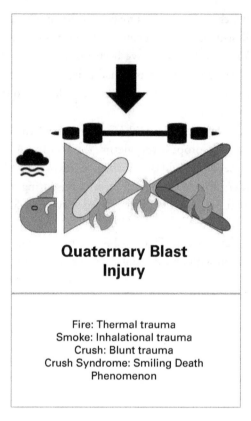

Quaternary Blast Injury

Fire: Thermal trauma
Smoke: Inhalational trauma
Crush: Blunt trauma
Crush Syndrome: Smiling Death
Phenomenon

FIGURE 12.8 Quaternary blast injury

internal and external thermal and/or chemical trauma, crush injuries secondary to building collapse, vehicular crash trauma, compartment syndrome, and crush syndrome.

Crush syndrome or traumatic rhabdomyolysis deserves special mention. It occurs when a heavy object lands on the large muscle masses of the body, such as thighs and the gluteus maximus. Based on the weight of the object, the amount of time it is on the body, and the amount of muscle mass that is impacted, there is compression and disintegration of striated myocytes and release of intracellular contents such as potassium, myoglobin, urates, and phosphates into the hypoxic, acidotic environment. Ultimately, this mélange of toxic material is deposited into the rest of the body once circulation is restored. Two results can occur. If the release of potassium into the circulation is significant enough, the hyperkalemia can lead to cardiac arrest. Otherwise, the dead or dying debris secondary to terminal injury to the muscle cells can lead to acute kidney injury and more multi-organ compromise. There have been situations where the victim's only trauma is one leg pinned under a massively heavy object for a period of time. In effect, the object is acting like a tourniquet, preventing any circulation to and from the involved leg. At that point, the victim may be feeling little, if any, discomfort, but lethal danger is lurking: Potassium, myoglobin, and other poisonous debris are pooling in the leg. Should the object be removed without prophylactic management, the sudden hyperkalemia can cause almost immediate cardiac arrest. This is the so-called smiling death syndrome.

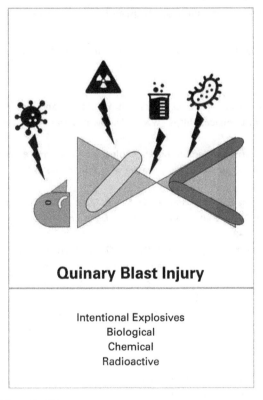

Quinary Blast Injury

Intentional Explosives
Biological
Chemical
Radioactive

FIGURE 12.9 Quinary blast injury.

Quinary blast injuries (Figure 12.9) are not relevant to this type of explosion and will be discussed in Chapter 13, which deals with intentional explosions.

KEY POINTS TO REMEMBER

- Determine whether the explosion was accidental or intentional and secure your ED accordingly.
- High-energy explosions generate both a blast wave and a blast wind.
- Blast waves produce over- and under-pressurization effects that negatively impact gas- and fluid-containing structures of the body.
- Low-energy explosions generate blast winds.
- Blast winds can cause both high-velocity penetrating and blunt trauma.
- Evaluate for both compartment and crush syndromes.

Further readings

Centers for Disease Control and Prevention. Explosions and Blast Injuries: A Primer for Clinicians. https://www.cdc.gov/masstrauma/preparedness/primer.pdf

El Sayed MJ. Beirut ammonium nitrate explosion: A man-made disaster in times of COVID-19 pandemic. *Disaster Med Public Health Prep.* 2020 Nov 18:1–18.

Hashim HT, Uakkas S, Reda A, Ramadhan MA, Al Mostafa MY. Beirut explosion effects on COVID-19 situation in Lebanon. *Disaster Med Public Health Prep.* 2021 Feb 16:1–2.

Li GQ, Hou SK, Yu X, Meng XT, Liu LL, Yan PB, Tian MN, Chen SL, Han HJ. A descriptive analysis of injury triage, surge of medical demand, and resource use in an university hospital after 8.12 Tianjin Port Explosion, China. *Chin J Traumatol.* 2015;18(6):314–319.

Li N, Wang X, Wang P, Fan H, Hou S, Gong Y. Emerging medical therapies in crush syndrome—progress report from basic sciences and potential future avenues. *Ren Fail.* 2020;42(1):656–666.

Liu Y, Feng K, Jiang H, Hu F, Gao J, Zhang W, Zhang W, Huang B, Brant R, Zhang C, Yan H. Characteristics and treatments of ocular blast injury in Tianjin explosion in China. *BMC Ophthalmol.* 2020;20(1):185.

Sever MS, Vanholder R. Management of crush syndrome casualties after disasters. *Rambam Maimonides Med J*. 2011;2(2):e0039.

Ur Rehman S, Ahmed R, Ma K, Xu S, Aslam MA, Bi H, Liu J, Wang J. Ammonium nitrate is a risk for environment: A case study of Beirut (Lebanon) chemical explosion and the effects on environment. *Ecotoxicol Environ Saf*. 2021;210:111834.

13 They're bombing the open-air market!

The triage nurse hurriedly comes over to you, leaving her post. There was breaking news on the waiting room TV: There was an attack in the open-air market a couple of miles away. According to the reporter, there were multiple assailants. One apparently was a suicide bomber who blew up a packed tour bus that just parked. Victim numbers are high, as well as the death rate on the bus. Search and rescue and EMS personnel are in the process of triaging and providing care. Police believe all the assailants have been neutralized, but they consider the scene as still active. As the nurse concludes her summary, the EMS phone goes off and the medic essentially confirms what was heard on Channel 5. Twenty are presumed dead and 50 or so have been wounded by bomb fragments, high-caliber bullets from a semiautomatic weapon, and machete hacks.

You are the only community hospital in a 25-mile radius.

What do I do now?

errorist attacks may not have received high priority in your community's hazard vulnerability analysis (HVA), but most assuredly, it will be in the future. Even though your community hospital may not be a high-level trauma center, certain disaster principles still apply (see Table 12.2 in Chapter 12). Figure 13.1 shows PGY I residents attending to the needs of a "patient" in a simulated bombing attack.

Additionally, with an intentional event, you should consider additional actions to safeguard your team, your patients, and you (Box 13.1).

Most suicide bombers can carry 25 kg of TNT in their backpacks. The detonation of that backpack will create 150 psi (pounds per square inch) peak overpressure for 2 msec at 3,000 to 8,000 m/sec (Box 13.2). In this regard, consider the possibility that the suicide bomber may have been chosen because they were infected with an infectious disease. An Israeli medical journal ran an article about a case in which the body parts of the suicide bomber embedded in the victims were positive for hepatitis. Prophylactic therapy was initiated in that case.

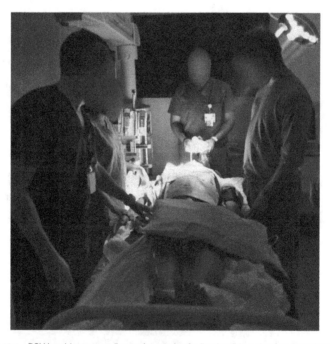

FIGURE 13.1 PGY I residents attending to the needs of a "patient" in a simulated bombing attack.

- Discourage freelancing by hospital personnel who wish to assist at the scene.
  - Likely they do not have the requisite pre-hospital training.
  - They may not be wearing the necessary PPE.
  - They may accidentally detonate a secondary explosive device meant to "take out" first responders.
  - Their expertise is better suited for the ED and ICU.
- Advise that lockdown must be as impenetrable as possible.
  - Hospital lockdown is notoriously porous and while you may not have any influence on this issue, it is advisable to discuss your concerns with security.
- Request appropriate security for the ED proper.
  - There is nothing guaranteeing that the perpetrators have all been "neutralized." They may be accidental victims of the firefight and escaped only to reappear as one of the first-wave or second-wave victims. Worse yet, they may actually be faux casualties. Part of their plan was to fake injuries, arrive at an ED, and "take it out" with as many additional victims as possible.
- Perform triage a certain distance away from the ED entrances.
  - This will provide a safety margin should a terrorist arrive for "treatment" and then decide to attack.
  - The triage process will include a swift pat-down for weaponry.
  - Security would be advised to monitor this area and assist with pat-down.
- Consider a Geiger–Müller counter at triage.
  - The hospital's radiation safety team should be at triage.
  - Scanning a radioactive contaminated victim may be the first time a radioactive "dirty bomb" was identified.
- Evaluate the victims and transporters (off-gassing) for any hazardous material syndromes.
- Try to keep the "reddest" of the Red victims in one area of the ED with all your ABC paraphernalia open and accessible.
  - This means there will be less running around if you need to needle the chest on Victim #1, insert three IOs in victim #2, and "tube" a third.

1.8 psi: Glass shards can penetrate the abdominal wall.
3.0 psi: Enough energy to lift a human body (1% mortality rate).
35 psi: Lung damage with a 1% mortality rate.
65 psi: Severe lung damage with a 99% mortality rate.

CASE REPORT: BOSTON MARATHON BOMBING, 2013

To appreciate how a hospital must go from zero to 60 when a sudden intentional MCI occurs, it is worthwhile studying the events at Brigham and Women's Hospital (BWH) on Patriot's Day, April 15, 2013, the day of the Boston Marathon bombings. It is worth remembering that no lives were lost when all those victims reached the hospitals.

Each year, up to 500,000 people arrive from all over the world to compete or participate in and attend the festivities associated with the Boston Marathon. One cannot find a more classic example of a mass gathering event. At BWH, it is standard procedure for the emergency management director to stand up the emergency operations center early that morning, given that BWH is only a little more than 2 miles away from the marathon's finish line near Copley Square.

The ED is a 55-bed set-up that is divided into four pods of 14 beds or so each. The charge nurse of Alpha Pod noted that, at 2:49 p.m., the ED was full up. There were 47 patients in the beds, six lined up in the hallways, another six in the waiting room, and four in triage.

At 2:50 p.m., two explosive devices shattered the 117th Boston Marathon. Reports of the bombings from the Boston Fire Department and EMS ignited the air in the ED at 2:54 p.m. Immediately, the Alpha Pod physician and charge nurse huddled together with the emergency management director and decided that the first item on the agenda was to clear the ED of as many patients as possible.

Another call came in from the Boston Health Commission's Medical Information Center and made two announcements: (1) Code Amber was being activated, which meant that there would be an all-hospital disaster response and (2) BWH would be receiving eight victims from the bombing site. Meanwhile, in the surgical area of the hospital, the perioperative nurse administrator immediately reviewed the caseload. Of the 42 operating suites, 30 were active and there were four patients still waiting to go in.

Interestingly, it was a senior emergency medicine resident who reminded the ED teams to consider the possibility of a HAZMAT situation. That was reasonable advice given the circumstances and one that should be in the front of an emergency physician's mind any time there is the threat of an intentional event. With that reminder, lockdown was activated as well as the decontamination unit. It is a little-known fact that when the 2008 Mumbai attacks were taking place, there was an attempted assault on one of the hospitals to which the victims were being transported. Thus, a hospital lockdown, no matter how porous, serves as another obstacle that could delay and frustrate a perpetrator seeking to add to the carnage.

One of the little-known heroes in the ED at that time was the chief of the Division of Medical Psychiatry. This physician entered the Alpha Pod area and immediately arranged disposition for eight psychiatric patients who were waiting for beds. This physician also worked closely with social services to calm each of the patients and to attend to their specific psychosocial needs. Also during this time, a team of internal medicine residents exited the elevators and began rolling the remaining ED patients to other wards.

Meanwhile, as the existing ED patients were being cleared out, swarms of trauma surgeons, anesthesiologists, and orthopedists were descending into the ED and formed ad hoc interdisciplinary teams to greet the incoming wounded. Bravo Team was prepared by 2:59 p.m. The nursing administrator, who in a past life was a U.S. Army major, began staging personnel and other resources.

At 3:08 p.m. the first victim arrived, and over the next 30 minutes, 19 more came through the ED doorways. As these patients entered their treatment areas in each of the pods, the healthcare team managed the intubations, the tranexamic acid (TXA) administrations, the blood transfusions, and other life-saving interventions. Five of the 19 went immediately to surgery.

As 3:15 p.m. rolled around, the OR medical director coordinated with the trauma and orthopedic surgeons in Alpha Pod concerning the triaging of their surgical patients to the operating suites. Who goes first? Second? Third? By 3:30 p.m. a thoracic surgeon was moving from room to room to see where his expertise was needed most. He was reliving his experiences at Hadassah Hospital in Israel, where he had cared for victims of multiple bus bombings.

Let's examine the care for one of these initial patients, an elderly man on warfarin who was admitted to Room 38 in Bravo Pod. He was in hemorrhagic shock and, besides burns and multiple facial wounds, he also had a compound fracture of the right ankle. The emergency physician performed a primary and secondary survey, the trauma surgeon inflated a blood pressure cuff tourniquet at the level of the right thigh to stem further hemorrhage, a second emergency physician performed the intubation, a plastic surgeon performed a lateral canthotomy, and the nurse infused blood and blood products.

Between 3:39 and 4:38 p.m., seven more victims arrived. At 3:45 p.m., the chief orthopedic resident was wheeling a young man to the OR. The 33-year-old's mangled legs had any further bleeding controlled with bilateral tourniquets. Although he survived, he did lose one of his legs due to the severe trauma. At surgery, he had loss of tissue along his right thigh and shrapnel consisting of nails and BB pellets.

More victims arrived over the next couple of hours. Of the 39 victims cared for at BWH, ranging in age from 16 to 65, all survived. Nine required emergency surgical intervention for open fractures, amputations, devascularized extremities, burn care, and shrapnel removal. Many of them required multiple surgeries for debridement, fasciotomies, tissue replacement, vascular reconstruction, and fracture stabilization.

Box 13.3 summarizes lessons learned from the Boston Marathon bombing. Box 13.4 gives four examples of other recent bombing events.

BOX 13.3 **Lessons learned from the Boston Marathon bombing**

- Lock down early.
- Cancel elective surgeries.
- Anticipate more victims coming in than what stated by EMS.
- Prepare the decontamination zone early.
- Medical admission teams work.
- Multidisciplinary resuscitation teams work.
- Tourniquets work.
- TXA works.
- Use mental health professionals to their best advantage.

---

14 "We're evacuating the hospital . . . now!"

You're working the night shift. It's relatively quiet: assorted colds, chest pains, bumps and bruises. Suddenly an explosion rocks the hospital literally off its foundation and sends all of you off your feet. The lights go out and the sprinkler system activates. The squeaks and pings of monitors and ventilators have suddenly been replaced by screams from both patients and staff. Debris is everywhere. False ceilings cover the floors. Both staff and patients are among the injured. The dazed and beleaguered Chief Nursing Officer has negotiated the ED entrance after going through the rest of the hospital and yells out to you to evacuate immediately: It has been determined that your hospital is in danger of imminent collapse. An illegal fireworks factory just 100 yards away has accidentally detonated, and the explosion had the force of 1,100 tons of TNT and will be registered as a 3.3M quake on the Richter scale.

What do I do now?

H as this happened in real life? Consider the San Fernando earthquake of February 9, 1971. Segments of the Olive View-UCLA Medical Center were impacted by the 6.5M tremblor and its aftershocks. There were three deaths at the hospital, two due to power failure of life-support systems and one due to falling debris. Interestingly enough, all three deaths occurred at the complex's new Medical Treatment and Care Building, which was said to be earthquake resistant. According to the after-action report, the building's power failed, its communications system was disrupted, and its elevators were out of action. The building "was on the verge of collapse."

The same earthquake caused more serious damage at the Veterans Administration hospital located at the base of the San Gabriel Mountains. Some of its buildings had been constructed before the 1933 earthquake mitigation code and some after. Four pre-code buildings collapsed entirely and those constructed after 1933 still sustained damage. There were 47 deaths, mostly from the collapse of the pre-code buildings.

More recently, wildfires triggered an emergency evacuation of the Feather River Hospital in Paradise, California. Over the course of a couple of hours, the decision was made to evacuate ("Code Black") because the hospital was about to be encircled by the inferno. Because ambulances, helicopter, and firefighting equipment were inaccessible, healthcare practitioners and other volunteers had to evacuate 80 patients, including 67 inpatients, in their own cars, with nothing more than oxygen cylinders in some cases. All but one patient survived the evacuation, including 200 personnel.

While it may be conjectured that American hospital administrators have learned and have largely applied technologically advanced mitigation measures to minimize nature's impact, we still need to remember that many emergency physicians volunteer with national and international disaster relief teams that deploy around the world when needs arise. They may inadvertently place themselves in harm's way as they are tasked with delivering medical assistance at hospitals that are vulnerable to quakes, floods, tornadoes, and cyclones.

EMERGENCY ED EVACUATION

With the distinct possibility that the four floors of your hospital can collapse on you like a sagging soufflé, your course is simple: Get out! Fortunately, most EDs are situated on the ground floor, so you are in an ideal position to evacuate everyone immediately. The priorities are your staff and patients. This is the time for "reverse triage." The ambulatory population is evacuated first because they require fewer resources and time expenditure. One or two staff people with booming voices, commanding presences, and flashlights (or even a smartphone flashlight app) can direct the ambulatory patients and their families quickly out of the threatened ED and well away from the potentially collapsing walls of the hospital.

While the ambulatory population is being evacuated, your staff are preparing the non-ambulatory Yellow and Red patients for a safer evacuation. This will take more time and more staff resources. Remember, the scene is not safe, so this is a "load-and-go" situation. The niceties and nuances of patient care take second place to speed and efficiency.

The Red and Yellow patients are encumbered by immobility, assorted pathologies, and all the attachments and equipment needed for the patient's well-being (ventilators, IV medications, monitors, chest tubes, Foleys, etc.). There is no time to "cap and clamp," so simply place what you can on the patient's gurney and move out. What you lose in the process can be restarted, but lives cannot. Probably, the one item that is essential is the ventilator. Unless it is a portable ventilator, disconnect it and "Ambu" the patient. There may not even be time to connect the bag to a portable oxygen source. If an oxygen D cylinder is immediately available, it can be thrown on the gurney and connected once the patient reaches a safe zone. "Bagging" the patient with 21% oxygen (i.e., room air) may be temporarily suitable in extreme circumstances. After all, you are still oxygenating and ventilating.

Gurneys have wheels that can be locked in a certain position so that they can be maneuvered by one person. Check to see if you have that type, and ensure that everyone on your team, especially the physicians, know how to work it. It will save resources and free up other team members to rescue others. If the passageways are unpassable, two rescuers can cocoon the patient in one or two bedsheets, slide them off the gurney onto the floor, and drag them to safety. The patient's entourage, if present, can assist unless you have already ordered them to evacuate.

There will be concerns about managing the patients and victims outdoors without meds and monitors, but we are talking about an extreme situation. Imminent collapse or destruction of your hospital is likely and any delay can endanger lives. Stick to the KISS method ("Keep it simple, stupid"): Save lives first, and worry about the rest later.

The initial paucity of resources can be soon eradicated as EMS arrives on the scene and provides you with their resources. One way to mitigate this initial lack of resources is to have the ED administration develop, with the team's input, an ED "Evac-Bag." It could be stocked with the essential airway, breathing, and circulation equipment needed to sustain life in the field. It can be stored right at the ambulance entrance to the ED so that it's easy to pick up on the way out.

Once outside, stay outside. Having people going in and out for supplies and such needlessly exposes them to recurrent dangers. However, you, as "captain of the ship," should quickly run through all the rooms to ensure no one is left behind. Use a marker to place a large "X" on the door or adjacent wall to convey to search and rescue people that the room has been cleared of all individuals.

EMERGENCY HOSPITAL EVACUATION

Exiting the ED emergently is considerably more straightforward than patient evacuation from the surgical suites, ICUs, and other patient care areas on the floors above. Elevators are off limits. The staircases leading to safety should be well demarcated as "Egress" or "OUT." One or two stairwells can be identified as "Ingress" or "IN" for incoming rescuers. There is no reason to add to the confusion by having those going up and those coming down collide in the same stairwell.

Here again, reverse triage is appropriate. The ambulatory or Green patients are quickly identified and are escorted down the stairs as a group with at least one staff member in front and behind with flashlights. To this group, I would add new mothers and their newborns as well as patients who have psychiatric or chemically dependent maladies. The types of patients suitable for reverse triage should be discussed at disaster preparedness meetings.

While all these patients are being evacuated, the nurses and physicians are readying their non-ambulatory patients for the journey to safety. Their evacuation is more problematic. More resources, critical decision-making, and decisive leadership are required. Virtually all these patients will have their individual "accoutrements" that need to be addressed. What must stay with the patient and what can be left behind are important decisions mandating immediate action. Stacking everything on the patient's evacuation conveyance adds weight and may impede rescuer movement and risk falls.

There is a plethora of conveyances to move patients in an emergency, such as stair-chairs, basket-litters, and simple backboards (Figure 14.1). They all work if the staff knows how to secure a patient to one and how to move a patient safely in one. That takes education, in-services, and periodic drilling. In your planning sessions, ask yourself and the committee members what would be an alternative if some obstacle was blocking access to the storage area where these devices are kept. The key in any of the disaster planning sessions is redundancy: If the initial plan cannot work, what's the alternative?

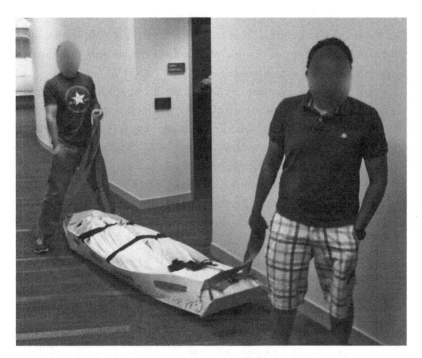

FIGURE 14.1 An economical method for evacuating hospitalized patients quickly.

1. Cocoon the patient in two of their bedsheets and top sheets.
2. Square-knot the sheets at both ends.
3. Encase any essential patient records, parenteral medications, tubing, and/or tanks within the patient's cocoon.
4. Discontinue any nonessential patient care devices or IV medications (e.g., antibiotics). These can be restarted later once the patient is in a safer location.
4. Rotate their mattress 90 degrees off the bed.
5. Slide the patient down the mattress onto the floor.
6. One team of two drags the patient.
7. Another team takes the mattresses from all the beds and lines them up end to end down the stairs.
8. The transporters drag the patient along the floor to the stairwell and then slide them down the mattresses on the stairs. Since the width of the mattress is usually less than the width of the stairs, the transporters can walk down the stairs as they slide the patient.

One alternative technique that can be quite serviceable during an emergency evacuation from any patient care zone in the hospital is the Iserson "cocoon and mattress" technique (Box 14.1).

The "cocoon and mattress" technique should be considered when the more traditional methods are unavailable. When a non-ambulatory patient requires immediate evacuation, encase them in a double bedsheet (two bedsheets provide strength) (Figure 14.2). Any necessary patient devices like Foley bags, drainage bottles, etc. can be secured and incorporated with the patient within the sheets. Tie a double square knot in each sheet separately at the head and the feet (Figure 14.3). Now the patient is fully wrapped in two sheets and any drips, tubing, and other devices are included within the sheets (Figure 14.4). Next, swing the patient and their mattress 90 degrees to slide the patient off the bed and onto the floor. As the patients are being pulled down the halls, any unused mattresses are appropriated to cover the stairs and act as "slides" (Figure 14.5). The "mattress slide" lessens the risk of caregivers harming themselves in lifting and also protects the patients from accidental head injuries (Figure 14.6). In many staircases, there is ample space to slide the

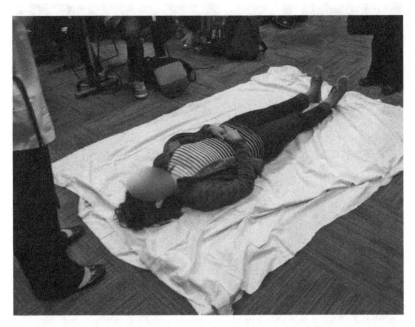

FIGURE 14.2 The patient is encased in a double bedsheet (two bedsheets provide strength).

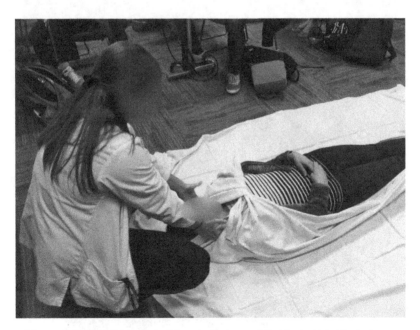

FIGURE 14.3 Tie a double square knot in each sheet separately at the head and the feet.

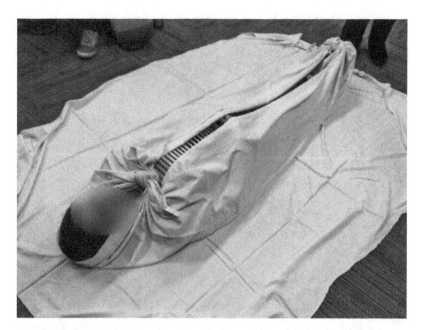

FIGURE 14.4 The patient is fully wrapped in two sheets, with any drips, tubing, and other devices included within the sheets.

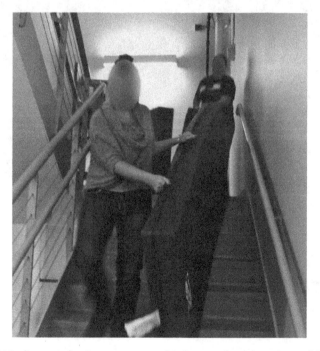

FIGURE 14.5 Any unused mattresses are appropriated to cover the stairs and act as "slides."

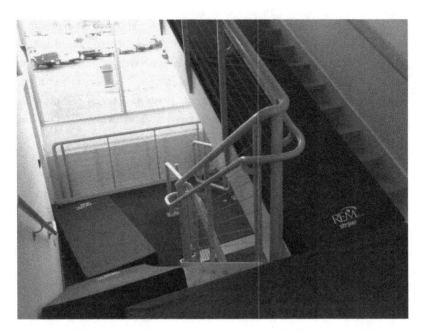

FIGURE 14.6 The "mattress slide."

patient down the stairs while the two caregiver-transporters are holding the sheets as they walk down the stairs beside the patient. To minimize injury, the transporters should not walk on the mattresses.

The idea of using the non-ambulatory patient's own hospital mattress as an evacuation mode has its advocates. In Germany, for example, an innovative design incorporating zippered retention and fixation belts into the mattress has been developed and is now being used in hospitals.

Continuous illumination of the stairwells would be ideal, and taping operational flashlights along the railings has been suggested.

Intubated-ventilated patients are always a logistical nightmare during evacuation. Ambu bags with or without an oxygen cylinder can be used in these circumstances, but to "Ambu" the patient going down the stairs can be dangerous for everyone concerned. One way to mitigate that situation is to hyperventilate on the stair landings and disconnect the bag while going down the stairs. This will minimize the risk of an accidental extubation.

At one New York City hospital that was evacuating all its patients at night during Hurricane Sandy, one morbidly obese patient could not be evacuated down flights of stairs due to the patient's weight. The patient was forced to stay the night with two nurse volunteers. The Iserson technique might have solved that problem. However, as spartan as this technique is, it is not fodder for just-in-time training. Pre-disaster education and drilling remains essential.

As was mentioned as a mitigation measure in the ED, an Evac-Bag could also be considered for the other patient care floors. Actually, there can be a couple of bags, one for patient care as mentioned earlier and another for the staff as they evacuate their patients. The components of such a bag could include:

1. Flashlights and batteries
2. Signage (IN/OUT; Ingress/Egress)
3. Markers to place an "X" on any empty room that has been cleared
4. Whistles
5. Hardhat

KEY POINTS TO REMEMBER

· Determine what hazards might force your hospital to emergently evacuate.
· Locate an area outside the hospital that can accommodate all the patients of the hospital.
· Once out, stay out.

Further reading

Abbasi J. Paradise's emergency department director recalls California's worst wildfire. *JAMA.* 2019;321(12):1144–1146.

Iserson KV. Vertical hospital evacuations: A new method. *South Med J.* 2013;106(1):37–42.

Kikta KJ. 45 seconds: memoirs of an ER physician. When the deadly EF-5 tornado struck Joplin, May 22, 2011. *Mo Med.* 2011;108(3):150–154.

Little M, Stone T, Stone R, Burns J, Reeves J, Cullen P, Humble I, Finn E, Aitken P, Elcock M, Gillard N. The evacuation of Cairns Hospitals due to severe tropical cyclone Yasi. *Acad Emerg Med.* 2012;19(9):E1088–E1098.

Okumura T, Tokuno S. Case study of medical evacuation before and after the Fukushima Daiichi nuclear power plant accident in the great east Japan earthquake. *Disaster Mil Med*. 2015;1:19.

Prokop A, Waiblinger B. Innovatives neues Evakuierungskonzept mit Rettungsmatratzen [Innovative new evacuation concept with emergency mattresses]. *Z Orthop Unfall*. 2018;156(6):723–724 [in German].

Rega PP, Locher G, Shank H, Contreras K, Bork CE. Considerations for the vertical evacuation of hospitalized patients under emergency conditions. *Am J Disaster Med*. 2010;5(4):237–246.

Sahebi A, Jahangiri K, Alibabaei A, Khorasani-Zavareh D. Factors affecting emergency evacuation of Iranian hospitals in fire: A qualitative study. *J Educ Health Promot*. 2021;10:154.

Steinbrugge KV, Schader EE, Moran DF *Building Damage in the San Fernando Valley, San Fernando, California, Earthquake of 9 February 1971*. Bulletin 196. California Division of Mines and Geology; 1975:323–353.

Sutherland S. 135 minutes. *NFPA Journal*. January 2, 2019. https://www.nfpa.org/News-and-Research/Publications-and-media/NFPA-Journal/2019/January-February-2019/POV/Perspectives

Zane R, Biddinger P, Hassol A, Rich T, Gerber J, DeAngelis J. *Hospital Evacuation Decision Guide*. AHRQ Publication No. 10-0009. Agency for Healthcare Research and Quality; 2010.

15 Zap, sizzle, and fizz: Contamination, irradiation, and trauma

A cryptic phone call comes into the ED and the charge nurse hands the phone to you. It is from the Chief Medical Officer. She has received word from the local FBI office that an assassination attempt on a national candidate who is in town has been interdicted by local and federal agents. The alleged assassin has been identified as a government-sponsored foreign agent who has been known to use stolen radioisotopes to assassinate political adversaries. In the process of arresting the agent, gunfire ensued, and the suspect was shot multiple times. During the shootout, several vials ruptured, contaminating the area and the alleged perpetrator. EMS will be in contact shortly. We are the closest hospital, she adds, and then hangs up.

As soon as she hangs up and before you can get a chance to process the news, the Bat-Phone rings. The EMT-P communicates that they are in load-and-go mode bringing in a middle-aged female patient who has been shot five times in the chest, head, and abdomen. According to the FBI, she may have been contaminated with polonium-210: In her hands are a couple of shattered vials, and her hands and face are wet. Her vital signs are pulse 124, respirations 6, BP 82/54, SaO_2 on 4 L nasal O_2 86%, and Glasgow Coma Scale (GCS) score 10.

What do I do now?

This is a radiological emergency. You activate the appropriate code from the hospital's disaster plan. Hopefully, your ED team and your radiological safety team have drilled a radiological mishap in prior exercises; if you have not, you should have. You are facing a rare situation in which the Radiation Safety Team will be managing the patient from an irradiated and contaminated viewpoint and your ED team will be managing the patient's primary and secondary trauma surveys.

A radioactive incident is any occurrence in which the environment and its flora and fauna, including humankind, are subjected to ionizing radiation. It could be as minor as an accidental spill of I_{131} in the radiology suite or as overwhelming as a nuclear war. A radioactive incident can occur in any number of ways. It may happen in a transportation accident or in a fixed establishment. It can be accidental or, worse yet, intentional. It can involve just one victim or entire populations. In any case, when most people think of a radiological incident, Hiroshima, Nagasaki, Chernobyl, and Fukushima come to mind.

Radionuclides or radioactive isotopes release ionizing radiation. There are two basic types: electromagnetic radiation and particulate radiation. Ultraviolet light, visible light, X-rays, and gamma (γ) rays constitute electromagnetic radiation. Gamma rays are the high-energy electromagnetic radiation emitted by certain radionuclides as their nuclei try to stabilize from a high- to a low-energy state. They have neither mass nor charge. Particulate radiation, on the other hand, has mass. The three fundamental particles are alpha (α) particles, beta (β) particles, and neutrons. Alpha particles consist of two protons and two neutrons and have a charge of +2. Beta particles, on the other hand, are electrons that have been ejected from a decaying nucleus; they have a charge of –1. Discussion on neutrons is reserved for a deeper analysis of a true nuclear detonation when there is the wholesale release of neutrons (see Chapter 16). Box 15.1 explains how radiation is measured.

Given the proper circumstances, ionizing radiation can damage and/or destroy living cells. While exposure to ionizing radiation may involve some combination of electromagnetic waves and particulate matter, each component will be discussed separately to clarify the similarities and differences.

ALPHA AND BETA PARTICLES

The deposition of radioactive α and β particles on the body (Figure 15.1).
is an example of radiological contamination. Radioactive contamination
occurs when a radioisotope (as a gas, liquid, or solid) is released into the
environment and then ingested, inhaled, or deposited on the body surface.

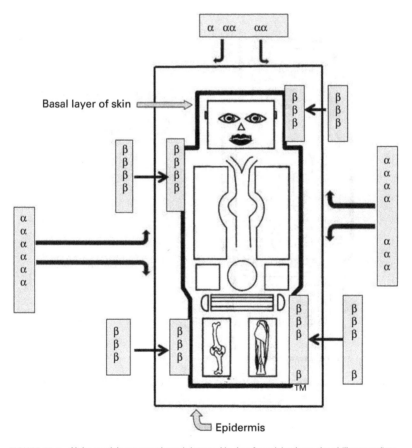

FIGURE 15.1 Alpha particles cannot breach intact skin, but β particles have the ability to radiate into skin, causing "beta burns."

Deposition of α particles on the skin really causes no injury. The skin is an excellent barrier to the radiation effects of these particles. Alpha particulate radiation cannot even penetrate paper. The problem with α particles occurs when they are accidentally or intentionally delivered internally into the body. Now there is no protective barrier, and the damage to internal systems can be both acute and chronic depending on the radioactive source material. Radon and polonium are both α emitters.

Beta particles, on the other hand, can penetrate skin and cause cutaneous damage (i.e., β burns). A single layer of clothes is sufficient to protect against the harmful effects of β particles. However, should β particles be internalized, they can cause considerable damage. There are no β barriers

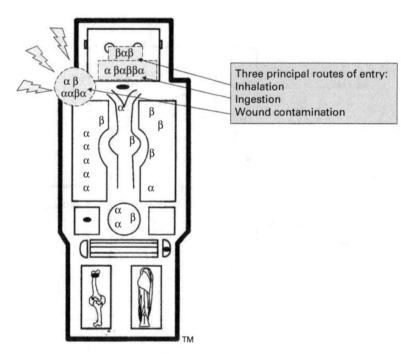

FIGURE 15.2 The purpose of decontamination is to prevent alpha and beta particles from entering the body and being incorporated into cells. Careful attention must be given to removing the α and β particles from eyes, nose, mouth, and wounds. Additionally, decontamination of the rest of the body must be accomplished in such a fashion so as not to recontaminate the wounds and facial areas.

once the skin is breached. So how does one contend with α and β particle contamination on the body surface? Decontamination. The decontamination process is meant to separate the contaminated victim from these particles (Figure 15.2). The act of radiological decontamination is the physical process of removing radioactive particulate matter (i.e., α and β particles) from the skin in a careful, meticulous process to prevent them from entering the body and being incorporated into the cells. Extreme caution must be taken to prevent the accidental entry of these particles into tear ducts, nasal passages, the mouth, and wounds. Conceivably, healthcare responders and caregivers can be secondarily contaminated from these patients, but donning appropriate PPE will minimize the risk, low as it is. Additionally, wearing film badges and dosimeters will keep a constant check on any irradiation mishaps.

GAMMA RAYS

Now, turning to γ rays, their impact on the body depends on the radioisotope emitting the rays and the amount of total body surface area (TBSA) that was exposed to the penetrating ionizing radiation. A person who was exposed only to γ rays is not a threat to anyone else, just like a person who gets a chest X-ray has momentarily been exposed to X-rays but is not radioactive (Table 15.1). This is an important concept for your people to appreciate because they may worry about their safety when caring for a patient who has been involved with a radiological incident. So, with γ rays, if the

TABLE 15.1 **Common radiation sources**

Natural background radiation:	300 mrem/year (North America)
Chest radiograph:	10 mrem
Lumbar spine radiographs:	70 mrem
CT head:	200 mrem
CT chest:	800 mrem
CT abdomen:	1,000 mrem

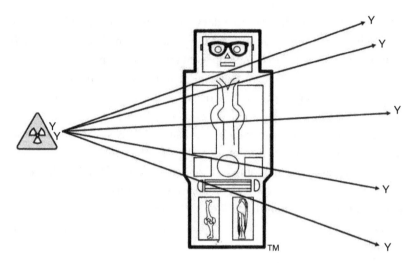

FIGURE 15.3 Gamma rays emanating from a radioisotope and traveling into and through an organism. Time, distance, and shielding will reduce the effects of the radiation.

exposure is long enough, the person is close enough (to the open source), and a significant part of the body has been exposed, then that person is at risk for acute radiation syndrome. It is all a matter of time, distance, and shielding, just like with any other hazardous material (Figure 15.3). Shielding can be accomplished by an inch of lead lining or a concrete barrier that is at least several inches thick.

ACUTE RADIATION SYNDROME

Acute Radiation Syndrome is the term for the sequence, degree, and types of manifestations that may occur once a human has been exposed to a given amount of γ rays. Once irradiated, a living cell will proceed to one of four outcomes. That outcome is, to a certain extent, still dependent on the principles of time, distance, and shielding.

- Outcome 1: Gamma rays strike the cell, but the amount was so slight that, apart from the initial impact, there are no lasting or permanent repercussions. The cell's DNA, the main target, remains unviolated.

- Outcome 2: Gamma rays strike the cell. The degree is more intense and there is cellular impact, but the cell's integrity and more importantly its DNA remain whole. Any clinical manifestations are short term.
- Outcome 3: Gamma rays damage the cell either because the time, distance, and shielding parameters have failed and/or because the cell is specifically sensitive to irradiation (Box 15.2). The cell doesn't die, but its DNA has been irreparably damaged, leading to mutative and carcinogenic alterations in the future.
- Outcome 4: A combination of the γ rays' characteristics and the cell type leads to the death of the cell.

An analogy may be of some use here. Think of a fighter in the ring. The fighter represents the cells, and the opponent's punch will represent γ rays. If the punch is delivered by a 1-year-old child to the fighter's chin, then there is virtually no impact, no damage. If a 7-year-old child delivers it, the fighter will feel it, shake it off, and walk away: no harm, no foul. If another fighter of equal ability delivers the punch, the recipient will feel its effects now and later, raising the possibility of concussive effects in the short and long term (namely, "punch drunk"). Finally, if the fighter receives a knockout blow, the internal damage can be severe enough to cause unconsciousness, coma, and death. Any and all of these outcomes can be seen with acute radiation syndrome (Figure 15.4).

BOX 15.2 **Radiosensitivity of human cells (from highest to lowest sensitivity)**

Lymphocytes
Erythrocytes
Spermatogenesis
Epidermal stem cells
Gastrointestinal stem cells
Myocytes
Osteocytes
Neurons

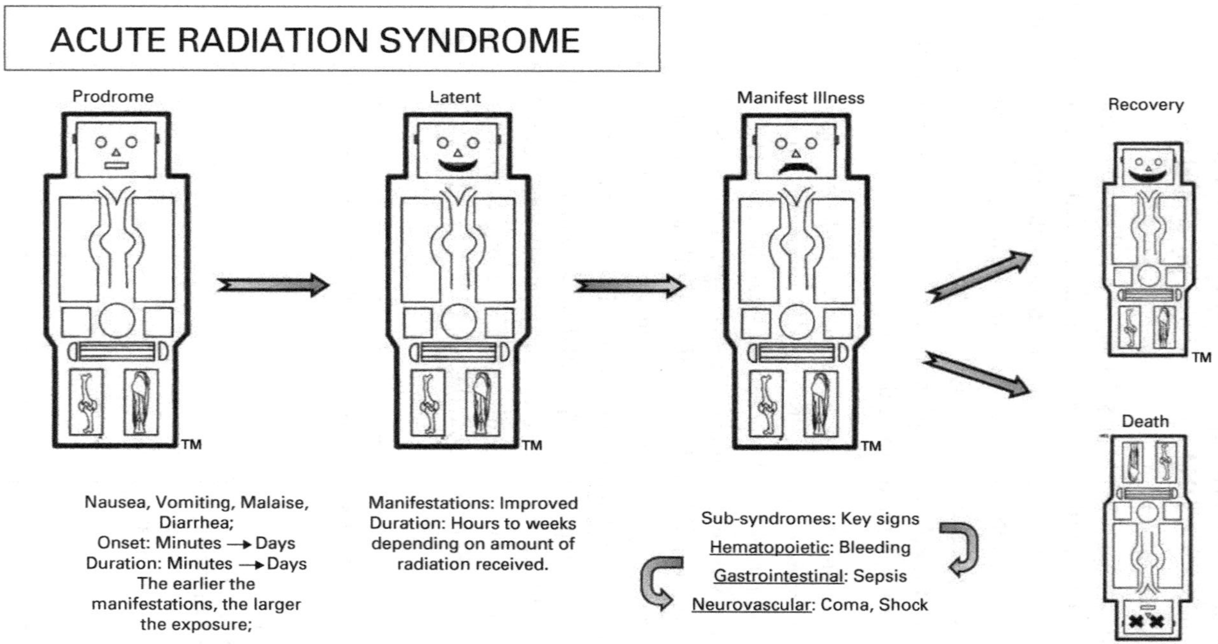

ACUTE RADIATION SYNDROME

Prodrome

Nausea, Vomiting, Malaise, Diarrhea;
Onset: Minutes ——→ Days
Duration: Minutes ——→ Days
The earlier the manifestations, the larger the exposure;

Latent

Manifestations: Improved
Duration: Hours to weeks depending on amount of radiation received.

Manifest Illness

Sub-syndromes: Key signs
Hematopoietic: Bleeding
Gastrointestinal: Sepsis
Neurovascular: Coma, Shock

Recovery

Death

FIGURE 15.4 Acute radiation syndrome usually develops when there is a significant or total body exposure to a radiation dose as low as 1 Gy.

Prodromal stage

The prodromal stage of acute radiation syndrome corresponds to the body's sudden exposure to γ radiation. The victim will be nauseated and may vomit. Malaise will be a dominant finding. When it manifests itself, its duration will depend on the amount of absorbed radiation. It can occur within minutes to hours after exposure.

Latent stage

In the latent stage, the victim feels clinically better. The nausea and vomiting have ceased, and the malaise has subsided. Yet, cellular changes can still be occurring, from transient to permanent. The duration of the latent stage is indirectly proportional to the amount of radiation absorbed.

Stage of Manifest Illness

In this stage, the clinical manifestations of the irradiated cells appear. The cells and therefore the body's systems will be affected based upon the cells' rate of division as well as cellular differentiation.

Within the stage of manifest illness is the *hematopoietic syndrome*, which typically occurs when a significant amount of the TBSA receives more than 2 Gy of penetrating radiation. The prodrome is usually less than a couple of days and the latent stage can last from 1 to 3 weeks. With the decimation of the hematopoietic cells, there will be episodes of bleeding and infectious disease vulnerabilities.

The *GI syndrome* can be seen when the body has been exposed to more than 6 Gy of penetrating radiation. Because the amount of radiation is so much greater, prodromal manifestations will occur within hours and the latent period will only last a week or less. Coupled with the disruption of the blood cell lines, there is also a denudation of the lining of the GI tract. The loss of the GI cellular barrier will enable the invasion of GI flora and fauna into the systemic circulation.

The final syndrome is the *neurovascular syndrome*. To arrive at this level, the victim has likely received more than 20 Gy of penetrating radiation. Altered mental status, seizures, coma, and death dominate the clinical picture. The prodrome may be seen within minutes of exposure and there may not even be a latent period as the patient quickly succumbs to the effects of the intense radiation.

The last stage is either partial or complete recovery or death.

Table 15.2 summarizes the phases of acute radiation syndrome and Box 15.3 provides an overview of its management.

Cutaneous radiation syndrome

Throughout all the phases of the acute radiation syndrome runs the Cutaneous Radiation Syndrome, which constitutes the pathologic changes seen in the skin when exposed to β radiation. It can range from erythema to bullae to extensive desquamation and ulceration.

In summary, the impact on a living being will depend on the radioactive material, its radioactive components, and the amount of living tissue exposed to the electromagnetic waves. Many of the severe effects can be mitigated by time, distance, and shielding. Keep in mind that while we are discussing irradiation and contamination as two separate entities, you

TABLE 15.2 **Phases of acute radiation syndrome**

Gy	Prodrome	Manifest illness	Survival
0.5–1	Up to 48 hours	Mild hematopoietic	Great
1–3.5	Up to 24 hours	Moderate hematopoietic	Very good
3.5–7.5	Within several hours	Severe hematopoietic Mild GI	Death within 2–6 weeks
7.5–10	Within a few hours	Severe hematopoietic Severe GI	Death within 1–3 weeks
>10	Within several minutes	Neurovascular	Death within 2–12 days

BOX 15.3 **Management overview: acute radiation syndrome**

- Isolation for patient protection
- Fluid/electrolyte replacement
- Avoidance of unnecessary invasive procedures
- Immediate surgery, if needed, while blood components are at their highest
- Anti-infection therapy
- Bone marrow stimulation
- Bone marrow transplant

should consider your patient as being both irradiated *and* contaminated unless your expert consultants declare otherwise.

THE ED RESPONSE

Which team's actions have priority, the radiation safety team, with its radiation safety officer, or the ED team, with you as the lead medical officer? You and your team are in charge. While a radiation event such as this may be considered a HAZMAT event, it differs from the other hazardous materials in that the patient's medical condition receives top priority. Decontamination comes second.

Time permitting, the radiation safety team starts prepping the treatment area and entrances with floor and wall coverings to minimize contamination spread. They check that the teams are in proper PPE plus a lead apron plus a radiation safety badge/dosimeter or both. You are either getting the trauma room ready as per standard operating procedure or adapting your decontamination area into a resuscitation room. Wherever this patient goes, she will need to be in an optimal environment to address the trauma caused by five bullet wounds.

You may be lucky if the radioisotope in this scenario is polonium-210; it is an alpha agent and its radiation power can easily be stifled by a piece of paper.

Wherever the patient winds up, ABCD & E come first: trauma's primary survey. Exposure is critical here because if there is any contamination on the patient, removal of the clothes will resolve a major percentage of the contamination. However, instruct your team to remove the clothes very deliberately so as not to aerosolize any entrapped embedded material (Box 15.4). Be judicious. You would not want to introduce surface contamination into any wounds or the patient's orifices (eyes, nose, mouth, wounds, etc.).

BOX 15.4 **Clothing removal guidelines**

Cut, do not pull off, clothes.
Cut from top to bottom.
Cut away from wounds.
Fold outer surfaces of the garments away from skin.
Change gloves after handling and removal of clothes.
Place clothes in marked plastic bags and secure.

Second, if you need to provide definitive airway control, decontaminating the oral areas first will help to minimize internalization of any radioisotope. Similarly, it would be prudent to wipe away any skin areas where you intend to start IVs or IOs—again, to limit internalization with your needles. Your radiation safety team will tell you where the sites of contamination are located using Geiger-Müller counters with alpha windows.

Once your patient has been stabilized as best as possible, your radiation safety team will be monitoring the level of contamination on the patient and the location. If there is contamination, rinsing the contaminated areas with tepid water should resolve most of the radioisotope on the skin. Cover the wounds and any other orifices with waterproof dressings so that any contaminated rinse water does not get internalized. Avoid using hot water to minimize superficial vasodilatation, and don't spray the water, again to avoid aerosolization. The radiation safety team will tell you how often to perform the decontamination procedure based on the counter's readings. Meanwhile, make sure that team has enough blood for any esoteric radiation levels in order to gauge internalization. They will also analyze debris, orifices, and any effluents of the patient (e.g., vomitus, urine, feces, or wound substrata). They will also record when and if the patient vomits, which may be a prognosticator of the acute radiation syndrome.

Box 15.5 summarizes management of the irradiated-contaminated patient.

At some point, with sufficient stabilization, the victim may be a candidate for further imaging in the radiological suite or may wind up going straight to the OR. It may be a team decision among you, the radiation safety officer, the trauma surgeon, and any other consultants. In any case, while the management of one traumatized radiation patient is hardly a mass casualty incident, it has been presented to underscore in a simplistic way the priorities that should be adhered to whether it involves one patient or multiple victims: *Treat the patient first and the radiation second.*

Box 15.6 presents some historical examples of radiation exposure.

General management of the irradiated-contaminated patient

- Primary survey: airway, breathing, circulation, disability, exposure
- Store clothes and personal articles in a double plastic bag and secure away from others
- Radiation survey (Geiger–Müller counter). Repeat after every decontamination procedure
- Uncontaminated wounds should be covered with waterproof dressings to prevent cross-contamination
- Wash down (soap/water) (may shower if ambulatory and uninjured)
- Use tepid water; too hot increases absorption, too cold increases entrapment
- Rule of thumb: Adequate decontamination is up to a level that is twice the background radiation level
- Contaminated wounds take decontamination priority
- Use gentle irrigation and avoid splashing.
- When performing a surgical sponge scrub, avoid abrading the skin.
- Debridement/surgical excision is done only as a last resort.
- Contaminated thermal burns
- Rinse gently
- Since there is no circulation in severely burned tissue, internalization of contaminants will not occur
- Contaminants will be removed with exudate
- Leave closed blisters closed
- For open blisters, irrigate as per burn protocol
- Oral/pharyngeal contamination: toothpaste/toothbrush, H_2O_2 gargles
- Eyes: Direct irrigation fluids from the inner canthus to the outer canthus to avoid washing contaminants into nasolacrimal duct
- Ears: Is tympanic membrane intact?
- Swab and survey each nasal passage and oropharynx
- Collect and survey bodily fluids (blood, vomitus, feces, wound and tissue samples, urine) to evaluate, mitigate, and prevent internal contamination/incorporation
- Bioassay sampling should be done after clothes removal and initial decontamination to minimize false positives
- Swabs from body orifices (saline-moistened)
- Swabs from wounds
- Swabs from intact skin
- Urine: 24-hour specimen
- Vomitus
- Feces: 24-hour specimen
- CBC/differential (may require repetition)
- BUN/creatinine

Continued

Continued

- Irrigating fluids
- Internal contamination therapy
- Pulmonary lavage
- Sputum induction
- Purgatives
- GI lavage
- Whole bowel irrigation
- Chelation therapy (EDTA, DTPA)
- Personnel performing decontamination should periodically change their clothing

---

BOX 15.6   **Historical examples of radiation exposure**

Location: Goiana, Brazil
  Date: 1987
  Radioisotope: cesium-137 (Cs^{137})

A couple of naïve individuals discovered a glowing blue rock (medical Cs^{137}) lost in the dismantling of a radiotherapy building. The rock was shared among friends and neighbors. Twenty of them eventually developed acute radiation syndrome, and four died. It is estimated that their total body radiation exposure was between 4.5 Gy and over 6.0 Gy. This public health emergency affected the entire country: More than 100,000 people were evaluated. Forty homes were found to be contaminated and required demolition. The entire country was in a state of unease. People from Goiana and their products were shunned

Location Yanango, Peru
  Date: 1999
  Radioisotope: iridium-192

A welder at a hydroelectric power plant found an unshielded ^{192}Ir industrial radiography source. He put it in the back pocket of his trousers. Over the course of the evening, he experienced irritation and redness at the contact site. It wasn't until a day later that the true significance of the incident was discovered and the radioisotope was secured. As soon as governmental agencies were notified (including the International Atomic Energy Agency), activities at the hydroelectric plant were curtailed and an epidemiological investigation was undertaken to determine further exposure to other contacts as well as the environment. The welder went on to develop acute radiation syndrome, with significant drops in leukocytes, lymphocytes, and platelets, and his gluteal area became ulcerated, necrotic, and infected. It is estimated that the local skin exposure to the radioisotope was nearly 10,000 Gy. The site could not be treated conservatively, and ultimately a hemipelvectomy was required to stop further death of tissue

Location: London, UK
  Date: November 2006
  Radioisotope: polonium-210 (^{210}Po)
  It is believed that on November 1 Alexander Litvinenko unwittingly ingested tea contaminated with ^{210}Po. Symptoms began with severe diarrhea and vomiting. Over the course of 23 days, Litvinenko had significant drops in his hematopoietic cells, leading to bleeding and infectious episodes. Ultimately, he developed multi-organ failure, seizures, shock, and coma, and died. Toxicology reports indicated that he received more than 10 times the lethal dose of radioactive polonium

KEY POINTS TO REMEMBER

- The ABCs supersede radioactive decontamination.
- The first priority for decontamination is areas of the body that may serve as conduits for the internalization of the surface contaminants (e.g., wounds, eyes, nose, and mouth).
- A systemic response requires communication, education, and drilling between ED and radiation safety teams.

Further reading

Ahn JS, Moon JD, Kang W, Lim HM, Cho S, Lim DY, Park WJ. Acute radiation syndrome in a non-destructive testing worker: A case report. *Ann Occup Environ Med*. 2018;30:59.

Avtandilashvili M, Dumit S, Tolmachev Sy. Ustur whole-body case 0212: 17-year follow-up of plutonium-contaminated wound. *Radiat Prot Dosimetry*. 2018;178(2):160–169.

Bybel B, Beebe W, Kim BY, Faiman C. Contamination of a bracelet following iodine-131 therapy: A case report. *J Nucl Med Technol*. 2000;28(4):257–258.

Centers for Disease Control and Prevention. Polonium-210. www.cdc.gov/nceh/radiation/Polonium-210.htm

Fojtík P, Malátová I, Becková V, Pfeiferová V. A case of occupational internal contamination with 241Am. *Radiat Prot Dosimetry*. 2013;156(2):190–197.

Hamawy G. The case of the radioactive pillow. *Health Phys*. 2001;81(5 Suppl):S62–S64.

Harrison J, Fell T, Leggett R, Lloyd D, Puncher M, Youngman M. The polonium-210 poisoning of Mr. Alexander Litvinenko. *J Radiol Prot*. 2017;37(1):266–278.

Högberg L. Root causes and impacts of severe accidents at large nuclear power plants. *Ambio*. 2013;42(3):267–284.

Iddins CJ, Cohen SR, Goans RE, Wanat R, Jenkins M, Christensen DM, Dainiak N. Case report: Industrial X-ray injury treated with non-cultured autologous adipose-derived stromal vascular fraction (SVF). *Health Phys*. 2016;111(2):112–116.

Jefferson RD, Goans RE, Blain PG, Thomas SHL. Diagnosis and treatment of polonium poisoning. *Clin Toxicol*. 2009;47(5):379–392.

Kaga K, Maeshima A, Tsuzuku T, Kondo K, Morizono T. Temporal bone histopathological features of a worker who received high doses of radiation in a criticality accident: A case report. *Acta Otolaryngol*. 2011;131(4):451–455.

Kairemo K, Kangasmäki A. Imaging of accidental contamination by fluorine-18 solution: A quick troubleshooting procedure. *Asia Ocean J Nucl Med Biol*. 2016;4(1):51–54.

Linet MS, Kazzi Z, Paulson JA. Pediatric considerations before, during, and after radiological or nuclear emergencies. *Pediatrics*. 2018;142(6):e20183001.

Liu Q, Jiang B, Jiang LP, Wu Y, Wang XG, Zhao FL, Fu BH, Istvan T, Jiang E. Clinical report of three cases of acute radiation sickness from a (60) Co radiation accident in Henan Province in China. *J Radiat Res*. 2008;49(1):63–69.

Nishiyama H, Saenger EL, Grossman LW, Lukes SJ. Accidental Cs-137 contamination. *Radiology*. 1985;154(2):513–517.

Stavem P, Brøgger A, Devik F, Flatby J, van der Hagen CB, Henriksen T, Hoel PS, Høst H, Kett K, Petersen B. Lethal acute gamma radiation accident at Kjeller, Norway. Report of a case. *Acta Radiol Oncol*. 1985;24(1):61–63.

Wolbarst AB, Wiley AL, Nemhauser JB, Christensen DM, Hendee WR. Medical response to a major radiological emergency: A primer for medical and public health practitioners. *Radiology*. 2010;254:660–677.

Yu NY, Rule WG, Sio TT, Ashman JB, Nelson KL. Radiation contamination following cremation of a deceased patient treated with a radiopharmaceutical. *JAMA*. 2019;321(8):803–804.

16 From fireball to mushroom cloud

"What was that?!" Everyone in the ED is looking at each other, but no one can make any immediate sense of it. It almost sounded like a clap of thunder, but it was somehow different. Besides, the weather was going to stay perfect over this holiday weekend in the tristate area. So, you all go about your business of saving patients' lives. However, in a matter of minutes, everyone is looking at their cellphones as breaking news commandeers the airwaves. Meanwhile, the agitated CEO of the hospital comes to you directly to tell you that he received word from a federal agency representative that a nuclear improvised explosive device was detonated in a major city nearby. Three pieces of news:

1. Building engineers, maintenance, and construction experts in consultation with local federal authorities agree that your hospital is nowhere near the zones of severe or moderate damage and is sound.
2. Your community and your hospital may still be in the fallout area and further information will be forthcoming.
3. Assuming your institution is away from the hot zone and the fallout areas, as part of the National Disaster Medical System, your hospital will be receiving victims.

What do I do now?

Arguably, if one evaluates most of the hazard vulnerability assessments created in the United States, one would find the perception that the risk of a nuclear improvised explosive device would be small. What cannot be argued, however, is that the impact locally, and even nationally, would be great.

With a nuclear detonation, nothing is immediately known. No one can tell you the magnitude of the detonation, its location, the extent of the damage zones, the size of the fallout damage zones, and whether this is the first of multiple detonations. Is it war or is it an act of terrorism? What is known immediately is that you've survived the immediate effects of the blast and now you and your hospital must consider surviving the effects of fallout. That is the immediate default action that has been advocated by experts. Evacuation is not an option since that option exposes one to radioactive fallout. The immediate answer to fallout is to shelter in place, preferably in the center of the building and/or the basement and to prevent the internal environment of your shelter from being contaminated by the possible radioactive fallout from the outside environment. That could involve shutting the HVAC system as well as instituting lockdown procedures.

The hospital incident command system, needless to say, has been activated and further action will be dictated by the findings of the state and federal investigatory agencies. It is time now to reassure both patients and staff, to encourage them to contact their loved ones, and to urge them to shelter and not to flee. It is also time to provide some just-in-time training about nuclear explosions.

Within a span of an hour or so, you have received official word that the structural integrity of your hospital is intact, that your community has been largely unaffected by the detonation 50 miles away (shattered windows and anxious poultry), and that the fallout zones are expanding in a northeasterly direction, which is 180 degrees from your location. You are open for business. Expect casualties. The numbers of casualties that may be coming your way is anyone's guess in the first couple of hours. It will depend on the size of the detonation, its geographic location, ground burst versus air burst, time of day, size of the local population near the detonation site and downwind from it, infrastructural integrity, and weather. For example, a ground burst (a detonation on land) will create more fallout as the ground is sucked into the fireball and is added to the fallout. On the other hand, an air burst (a detonation in the sky) will cause less fallout, but it will increase exposure to both thermal and radioactive energy.

When those casualties will be coming will, to a large extent, depend on the proximity of your hospital to ground zero. In any case, don't be too surprised that many local inhabitants will be arriving shortly because of perceived exposure to the bomb or because of anxieties related to the bomb. The event can also exacerbate common maladies such as fear-provoked myocardial infarctions or multiple-vehicular collisions related to erroneous evacuation strategies. In the meantime, radiation safety personnel may soon be doling out film badges and dosimeters to key staff. Once you are open for business, it will also be prudent to check incoming people/patients for contamination. Maintaining lockdown and funneling visitors to limited sites will expedite the radiation monitoring process.

For the purposes of this discussion, the detonation was a 10-kiloton (kT) explosion. Why 10 kT? Much of the literature and damage and casualty estimates are based on a 10-kT explosion. It is also the size of the bomb that has usually been employed when executing preparedness and response plans (e.g., national planning scenarios). The term "10 kT" relates to the number of kilotons of conventional TNT that has to be detonated to create the same nuclear effect.

The energy that is released from a nuclear explosion is divided into multiple parts:

- Fireball
- Blast effects (both wave and wind)
- Prompt radiation
- Thermal
- Nuclear electromagnetic pulse (EMP)
- Delayed ionizing radiation (i.e., fallout)

Nuclear radiation will have components of electromagnetic radiation such as UV, IF, visible, gamma, and X-rays. It will also contain particulate radiation such as alpha, beta, and neutron particles.

TYPES OF INJURIES

Expect your patients from within the detonation area to exhibit varying degrees and severities of injuries based on the different types of energy that impacted the victims (Box 16.1). Modeling studies reveal that the victims could number in the thousands. Their trauma will depend on the varying degrees of blunt and penetrating trauma, burn severity (TBSA), and acute radiation syndrome (ARS). The number of casualties will be higher with an air burst compared to a ground burst. Finally, those with combined trauma will always fare worse.

Fireball

A fireball is an example of visible light energy. It consists of incandescent gas and vapor and has been described as more intense than sunrays at high noon. Fireball witnesses whose eyes are not protected are subject to permanent retinal burns and transient flash blindness. During daytime hours, flash blindness can occur up to 12 km away from the blast site. During the night, flash blindness can be experienced as far as 24 km from the blast site. On the other hand, victims can sustain retinal burns up to a distance of 110 km. It is obvious that a sudden injury like this can lead to further trauma— for example, a vehicular accident.

BOX 16.1 **Summary of nuclear detonation injuries**

Flash blindness
Flash blindness + retinal burns
Acute radiation syndrome (ARS)
Primary (1°) blast injuries (overpressure trauma)
Secondary (2°) blast injuries (penetrating trauma)
Tertiary (3°) blast injuries (blunt trauma)
Quaternary (4°) blast injuries (burns, crush, etc.)
Quinary (5°) blast injuries (nuclear contamination)
ARS + 1° and/or 2° and/or 3° and/or 4° and/or 5° blast injuries
Fallout + ARS + 1° and/or 2° and/or 3° and/or 4° and/or 5° blast injuries
Fallout + ARS
Behavioral health issues
Fallout +/- ARS +/- 1° and/or 2° and/or 3° and/or 4° and/or 5° blast injuries and behavioral health issues

---

Electromagnetic pulse

This sudden pulse of energy that occurs with nuclear explosions does not affect people directly, but following a 10-kT explosion, the EMP can cause disruption of communications and electrical equipment for a radius of up to 4 km. It has been suggested that up to 65% of electrical medical equipment can also be adversely affected. There is a possibility that cell-phones and handheld radios may still function due to the length of their antennae.

Thermal energy

The initial thermal pulse can be intense enough to incinerate buildings near ground zero and cause flash burns on victims. These burns can be directly on the skin itself or can result from the ignition of the person's clothes or jewelry.

Blast effects

These are injuries associated with the blast wave and blast winds and were previously described in the chapter on high-energy explosives. Blast wave injuries involve the gas-containing and fluid-encapsulating structures of the body. At ground zero, the overpressure will be as high as thousands of pounds per square inch, and it will expand outward at speeds exceeding hundreds of miles per hour. Blast winds will achieve speeds of more than 160 mph. Blast wind injuries involve not only penetrating and blunt trauma, but also the explosion's secondary impact such as burn trauma. Quinary blast effects are related to exposure to ionizing radiation either in terms of electromagnetic waves or radioactive particulate matter. It has been estimated that the LD_{50} (i.e., the radiation dose that kills half of an exposed population who received no medical intervention) is 350 centigrays (cGy). However, that number can easily change for the worse depending on the age of the patient, total body surface area exposed, past medical history, concurrent medical conditions, etc.

Prompt radiation

With the detonation, victims will receive an unknown amount of electro-magnetic radiation, the principal one being gamma rays. Three factors—time, distance, and shielding—will determine whether an individual has been irradiated sufficiently enough to develop ARS. The victims can also be contaminated with radioactive particles such as alpha particle, beta particles, and neutrons. Exposure of objects to neutron bombardment can also make them radioactive. Therefore, each victim can have varying degrees of irradiation and radioactive contamination.

Delayed radiation or fallout

This is the main source of radioactive contamination. Immediate sheltering following detonation will minimize exposure to fallout and the incorporation of alpha and beta particles into the body. That act will lessen the possibility of developing ARS. Maximal danger of fallout occurs in the first 1 or 2 hours after detonation. Then it will drop by 90% for every sevenfold increase in time. To put this more simply, consider that the dose rate is given the value of 100. At 7 hours that value drops to 10. At 49 hours, it drops down to 1 and after 2 weeks it is down to 0.1. The mapping of fallout and any other pertinent information associated with it will be within the province of the Interagency Modeling and Atmospheric Assessment Center (IMAAC).

To appreciate the potential impact of a nuclear detonation on individuals, models have been created that evaluate the degree of damage and fallout expanding from ground zero and how it can impact any response effort. Regardless of the size of detonation, three zones of damage have been described as well as fallout perimeters:

1. The *severe damage zone* (SDZ) comprises ground zero and the adjacent surroundings. This is the "no-go" zone. It is the hottest of the hot zone and carries with it the dubious distinction of having the lowest rate of victim survival as well as being a real threat to first responders. The zone can be as small as a quarter-mile radius with a 0.1-kT detonation, up to a half-mile radius with a 1-kT explosion, and 1 mile in a 10-kT explosion.
2. With a 10-kT explosion, the *moderate damage zone* (MDZ) will extend beyond the 1-mile radius and will have survivors. While some buildings will remain standing, there will be significant damage, multiple structural fires, and ruptured water and utility lines.

3. The *light damage zone* (LDZ) will extend out as far as 10 miles with a 10-kT detonation. Structural damage will be minimal to moderate, with broken windows and shattered glass. This zone will have the largest number of survivors.

Apart from the damage zones, another topographical event that must be identified within nuclear detonations is the fallout zone. It is divided into two levels of criticality: the dangerous fallout zone (DFZ) and the radiation caution zone (RCZ). The boundary between zones is determined by the radiation exposure rate (RER): An RER of 10 R/hour and higher is considered the DFZ.

With a 10-kT detonation, the DFZ will expand in the first hour of detonation up to as much as 20 miles from ground zero. The RCZ will also continue to expand. Over the next couple of hours, the DFZ will shrink to about 11 to 12 miles from ground zero while the RCZ will continue to grow due to prevailing air currents. The expansion of the entire fallout zone can reach a maximum of several hundred miles in only a matter of days before its inevitable dissipation.

PLANNING YOUR RESPONSE

As you are preparing to receive victims from the nuclear blast, there may be some comfort in knowing that you have a plan to retrieve them and provide them with the care and support needed. It is also useful to appreciate exactly where your hospital fits into this regional response effort.

The term to remember is the RTR response system, which stands for the Radiation Triage, Treat, Transport System (Box 16.2). Essentially, it is a medley of diverse medical venues with varying capabilities that have been identified to care for victims of a nuclear detonation. It is likely that your hospital, if it is outside the major damage and fallout zones, will likely be considered a medical center for nuclear detonation victims.

In addition to the RTR response system, there is also the Radiation Injury Treatment Network (RITN). There are approximately 80 institutions within the RITN. Guidelines, communications, and transportation links will be crucial in identifying patients within the RTR response system who will be better served at one of the specialized RITN hospitals. For example,

RTR 1: This venue with any stockpiled resources is located virtually at the perimeter of the SDZ. Because of its theoretical location, it may not be established and ready to render aid for at least several days. In all likelihood, the victims will have sustained the most severe combined trauma. Personnel must be in appropriate PPE and wear radiation detectors.

RTR 2: This venue is intended to be located outside of the MDZ, but it may still fall within the DFZ. The survivors coming here to be treated may have very survivable trauma. They may even be ambulatory. Here, too, the personnel must be in appropriate PPE and be monitored for radiation exposure.

RTR 3: These sites are located in the LDZ. The plan is that victims coming to these sites will have no immediate acute medical needs. The goal is mainly to assess them rapidly and to send them out to more sophisticated healthcare venues.

Medical care: These are the hospitals and other established healthcare facilities in the nearby safe area that have been identified to supply the appropriate medical, trauma, and radiation care to victims coming from RTR 1–3 or who made their own way to the facility.

Assembly centers: These are mainly venues for victims who have minimal, if any, acute medical needs but who require shelter as they await final disposition (e.g., Red Cross shelters).

Evacuation centers: These venues are specially developed to document, facilitate, and track displaced individuals who require more permanent housing.

---

the best candidates are those who sustained a radiation dose between 1.5 and 8.3 Gy. They can receive outpatient monitoring and specialized supportive care, up to and including bone marrow transplants. These hospitals may also be of limited service to victims who have combined trauma and radiation injuries.

In addition to caring for patients in your current place of work, you may have volunteered to assist at any of the healthcare centers in the RTR response system. Regardless of where you might be, your patients can have varying degrees of medical, surgical, radiation, and behavioral trauma. Victims who evacuated during the first hour and exposed themselves to fallout may manifest no symptoms. Nevertheless, you may be seeing them during their latency period and in a matter of days will begin to exhibit the ARS hematopoietic syndrome.

Box 16.3 lists some essentials that should be considered when evaluating any victim of a nuclear detonation. These essentials address the myriad issues associated with this unique event and are not well known.

Finally, an issue that needs to be resolved before such an event actually occurs is the concept of "allocation of scarce resources." Murmurings about which type of patients should receive what type of insufficient resources have been growing louder and louder since the SARS-CoV-1 outbreak in 2002 and it has become overpowering during the COVID-19 pandemic. However, with any pandemic, since it is one of those slow, relentless disasters, there is time to consider how best to manage the scarcities within a framework of legal rulings and ethical guidelines. The operative word is "time." With a nuclear detonation, there is no time to discuss this issue in a fair and transparent manner. Therefore, this issue must be discussed now, not right after the first mushroom cloud is visible.

- A sudden white flash in the sky, brighter than the sun at high noon, could signify a fireball. Avert your eyes immediately to avoid retinal burns and transient blindness.
- The first action to take after detonation is to shelter in place, not evacuate. Immediate sheltering limits one's exposure to fallout and the possibility of ARS.
- Victims may have sustained varying degrees of irradiation, radioactive contamination, primary to quinary blast injuries, and mental health issues.
- Ascertain where your institution fits into the RTR response system.

Further reading

Coleman CN, Knebel AR, Hick JL, Weinstock DM, Casagrande R, Caro JJ, DeRenzo EG, Dodgen D, Norwood AE, Sherman SE, Cliffer KD, McNally R, Bader JL, Murrain-Hill P. Scarce resources for nuclear detonation: Project overview and challenges. *Disaster Med Public Health Prep.* 2011;5(Suppl 1):S13–S19.

Coleman CN, Weinstock DM, Casagrande R, Hick JL, Bader JL, Chang F, Nemhauser JB, Knebel AR. Triage and treatment tools for use in a scarce resources-crisis standards of care setting after a nuclear detonation. *Disaster Med Public Health Prep.* 2011;5(Suppl 1):S111–S121.

DiCarlo AL, Maher C, Hick JL, Hanfling D, Dainiak N, Chao N, Bader JL, Coleman CN, Weinstock DM. Radiation injury after a nuclear detonation: Medical consequences and the need for scarce resources allocation. *Disaster Med Public Health Prep.* 2011;5(Suppl 1):S32–S44.

Federal Emergency Management Administration. *Radiological Emergency Preparedness: Program Manual.* FEMA P-1028; 2019.

Hick JL, Weinstock DM, Coleman CN, Hanfling D, Cantrill S, Redlener I, Bader JL, Murrain-Hill P, Knebel AR. Health care system planning for and response to a nuclear detonation. *Disaster Med Public Health Prep.* 2011;5(Suppl 1):S73–S88.

Knebel AR, Coleman CN, Cliffer KD, Murrain-Hill P, McNally R, Oancea V, Jacobs J, Buddemeier B, Hick JL, Weinstock DM, Hrdina CM, Taylor T, Matzo M, Bader JL, Livinski AA, Parker G, Yeskey K. Allocation of scarce resources after a nuclear detonation: Setting the context. *Disaster Med Public Health Prep.* 2011;5(Suppl 1):S20–S31.

Mercer JC. *Federal Response to a Domestic Nuclear Attack.* Counterproliferation Paper No. 46. U.S. Air Force Counterproliferation Center; 2009.

Murrain-Hill P, Coleman CN, Hick JL, Redlener I, Weinstock DM, Koerner JF, Black D, Sanders M, Bader JL, Forsha J, Knebel AR. Medical response to a nuclear detonation: Creating a playbook for state and local planners and responders. *Disaster Med Public Health Prep.* 2011;5(Suppl 1):S89–S97.

Radiation Emergency Medical Management. Nuclear Detonation: Weapons, Improvised Nuclear Devices. https://www.remm.nlm..gov/nuclearexplosion.htm

Radiation Emergency Medical Management. Radiation Triage, Treat, and Transport System (RTR) After a Nuclear Detonation: Venues for the Medical Response. https://remm.hhs.gov/RTR.htm

Radiation Injury Treatment Network. RITN Concept of Operations. https://ritn.net/about/

Tan CM, Barnett DJ, Stolz AJ, Links JM. Radiological incident preparedness: Planning at the local level. *Disaster Med Public Health Prep.* 2011;5(Suppl 1):S151–S158. Erratum in: *Disaster Med Public Health Prep.* 2011;5(2):97.

U.S. Department of Health & Human Services, Office of the Assistant Secretary for Preparedness and Response. *A Decision Maker's Guide: Medical Planning and Response for a Nuclear Detonation.* (2nd ed.). https://remm.hhs.gov/decisionmakersguide.htm

17 Pandemic: Hospital preparedness and response for the future

The recovery from COVID-19 has been an arduous one, not only for your hospital, but for the global population as well. The most vulnerable of us have paid the ultimate price. While that may have been "breaking news" for a great many of the literati and glitterati inhabiting the myriad media outlets, it comes as no surprise to those of us who have spent decades fighting in the trenches of emergency medicine.

With the pandemic fresh in everyone's mind, the administration has asked you to evaluate the hospital's preparedness and response activities so as to be better prepared for the next pandemic. They want you not only to identify the successes but more importantly to home in on the unexpected challenges that might be able to be mitigated in the future.

Their request could not be timelier. There are ominous signs of a killer infectious disease outbreak in Mexico that could easily get out of control and become the next pandemic of the 21st century. The news media continue to regurgitate the reassurances of pundits and politicians that what is happening in Mexico is nowhere close to what developed with the SARS-CoV-2 virus. Besides, the nation is better prepared now than ever. And yet, people in Mexico are dying every day from this novel disease. It is only a matter of days before the outbreak jumps the barrier walls and infects the United States.

What do I do now?

According to the World Health Organization, there is one new emerging disease every year. Some of them will exhibit human-to-human transmission. Some of the current threats that are most worrisome since they have no proven therapy or vaccine include MERS-CoV, Zika virus, and specific viral hemorrhagic fevers.

As the analysis of the hospital's COVID-19 response begins, it would be helpful to break down the institution's preparedness and response in terms of "surge capacity." That term can be defined as the maximum supply of resources that are available to address a given contingency. Box 17.1 outlines the three levels.

You are in Stage 1, conventional capacity. The threat is real. It is looming. The first cases may even be arriving, but the system has the resources to meet the challenge. Since you are on the disaster committee and are heading the hospital's preparedness and response effort, you now have two obligations, one to your hospital or hospital system and one to your ED.

Let's consider the ED first. Much of the planning, needs assessment, and education should have occurred during the inter-pandemic period. If the challenges and failures were not addressed during that period, then it will have to be done during Stage 1. Review any official notes, documents, and

---

BOX 17.1 **The three levels of capacity**

Stage 1 (conventional capacity): Supplies, staffing, and venues are available for and consistent with the usual daily practices within an institution.

Stage 2 (contingency capacity): Supplies, staffing, and venues are available but are not at a level that would be consistent with the usual daily practices. However, they are functionally equivalent to typical patient care practices.

Stage 3 (crisis capacity): The adaptive supplies, staffing, and venues are not sufficient to maintain the usual practices of daily healthcare. Therefore, while practices could be different from the usual standards of care, there is every attempt to provide a "sufficiency of care" during catastrophic circumstances. The objective is to provide the best possible care to all patients given a dearth of resources. A synonym is "altered standards of care."

after-action reports that were written during the COVID-19 pandemic. Each ED will have its own set of successes and challenges. Keep what was successful, but home in on the challenges or even the failures that were in evidence during the COVID-19 pandemic. Certain themes came to light during the last pandemic that require further investigation:

1. PPE: Beg, borrow, or steal as much PPE as your hospital's budget allows. The operative term is "stockpile." There is no need to remind ourselves how the American system failed its healthcare providers in terms of PPE supplies. The ED staff should be considered a funding priority.

2. Training: Your ED team and the rest of the hospital staff should have been receiving PPE training during the inter-pandemic period. However, as we enter Stage 1, that training should be more frequent and more rigorous. Use luminescent powder and a black light to determine whether an individual nurse or physician self-contaminated when they doffed their PPE gear. Such self-contamination makes them an automatic "hot zone" and a threat not only to themselves but also to the colleagues, their patients, and their families. Have them tested and retested until they pass.

3. Review the peer-reviewed medical literature and the valid news services on a regular basis and share that information with the ED team (Figure 17.1). This is only one means of communication that will enhance camaraderie and lessen individual stress.

4. Survey your team, all the shifts. What are their concerns and anxieties? More to the point, several years after the SARS-CoV-1 outbreak ended in Toronto, some ED nurses were unwilling to attend to patients who presented with cough and a fever. Begin this activity during Stage 1 and continue it throughout all three stages. If these conversations are begun during Stage 1 they will be regarded as another normal function of the ED throughout all the potential stages. This will pay dividends in the future.

5. Create a website or a weekly newsletter for the ED or even the entire hospital to enhance communications among the staff and other personnel. Based on the COVID-19 crisis, having

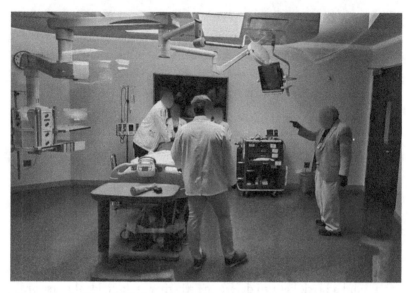

FIGURE 17.1 Amid the COVID-19 pandemic and the pre-vaccine period (2020), medical education continued, albeit with social distancing and masking measures in force.

Credit: Jeff Schneiderman, EMT-P

the ability, in a timely fashion, to confront and invalidate misinformation will become one of the major objectives of this type of communication.

6. Begin developing a plan for triaging patients in light of this new infectious disease threat. Many of the triage decisions will depend on the interim case definitions being developed by the Centers for Disease Control and Prevention and the current resources of your hospital. Will triage be divided into sorting out individuals with fever and upper respiratory symptoms into one area and everyone else into a "clean zone"? In Toronto, "fever clinics" were developed in some of the hospitals. The goal was to assess large numbers of patients while minimizing the risk of SARS-CoV-1 transmission. These areas had dedicated entrances and exits, and seating between individuals was more than 1 meter apart. These areas all had excellent ventilation. Can all areas of the ED become a negative-pressure environment to limit transmission? While performing the

triage process, how will you manage accompanying friends and families? Consider measures that have been published. In Toronto during the SARS-CoV-1 crisis (2003), a triage screening tool was used to identify possible transmissible disease patients, everyone had a temperature check, hand hygiene was mandatory for all, and everyone was masked.

7. Develop a buddy system between fellow workers. This is a tried-and-true conceit that worked well with the members of Disaster Medical Assistance Teams (DMAT). One member of a particular shift connected with one other person on the same shift and made sure each was OK both mentally and physically. More importantly, they were all empowered to come to the command leaders about any concerns they had about their buddy.

As for the hospital, create a pandemic subcommittee within the disaster committee. This subcommittee will work on pre-pandemic planning and report at regular intervals to the disaster committee. This committee will concern itself with the following issues.

Clinical issues

Clinical issues should include the triggers that suspend elective surgery, cancel well-checks in clinics, and manage patient care in alternate care facilities (ACFs) within the hospital complex. There are also clinical issues that may pertain to only a minority of hospitals in a minority of communities. For example, in some areas there are pediatric hospitals. Many of the moderately to severely ill and traumatic pediatric cases bypass general hospitals and are transported to these hospitals where pediatric expertise is concentrated. Over time, that could suggest that these other hospitals may have allowed their pediatric resources to wane. This could be detrimental if they are called upon during a pandemic to absorb these kinds of critical cases should the pediatric institutions become overwhelmed with cases. Therefore, it is worth assessing the pediatric capabilities of these general hospitals now and then decide how best to handle these types of patients should it be necessary. Pediatric resuscitative supplies, simulation training, pediatric transportation requirements, and immediate consultation services with pediatric specialists may be enough to resolve that issue.

A similar conundrum can occur with trauma patients during a pandemic. That would especially be an issue during a trauma-related mass casualty incident. There is no guarantee that during a pandemic, there will not be an earthquake, a tornado, or even a flood. So, while your hospital is currently not likely to receive trauma patients with severely elevated Injury Severity Scores, EMS may be forced to come your way for stabilization of trauma patients should Level 1 Trauma Centers become overwhelmed. Therefore, a discussion about resources, training, and communications for these situations should have begun even before Stage 1 capacity has been reached. All these solutions cannot be developed in a vacuum or, worse yet, in secrecy. The problem and possible solutions should be identified and shared with the community at large. Assign a hospital liaison to fulfill that role.

Infection control issues
Infection control issues will involve access to patients by visitors and families, masking procedures, personal hygiene measures, etc.

Resource issues
Resource issues are concerned with management of scarce patient care supplies such as medications, blood products, extracorporeal membrane oxygenation (ECMO), and ventilators.

Personnel issues
Handling personnel issues involves more than surge capacity strategies such as tightening contractual terms with nursing- and physician-for-hire agencies and recruiting medical volunteers from within the community and the local Medical Reserve Corps. It is also a matter of maintaining the team's physical and mental health over the long haul. Contacting human resources and the psychiatry department is essential.

Determine whether there is a role for an internal or closed point of distribution (POD) and an ACF at your hospital. During the early vaccination phase of the COVID-19 pandemic, hospitals developed closed PODs to vaccinate their personnel, for example. Similarly, there may be an entire building on campus that could, for instance, serve as an ACF for acute Green patients (i.e., those with lacerations, sprains, and tummy pains). The same principles and procedures that would apply to a community ACF will apply to a hospital ACF, except that it would be easier to accomplish. Establishing ACFs for severely ill people or pandemic patients may be counterproductive since their specialists would, arguably, be most efficient caring for their complex patients in more comfortable and familiar surroundings. Emergency physicians, on the other hand, can function anywhere with any type of patient.

Structural issues

The "nuts and bolts" people—namely, the department that manages facilities and construction—will have three major tasks: preserve the integrity of the hospital now and in the future, determine what sites can best serve as PODs or ACFs without impairing ongoing operations, and identify the areas of the hospital that can easily be converted into negative-pressure environments for overflow of pandemic cases.

Ethical issues

The ethics group of the committee, given their importance during COVID-19, are no longer "mushrooms in a cavern." The members must confront issues of allocation of scarce resources and withdrawal of care within a catastrophic setting. To accomplish these tasks competently, they must continue their education on these issues, adopt best practices from other institutions, communicate with their peers from other local hospitals or healthcare systems, and, hopefully, agree to a common set of principles that can be shared transparently with local stakeholders and the public. The goal is to have a document written by representatives from all the local healthcare institutions explaining how, during Stage 3 of capacity, scarce resources will be apportioned within a given ethical framework and legal mandates.

There should also be scheduled meetings between this committee and a select cohort of healthcare providers from the ICUs and EDs. Much of the legwork has occurred during the COVID-19 pandemic, but self-interest and other lapses in judgment occurred nevertheless. Having practitioners and theoreticians work this out together will be important to address the problems and work out the solutions. Tabletop exercises can get to the heart of the problem. A simple one that will get everyone to focus on the issue would involve three patients (complete case histories provided), all of whom require a ventilator—but there is only one ventilator free. Who gets it? A more ominous scenario would be one in which (1) no ventilators are free, (2) a patient in the ED needs a ventilator now, and (3) there is a patient in the ICU on a ventilator, but their sequential organ failure assessment (SOFA) scores not only are not improving but are in fact worsening. Can that ventilator be withdrawn from the ICU patient and given to the more viable candidate in the ED?

THE NEXT PANDEMIC

At this stage of the game, we really have no idea how the next pandemic will be handled. In fact, it may not even be a new pandemic, but, after a long latency period, another resurgence of the SARS-CoV-2 pandemic may be developing. If it is, it's easy to see that the first generation of the SARS-CoV-2 isn't working.

As an emergency physician, you have a responsibility to share those concerns with the ED staff, the hospital administration, and even the community. Whether those concerns will be addressed in a timely fashion is certainly problematic, especially coming off the COVID-19 pandemic. Nevertheless, there is much you can do while the events begin to clarify themselves. Meanwhile, to paraphrase George Santayana, whoever doesn't know history is condemned to repeat it.

KEY POINTS TO REMEMBER

- There will be another pandemic. Prepare for it now.
- To paraphrase John Donne, "No disaster is an island." While preparing for a pandemic and guided by your community's hazard vulnerability analysis, plan your response should another disaster occur during a future pandemic.
- Strategize multiple ways to maintain the health and mental well-being of your ED and hospital staffs over the long haul.
- Investigate how PODs and ACFs can be integrated into your hospital's pandemic response.
- Work with similar community institutions and other stakeholders to develop a consistent strategy for the ethical and legal allocation of scarce resources.

Further reading

Cable J, Heymann DL, Uzicanin A, Tomori O, Marinissen MJ, Katz R, Kerr L, Lurie N, Parker GW, Madad S, Maldin Morgenthau B, Osterholm MT, Borio L. Pandemic diseases preparedness and response in the age of COVID-19: A symposium report. *Ann N Y Acad Sci*. 2021;1489(1):17–29.

Iserson KV. Alternative care sites: An option in disasters. *West J Emerg Med*. 2020;21(3):484–489.

Iserson KV. The next pandemic: Prepare for "Disease X." *West J Emerg Med*. 2020;21(4):756–758.

National Academies of Sciences, Engineering, and Medicine. *Emergency Evacuation and Sheltering During the COVID-19 Pandemic*. National Academies Press; 2021. https://doi.org/10.17226/26084

18 They want you!: A regional response to a future pandemic

There is something brewing in a not-so-far-off land. It has all the earmarks of another pandemic. You have been a major factor in preparing your hospital, even cajoling the "suits" into believing that another pandemic in our lifetime is not impossible. Because of your relentless Churchillian warnings, your hospital is grudgingly on board. Within certain unavoidable economic restraints, leadership and staff have begun the initial preparations, stockpiling, and training. As a result, your reputation in the community has not gone unnoticed. The regional public health authorities and their associates have received permission from your hospital to invite you to become a vital part of the regional pandemic plan.

What do I do now?

Accept with humility, but keep your eyes open and count your fingers after you shake hands.

The 21st century has witnessed the H1N1 and the COVID-19 pandemics. It will take another generation of historians to capture the essence of preparedness and response efforts to COVID-19. Regardless of how we eventually overcome the SARS-CoV-2 virus, the emergency physician will need to evaluate the events of 2020 and 2021 and use the lessons learned for the next pandemic.

However, to place the COVID-19 pandemic in some sort of context, it is always worthwhile to study past epidemics and pandemics in American history. In my third life as an educator in emergency medicine and public health, I developed a 3-credit postgraduate course entitled *Pandemic Preparedness and Response*. I taught that course during a 10-year period, and a review of the roots of the global efforts, and America's in particular, in combating pandemics prepared me to comprehend the events as they unfolded in 2020. In the following we will review the responses associated with selected American infectious disease outbreaks.

Smallpox: Boston, 1775

During the Revolutionary War time, smallpox was at epidemic levels in the colonies. It is estimated that 100,000 people died of the pox between 1775 and 1782. During this time, there were two strategies to fend off the disease: isolation and variolation. In South Carolina, sentinels were placed outside of pox houses to reinforce isolation. Off the coast of Newport, Rhode Island, an island was repurposed as a smallpox island. Across the colonies, any ships coming from diseased lands were kept in quarantine. That included slave ships.

Jenner's concept of vaccination was still on the horizon. However, over the centuries, from Europe to Africa and now into the colonies, variolation was practiced as another way to cut down on morbidity and mortality. The technique consisted of taking a small amount of live pox from a smallpox survivor and introducing it into an unexposed individual by means of a small incision on the hand or arm. Variolation was popularized by Cotton Mather, a New England Puritan minister. It caused fewer lesions and less scarring. Did it have an impact on the death rate? It was recorded that in Boston in 1791, 15% of the population died from the pox as opposed to only 2% who were variolated. Further refinements to the basic technique occurred. For example, as preparation, 1 week prior to the variolation, a person was subjected to a milk diet, ipecac, and mercurial ministrations. Another refinement was the Sutton method: Instead of taking pox material from an actual pox survivor, the material was taken from a variolated inoculee, presumably to avoid as much as possible any adverse effects.

However, this was also a time for the anti-variolators. These were individuals who feared the technique because for some the cure was worse than the disease. There were riots. In 1774, inoculation hospitals in Salem and Marblehead were razed and closed down. Towns like Charlestown and New York passed laws forbidding variolation within their borders.

So, within this colonial environment, during July 1775, Boston was experiencing a smallpox outbreak. At that time, Boston was a city of 13,000 inhabitants that was under occupation by the Redcoats. George Washington had ringed the city with his troops as part of a siege strategy. Bostonians were trapped. They were witness to 30 funerals on some days.

The general of the Continental Army knew that his troops were susceptible to smallpox (i.e., no pox scars), but he did not want to variolate his troops for fear of initiating the pox within his army. Faced with this conundrum, he provided his own version of isolation and quarantine: Any Bostonians escaping to his escarpment were quarantined in Brookline, and any of his troops who came down with the pox were isolated in Cambridge.

During the waning months of 1775, the citizens of Boston continued to fare poorly. Any British troops who took sick were ferried to their smallpox ships for care. The civilians were abandoned to their own devices. They remained without adequate food stores. The very sick were prevented from going through Washington's siege lines and had to be ferried to hospitals in Salem and Chelsea. Sentinels were deployed to the exit roads of the city. The Council of Massachusetts finally allowed the public to be variolated. In time, about 5,000 citizens were variolated. Smallpox houses were smoked and cleansed. It took until the end of August and the beginning of September before smallpox was on the wane and its siege of Boston was lifted.

Parenthetically, while our history books mention how the British general Amherst gifted smallpox-infected blankets to decimate Native American tribes, we cannot ignore that not only did the British leaders try to direct infected Bostonians to Washington's siege lines in 1775, but during the

Battle of Yorktown, the British released smallpox-infected ex-slaves from their encampment so as to infect the Continental Army. Apparently, biological warfare has deep roots in American history.

Yellow fever: Philadelphia, 1793

In 1793, Philadelphia, then the capital of the nascent United States of America, had a growing population of 51,000. The epidemic started as a French sailor took ill and began to seize. Within a couple of days, he died. However, the fever spread throughout the house where he lay, to neighbors down the street. Eight died from two houses on the same street, all within 1 week. The alarum of yellow fever was sounded when Dr. Benjamin Rush, upon attending to a 33-year-old female with fever and abdominal pain who was vomiting black bile, declared, "All is not right in our city."

During the third week of the epidemic, as scores of inhabitants were dying, "dead carts" were circulating through the neighborhoods to carry off the unfortunate to final resting places. By the fourth week, an exodus from Philadelphia began. It is estimated that ~20,000 fled. The infrastructure was hobbled. As others fled, the mayor and Dr. Rush remained to manage their obligations as best as possible. The College of Physicians was convened to provide its expertise to the situation that was inevitably growing out of control. Their best advice to the citizenry was to avoid the sick, clean the streets, establish a hospital, limit wine and beer, moisten handkerchiefs with vinegar to ward off disease, and burn gunpowder to purify the air.

Meanwhile, stores and schools closed as those too poor to evacuate walked the streets chewing garlic, smoking cigars, and sniffing camphor to ward off disease. By the end of August, as a score or more people were dying every day, the government was at a standstill and fear gripped the city. Street sanitation and ship inspections in this port city died out. Farmers no longer brought their produce into the city. Pennsylvania Hospital refused to admit "fever" patients.

As one of the first examples of an alternate care facility (ACF), a number of individuals, the self-proclaimed Guardians of the Poor, seized Bush Hill mansion to care for the ill. While initially overwhelmed by the increasing number of ill and dead, this site, with proper organization and planning, eventually became an adequate source of care for the underserved. Meanwhile, in the heart of Philadelphia, the dead were lying in the streets as the bidding for nursing services skyrocketed and price gouging and profiteering became rampant. During this time the federal government, too, abandoned the Philadelphia confines. Washington and Jefferson took to their estates, accidentally leaving behind important federal papers.

At the request of Benjamin Rush, the Free African Society volunteered to help their brethren. According to the Elders, "It was our duty to do all the good we could to our fellow mortals." Their duties consisted of nursing and staffing Bush Hill and buying food, medicines, and sundries for the stricken.

By September 14, Bush Hill became an exhausted shell despite everyone's good intentions. It housed 100 patients with no physicians in attendance, and the dead remained unburied. In the city, the courts and taverns were closed. The markets were empty. The College of Physicians no longer convened to manage the emergency as one unified group of professionals. Instead, physicians were freelancing, publishing their own contradictory opinions in the one newspaper remaining.

Faced with more than 60 deaths per day, the mayor organized a "Committee by Twelve only." These were 12 ordinary citizens, among them a tavern owner, a mechanic, and an umbrella maker. This committee arranged care for the sick and burial of the dead at Bush Hill. An Orphan Committee was organized to care for the 192 children left homeless and uncared for. They spent $37,000 of their own money to arrange for professional care and to buy food, medicines, and coffins, and they appropriated land for burials. That is said to be equivalent to $1 million in 2021 dollars.

At Bush Hill, flooded with the inspirational and financial support of the Committee, two individuals took over. Peter Helm managed the events on the grounds of Bush Hill while Stephen Girard managed the inside of the building. They developed systems for triaging the incoming patients (i.e., "dying" and "not dying"), systems for caring for the sick, systems for rehabilitating the recovering, and systems for constructing coffins and burying the dead.

As Philadelphians began to have confidence in Bush Hill as a sanctuary for the ill and repose of the dead, the municipalities surrounding the city had a different outlook. They too were scared of spread. Any outgoing mail was dipped in vinegar first. There were armed patrols circumnavigating the City of Brotherly Love. Stagecoaches were turned back. In one situation, a female evacuee was tarred and feathered before being "returned to sender." However, there were also signs of humanitarianism: Communities donated food, clothes, and money to the beleaguered.

Through October, the daily death toll in Philadelphia often grew to over 100 (e.g., 10/12/1793: 111 deaths; 10/13/1793: 112 deaths). Crime increased in the city and rioting was reported. Night in Philadelphia became a black abyss. There was no whale oil brought in to fuel the oil lamps in the streets. People shunned each other as the disease was spreading into suburbia.

Then, as October transitioned into the cooler month of November, the daily death toll started to drop. Confidence grew and citizens returned to their city. Now, however, they saw that the streets were empty of garbage and bodies. Beggars and homeless children roaming the streets were no longer plentiful. They also saw survivors with yellow-tinted skin and black teeth due to mercury purges.

By the time the yellow fever epidemic was deemed to be concluded, between 4,000 and 5,000 people had died. However, this breakout was the inciting event to create laws to keep streets and markets clean and to improve potable water sanitation.

Yellow fever: New York City, 1858

Yellow fever outbreaks were frequent in New York City, occurring almost like clockwork from 1702 through 1821. However, when the disease struck in 1858, there had not been a recorded outbreak for 37 years. In the interim, the time was put to good use. A quarantine hospital was established on Staten Island. It was considered state of the art. Its physicians and staff were considered to be leaders in the management of infectious diseases. It was clean and safe, having been constructed in a residential area of the island. Since, at that time, it was thought that yellow fever was being brought to the New World by the new wave of poor Irish immigrants coming by trans-Atlantic shipping, it was an accepted practice to weed out the probable yellow fever immigrants by quarantining them at that hospital.

However, in 1858, with fear gripping the city, the residents of Staten Island were resentful that immigrants were being sequestered in their neighborhood, possibly bringing a lethal infectious disease into their midst. So, on September 1, 1858, a group of the hospital's neighbors advanced onto the hospital grounds and burned the two hospitals and the doctors' residence to the ground. They were careful enough to remove the patients first. Even after the New York Fire Department came to extinguish the fire, the neighbors came back the next day to put the finishing touches on the conflagration.

Cholera: New York City, 1892

By 1892, the world had witnessed global cholera outbreaks that verged on the levels of a pandemic (1832, 1849, 1866). Cholera had become a reasonably well-understood disease in terms of its etiology, mode of transmission, and incubation periods. Yet, in New York and the rest of the country, the science of cholera was sidestepped by the art of politics and the grip of fear as a new wave of cholera hamstrung the world. For 5 years, it held Europe, Russia, India, and the Middle East in its grip. More than 300,000 deaths were reported in Russia alone. By 1892, it had not made itself known to the New World. Nevertheless, there was concern in the United States especially since there has been a growing influx of immigrants from Europe, most of whom were embarking from Hamburg, Germany, the largest embarkation port in the world. This exodus was a trickle in 1880, when about 6,000 immigrants per year came to America, but by 1892, that trickle became a torrent as 75,000 immigrants came to the U.S. shores annually. Even the *New York Times* on 8/29/1892 labeled these people "human riff-raff."

This anti-immigrant fervor became more pronounced when it was announced, on August 23, 1892, that Hamburg had become another center of a cholera epidemic. The River Elbe was said to be teeming with *Vibrio cholerae*. While that announcement was being made, many of the ships leaving the port city of Hamburg were already at sea heading for the "Promised Land." Government at all levels, as well as the fourth estate, raised concerns about what was to come in a few short weeks. Boston, Chicago, Detroit, Cleveland, and Baltimore established a blockade of their ports of entry. Through some sort of political manipulations, wealthy immigrants, who were thought to be less of a risk, embarked on faster ocean liners while the poor immigrants had to settle for slower ships. The reason was that should there be an outbreak among the poor, it would happen while the ships were still sailing across the Atlantic and the stricken could simply be buried at sea and not infect the "glitterati" of the Big Apple. On one ship at sea, 22 Russian Jews died between August 19 and 29 and were buried at sea. By the time the ship docked in New York, the trans-Atlantic quarantine worked: Only two passengers were ill.

By the end of August, as these ships began arriving in New York Harbor, a new inspection policy went into effect. Steerage passengers, after their initial inspection, underwent disinfection with steam heat and bichloride of mercury baths. For the first-class passengers, after their luggage was fumigated, they were allowed to disembark without delay. Even President Benjamin Harrison got into the act: He issued an executive order that steerage passengers and their ship had to be quarantined for 20 days. That order was not extended to the cabin passengers, who were allowed to disembark early. By September 3, there were 20 ships stuck in the harbor, and teams of city public health professionals from the Quarantine Station and the Swinburne and Hoffman islands centers handled the inspection of the ships and their passengers. Cholera mini-epidemics did break out on these ships.

The SS *Normania* illustrates a situation when infection control practices went awry. She arrived on September 3 with 308 crew, 482 steerage passengers, and 573 cabin passengers. The entire ship was quarantined, leaving both the ill and the healthy to congregate on one ship. During that time, 53 individuals fell ill and died. Similar catastrophes were occurring at the infectious disease installations on Swinburne and Hoffman islands. In early September, all 900 beds were filled. Quarantine and isolation segregation fell apart. The ill and the exposed were herded together, sharing common areas, water supplies, and privies.

As ships were stacked up in New York Harbor, on September 9, a National Quarantine Station was erected on Sandy Hook, New Jersey. Meanwhile, decisions were reversed and it was decided to allow the *Normania* passengers to disembark. The steerage passengers were sent to the overcrowded Hoffman Island facility while the cabin-class passengers were escorted to a hotel on Fire Island. The term for this separation was "class-oriented quarantine." The inhabitants of Fire Island did not take this decision lightly and, fully armed, resisted the landing of the passengers. The governor had to send in the National Guard and the Naval Reserve to resolve the situation.

Smallpox: Milwaukee, 1894

In 1894, a smallpox outbreak stuck Milwaukee, Wisconsin. Arguably, if it had to happen, it could not have happened at a more convenient time. Eleven months earlier, Walter Kempster was hired as the new public health commissioner. He was well grounded on the principles of public health, and he began to reorganize the department, hiring people for their competence—not their politics. So, when the outbreak occurred, he sprang into action. He initiated a vaccination campaign and opened up an "isolation" hospital. Unfortunately, class consciousness reared its ugly head. The action plan he developed was that the upper and middle classes of Milwaukee could quarantine at home, while the poorer classes, namely the immigrant population, had to go to the hospital. That stirred up controversy and resentment.

The vaccination campaign did not go down well either. The Milwaukee branch of the Anti-Vaccination Society spread information that not only was the vaccine useless, but it also spread syphilis. One third of the local medical society agreed with the anti-vaxxers. As for the hospital, the community believed it was a pesthouse, a slaughterhouse, and a menace to the communal health. As a result, if there were any cases circulating in the community, it was better to hide them than to condemn them to the hospital.

The situation got so out of control that riots developed. It was the immigrants versus the health department. Pomeranian and Polish women would ambush the horse-driven smallpox transportation vans and douse the horses with hot water and pepper spray. They would attack the public health officers with sticks and bats. Eventually, when cooler heads prevailed, Kempster was impeached and thrown out of office. The end result? There were 1,079 smallpox cases and 249 deaths.

Plague: San Francisco, 1907

Plague struck the City-by-the-Bay in 1907, possibly as a result of a couple of recent immigrants to the city or perhaps a foreign sailor. The city government could not meet the crisis and President Roosevelt offered assistance. At this point, local, state, and federal authorities were working together in coordination with local humanitarian groups and medical experts. The strategy was to keep the public well informed; to educate the populace; to rely on peer pressure to ensure that everyone did their duty; and to obtain concordance with the city's business and community leaders. Behind all this was the Roosevelt-ian threat that if San Francisco did not accomplish what was expected of it, then the arrival of the Great White Fleet of the U.S. Navy would not anchor in the Bay. That would be an enormous political and economic tragedy for the city.

A Citizen's Health Committee was formed to work with the U.S. Public Health Service and the Marine Hospital Service. The committee comprised 11 civilian leaders and 11 physicians. The Citizen's Health Committee was successful. Its major achievements were to enforce sanitary regulations; improve sanitation of schools, buildings, and the waterfront; work with the media delivering frequent and consistent messaging; eliminate the rats; and educate the public. The committee invited women's clubs to recruit their children to collect trash and dead rats from the traps. The city was divided into 12 medical districts, each with its own medical inspector. Plague victims were cared for in public health tents (additional examples of ACFs). In the meantime, funds were made available to build an isolation hospital with rat-proof fences. The federal response was directed at fumigating ships as they entered the harbor. The agreed-upon strategy was to kill the rats; vaccination was not the priority. As plague cases climbed to 25, public health laid out more than 1 million rat traps. They even had bounties on the rodents: 10 to 25 cents per each male rat and up to 50 cents for a female rat. Inspectors were recruited to inspect homes and businesses. Any miscreants were tried and convicted and their names published in the newspapers for public ridicule.

Meanwhile, the *San Francisco Chronicle* disputed the severity of the crisis and felt it was a manufactured motive for medical profiteering. However, over the next several months, the war against plague was won. It was declared that the last plague rat in San Francisco was exterminated on October 23. Cases dropped from 60 in September to just 11 in December.

Influenza pandemic: Philadelphia, 1917–1918
In 1870, the population of the United States was 40 million. By 1917, it had surged to 105 million and the nation's attention was on the Great War. Resources, propaganda, and laws were directed toward winning the effort, and everything else was put on the back burner. Consider the lowly sauerkraut: Its name was changed to "Liberty Cabbage" as a way to limit any Teutonic references. As American troops massed together prior to

embarkation, the stirrings of a significant disease were beginning to be felt in barracks and soon in the civilian population.

Philadelphia was no exception. The City of Brotherly Love had a population of 1.75 million in 1917. To say it was overcrowded is an understatement. In some cases, four families were bundled into one apartment and slept in shifts. The slums of the city were said to be worse than New York. Yet the political machine that governed the city was virtually ineffectual on a daily basis. Graft and corruption were rewarded and social services were ignored. Lincoln Steffens, a Progressive investigative journalist, declared that Philadelphia was "the worst-governed city in America."

The pandemic in Philadelphia started on September 7, 1917, as sailors bound for Europe established themselves in the Philadelphia Navy Yard. By September 15, 600 sailors were bedded down at the Naval Hospital and the overflow patients were admitted to the civilian Pennsylvania Hospital, which set the stage for spreading the flu among the civilian population. As September was drawing to a close, not much was done as civilians and sailors were dying with increasing regularity. Manifestations in the severely ill consisted of fever, chills, headaches, pulmonary congestion, nausea, and vomiting. There was intense cyanosis as patients gasped for breath. Blood emanated from the conjunctiva, mouth, nose, and GI tract. Patients became delirious and died. Autopsies revealed that no organ was left untouched by the virus. There was marked hyperemia of the brain, pericarditis, and myocarditis. The lungs looked like those destroyed by toxic gas or the plague. Public health officials agreed to monitor events and soon declared that the flu was a reportable disease. Meanwhile everyone should stay warm, keep their feet dry and their bowels open, and avoid crowds. That last advisory conflicted with the fact that on September 28, the Great Liberty Loan Parade was scheduled for the city, an event designed to boost public morale and popularize the nation's war effort. Local infectious disease experts and physicians wanted it canceled, but it wasn't. Their concerns did not hit the newspapers.

Several hundred thousand lined the streets to view the parade. Two days later, the Public Health Commissioner declared a citywide epidemic, and on October 1, the beds in all 31 Philadelphian hospitals were filled. More than 100 people were dying each day. People were waiting on lines for admission into Pennsylvania Hospital. Nurses were offered $100 bribes for care.

By October 3, the public health commissioner reacted to the crisis. All public meetings were banned. Schools, theaters, courts, and places of worship were closed. Public funerals were canceled. The saloons were allowed to stay open, but that was because they were owned by the politicos in power. The state health commissioner shut them down the next day.

The first ACF (Emergency Hospital #1) was established at the City Poorhouse on October 3. Its 500 beds were filled in 1 day. Ultimately, 12 similar facilities were opened at the height of the pandemic. As people were falling ill and dying by the hundreds each day, placards were disseminated throughout the city with instructions such as "Use handkerchiefs," "Avoid crowds," and "Spitting Equals Death." Anyone caught spitting in public was subject to arrest. Sixty were arrested in 1 day.

The first couple of weeks in October were intense: The daily death rate exceeded 300 on many of those days. It reached 428 on October 9, but that number would be eclipsed as nearly double that figure died on a daily basis over the next couple of weeks. Two thirds of those deaths were under 40 years of age. What was to be done with the dead? The city morgue was bulging with cadavers. Its normal capacity of 36 was overwhelmed at one time with 200 bodies. Bodies piled up not only at the morgue but also throughout the city. Individuals who died at home were packed in ice and deposited on porches to await the "dead wagons" to cart them off. Where? That was problematic, since gravediggers refused to bury them and, besides, the coffin shortage was so acute that guards were posted to prevent thievery.

Communal mental health must have been at serious risk with all the social amenities and the congregate bonhomie placed on hold. Even phone calls were banned unless there was a true emergency.

Philadelphia General Hospital's surge capacity was extremely limited. During one period, eight of their physicians and 54 nurses required hospitalization. Ten of the nurses subsequently died. The Board of Health asked retired nurses and physicians to assist. That was a double-edged sword when it was discovered that one elderly doctor was performing purging and venesection to cure his patients. Medical students and pharmacy students were recruited to lend a hand. In fact, at one of the ACFs, one medical student was in charge of an entire floor of patients. Consider his short- and long-term mental health as each day 25% of his patients died!

With little to no assistance coming from state and national agencies like the American Red Cross, local civilian stakeholders filled the vacuum that was created by the ennui and incompetence of local government. Much of the reorganization of aid was handled by local societal organizations like the Council of National Defense and the Emergency Aid Society. The leadership of these local branches came from the wealthy women of Philadelphia, who already had been making considerable contributions to the citizens of the city even before the pandemic. These doyennes of Philadelphia already had in place a system that provided leadership, organization, and money. For example, the Emergency Aid Society, using its preexisting system, delivered food, care, and physicians across the city's seven districts. They opened soup kitchens. They started a 24-hour phone bank to provide information and obtain referrals. They drove the doctors in their own cars to visit homebound patients and, if the need was there, they drove patients to hospitals, in effect serving as ambulances. Inspired by these women, the city's public health commissioner was revitalized. He redirected $120,000 to pay for more doctors, to gather more supplies for the resource-strapped hospitals, and to improve sanitation services for the city streets.

All the infrastructural innovations began during the second week of October, but by mid-October 33 police officers died from the flu as they, priests, and seminarians volunteered to move and bury the dead. By this time, there were six alternative morgue sites and public health officials recruited mortuary science students and morticians from 150 miles away to manage the influx of bodies. On October 10 alone, the death toll was 759. That number is all the more impressive when we consider that before the pandemic, the *weekly* death rate in Philadelphia was 485 from all causes. The worst week of the pandemic was the week of October 16, when there were over 4,500 deaths. Care and feeding of orphans rapidly became a priority.

Then, the numbers began to drop. Fewer people died and fewer people required hospitalization. On October 26, the ban on social gatherings was lifted, and by November 11 the flu in Philadelphia was officially ended.

Smallpox: New York City, 1947

It was 1947. New York City had not seen a case of smallpox in a generation. It is believed that in 1947, only about 2 million out of the 7.5 million inhabitants had any immunity to the contagious disease. Then on March 1, a man on his way from Mexico to Maine fell ill. He was transferred from Bellevue Hospital to Willard Parker Hospital with an "infection of unknown etiology." He died by March 10, but by then two other patients had also died and smallpox jumped to the top of the diagnostic list. Willard Parker staff were then receiving smallpox vaccinations. On April 4, laboratory reports confirmed that the dead patients had died from smallpox. On April 5, in keeping with the goal of transparency, the city's public health commissioner, Weinstein, and the Hospital Commission announced that cases of smallpox had been discovered in New York City, that the threat to the general public was small, and that vaccination of the public was important to keep the disease at bay. Meanwhile, the strategy for Weinstein was not only a mass vaccination campaign but also contact tracing. Fortunately, given the size of the population, the U.S. Public Health Service was also there to assist. To keep the public's confidence and trust high, daily press conferences were held reporting the numbers of suspected and confirmed cases, and a media blitz was initiated with placards and buttons saying, "Be safe. Be sure. Be vaccinated." Radio broadcasts instructed the listening public about the disease. It was said that some pharmaceutical companies were hesitant in supplying the vaccines because of cost. This was at a time when a mayor had some degree of power. Mayor O'Dwyer invited the reluctant individuals to City Hall, escorted them into a room, and delivered an ultimatum: "Make more vaccine, make it cheaply, or you won't get out of the building!"

With that problem out of the way, the vaccines arrived. The program was free and it was voluntary. No coercion was used. Volunteer groups assisted public health officials with the vaccination program. In fact, as in the past, points of distribution (PODs) were developed in police stations, clinics, and schools to vaccinate the public. In the first 2 weeks, 2 million New Yorkers were vaccinated. In the next couple of weeks the count increased up to more than 6 million people vaccinated. The mayor was vaccinated as well as President Truman. In the end, it was suspected that there were 5,000 smallpox cases in the city resulting in 12 proven cases and only two deaths.

This epidemic is considered a true success story for public health. Everyone was on the same page. The public was informed early and kept informed, and all the agencies, from the local to the state to the federal, banded together to make things happen. Much of the success is said to be due to the fact that this was part of the "Greatest Generation" who had survived the Great Depression together and who had won a world war together. Compared to those challenges, smallpox was "small potatoes."

Box 18.1 describes public health issues and the epidemics and pandemics in which they were prominent.

BOX 18.1 **Public health characteristics of selected infectious disease outbreaks**

Patient abandonment
. Yellow fever: Philadelphia, 1793

Overwhelmed infrastructure
. Yellow fever: Philadelphia, 1793
. Influenza: Philadelphia, 1917

ACFs
. Yellow fever: Philadelphia, 1793
. Yellow fever: New York, 1858
. Influenza: Philadelphia, 1917

PODs
. Smallpox: New York City, 1948

Isolation as a public health measure
. Smallpox: Boston, 1775
. Smallpox: Milwaukee, 1894
. Yellow fever: New York, 1858
. Cholera: New York City, 1892

Quarantine as a public health measure
. Smallpox: Boston, 1775
. Yellow fever: New York, 1858
. Cholera: New York City, 1892

Public fears
. Yellow fever: Philadelphia, 1793
. Smallpox: Boston, 1775
. Yellow fever: New York, 1858
. Cholera: New York City, 1892
. Smallpox: Milwaukee, 1894

Continued

BOX 18.1   Continued

Violence
- Yellow fever: Philadelphia, 1793
- Yellow fever: New York, 1858
- Smallpox: Milwaukee, 1894

Media misinformation
- Smallpox: Boston, 1775
- Plague: San Francisco, 1907
- Influenza: Philadelphia, 1917

Discrimination (real/perceived)
- Yellow fever: New York, 1858
- Cholera: New York City, 1892
- Smallpox: Milwaukee, 1894
- Plague: San Francisco, 1907

Intergovernmental cooperation
- Plague: San Francisco, 1907
- Cholera: New York City, 1892
- Smallpox: New York City, 1948

Crisis leadership (presence/absence)
- Yellow fever: Philadelphia, 1793
- Smallpox: New York City, 1948

Civilian volunteerism
- Yellow fever: Philadelphia, 1793
- Influenza: Philadelphia, 1917

Civil rights issues
- Yellow fever: New York, 1858
- Smallpox: Milwaukee, 1894

The lessons learned from these outbreaks were as follows:

Development and use of PODs

Establishment of quarantine stations

Validation of isolation precautions

Validation of quarantine precautions

Importance of volunteerism

Surge capacity development and utilization

Importance of the media

Mass fatality management
Mental health needs

And some of the challenges that occurred during these outbreaks were as follows:

Stigmatization
Weaponization of natural infections
Racial discrimination
Socioeconomic discrimination
Politics overshadowing healthcare
Failure of local government
Failure of the federal government
Societal inequality
Physical attacks on healthcare personnel and resources
Inaccurate and conflicting medical advice from "experts"
Profiteering

Emergency physicians are in a unique position to lend their expertise during any crisis—local, regional, national, and even international. Speaking regionally, they are the eyes and ears of both the hospital and prehospital infrastructure. They occupy a specific healthcare niche in providing emergency and disaster care to all segments of society at a level that cannot be replicated by any other discipline. Therefore, it stands to reason that the members of this specialty would be asked to contribute their expertise beyond patient care and into the realm of policymaking.

Having said that, it is important that you are not simply window dressing or the new flavor of the day. Accept this new role, but go into it with your eyes wide open. Consider the following:

1. Is there a regional incident command system (ICS) in place (Figure 18.1)?
2. If so, ask to see the ICS organization chart (Figure 18.2).
3. Attend one of the meetings to see the regional ICS in action.
4. What is your title and position in the ISC framework? "Medical specialist" is a reasonably good title. Ideally, you would want your position to be at a level that is as high as possible on the organizational chart. This way your counsel and expertise will

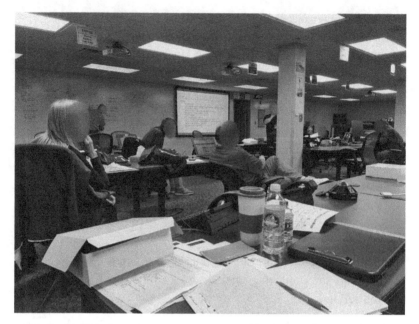

FIGURE 18.1 The Emergency Operations Center during the early stages of the COVID-19 pandemic. Note the signage on the ceilings that designates the location of each of the emergency support function (ESF) personnel in the ICS.

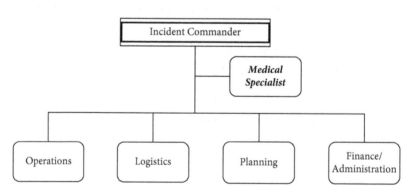

FIGURE 18.2 This organizational chart is an example of how the "medical specialist" can fit into the ICS system. Basically, this would indicate that the medical specialist answers only to the Incident Commander and has immediate access to the command system without any major communications disruptions.

have a greater opportunity of being heeded rather than ignored or diluted by lower-level bureaucratic naivete.

5. Document exactly what the role of the "medical specialist" is and exactly what responsibilities they would have. Obviously, this would be altered or modified as the events change. Keep it all in writing so that it is known to all and that accountability is maintained.

6. Preserve all communications between you and everyone else. That means emails, letters, tweets, etc. You are serving during an emergency. You are accountable, as is everyone else. Therefore, any correspondence that occurs should be considered sacrosanct for the purposes of posterity as well as protecting yourself in the clinches.

7. Unless you receive permission from the public information officer (PIO) or joint information command (JIC), do not communicate with the media. You may not have the total picture of the current events, and you must avoid transmitting misinformation. As a physician, whatever you say will carry significant weight in your community. Providing incorrect information or your own personal beliefs could undermine the integrity of ICS. You want to build trust in the system, not damage it.

While you are serving as the "medical specialist," lobby the incident commander for a medical advisory team of local, respected healthcare professionals to serve as your "think tank" (Figure 18.3). What worked well for FDR should serve you well also. These professionals would come from various specialties and disciplines and would include physicians, physician assistants, nurses, psychologists, etc. Other than their normal day-to-day practice, they would also, in a nonpartisan manner, review and provide counsel to the medical specialist concerning the pandemic from a medical and psychological perspective. Their recommendations would go through you to the incident commander for consideration.

If we review the events of the COVID-19 pandemic, we may, arguably, entertain the notion that more could have been done from a medical point

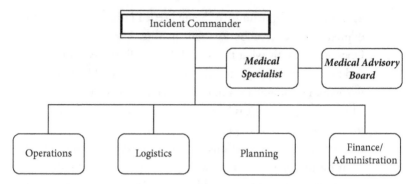

FIGURE 18.3 This is an ICS organizational template that places the medical advisory board at a key level to provide advice and counsel to the medical specialist.

of view to lessen the impact of the virus on vulnerable populations. For example, initiatives regarding vitamin D and monoclonal antibodies might have been more forceful had there been greater advocacy on the part of the medical community. Usually, the fields of public health and medicine work hand in glove, but in dire situations, public health officials can be well served if they receive counsel not just from one medical advisor but from a local body of medical experts who can review events, study the pertinent literature, and present to the incident commander recommendations on how pandemic management can be improved on the local level.

To assist the medical advisor on the major issues as the region goes from pandemic planning to pandemic response, consider the following issues to see if they are being accomplished satisfactorily. Think about how you could be of service in ensuring that they are being managed successfully:

1. Personal non-pharmaceutical interventions
    a. Personal hygiene
    b. Social distancing
    c. PPE
2. Societal non-pharmaceutical interventions
    a. Quarantine
    b. Isolation
    c. Social distancing

3. Prophylactic pharmaceutical interventions
   a. Vaccines
   b. Safe and effective
   c. Safe and possibly effective
4. Therapeutic pharmaceutical interventions
   a. Inpatient
   b. Outpatient
5. Altered standards of care

   a. Surge capacity
   b. PODs
   c. ACFs
   d. Allocation of scarce resources
   e. Mass fatality management

Several aspects of these activities require further elucidation.

Community pharmaceutical interventions

The field of public health, as we have noted, has been consistent in its messaging about masking, social distancing, personal hygiene, testing, contact tracing, isolation, and quarantine. However, it is within the medical sphere of influence to research, discuss, and present advisories to the local ICS concerning certain medical measures that may work synchronously with public health measures and, more importantly, which measures should be avoided.

Regarding the recent pandemic, community discussions regarding vitamins C and D, outpatient monoclonal antibody infusions, hydrogen peroxide gargles, etc. may have added layers of protection and care to the more traditional measures. However, interventions were advanced that could have been detrimental to certain patient populations (e.g., hydroxychloroquine, ivermectin).

The point is that having a local, expert, and unbiased medical advisory committee to research the literature, study data, assess benefits versus harm, and reach an informed opinion about these matters would be a much-needed complement to the public health actions. It would not be inappropriate to have an emergency physician lead that type of committee. At the very least, an emergency physician should be on the committee.

PODs

PODs are venues where a specific resource is provided to community members who have been impacted by an adverse event. It is a concept that has been used in the past after hurricanes, tornadoes, and other disasters. One example occurred during the New York smallpox outbreak in 1947: To vaccinate millions of vulnerable people as quickly as possible, vaccination PODs were opened in doctor's offices, police stations, and schools. More recently, the Federal Emergency Management Administration (FEMA) and local authorities have activated PODs to provide bottled water and "Meals-Ready-To Eat" (MREs) to survivors in Galveston, Texas, after Hurricane Ike (2008) and influenza vaccinations during the H1N1 pandemic (2009). The COVID-19 pandemic saw the development of PODs that, depending on the time period, facilitated mass SARS-CoV-2 testing and vaccinations (Figure 18.4, 18.5, 18.6, 18.7, and 18.8).

There are multiple types of PODs that could be beneficial to your needs (Box 18.2).

The success of a POD depends on how well the ICS can accomplish the POD's operational purpose. For example, if a POD has been created to distribute water, different personnel would be needed than in a POD intended to provide vaccinations or prophylactic medications for an airborne anthrax attack. Box 18.3 lists generic POD considerations (Box 18.3).

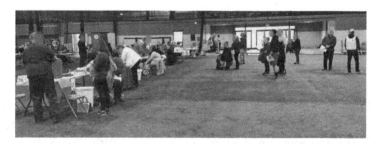

FIGURE 18.4 Lucas County, Ohio, COVID-19 vaccination POD. This an example of a fixed POD that was open to those who fit the criteria of a specific, vulnerable population while the vaccine supplies were ramping up.

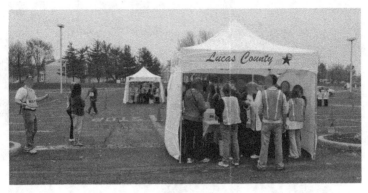

FIGURE 18.5 H1N1 influenza vaccination POD (2009). The set-up with just-in-time training.

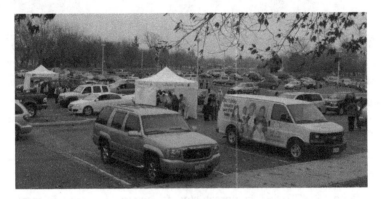

FIGURE 18.6 H1N1 influenza vaccination POD (2009). Vaccinations in progress by four teams at four stations. Each stationed was manned by University of Toledo healthcare students and their faculty.

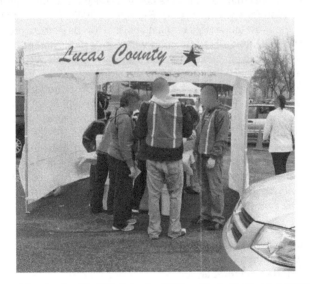

FIGURE 18.7 A functional mobile POD during the H1N1 pandemic. Healthcare students and their faculty managed several of the mini-stations at this mobile POD. It was managed principally by the local health department with the university personnel, grounds, and resources. The clients in the vehicles would follow preset traffic patterns to reach one of four vaccination stations. Ordinarily, they would receive the flu vaccine while in their cars, wait for 15 minutes near the EMS station, and then drive off. Those who brought dogs with them were asked to get out of their car to receive their shot to avoid having the vaccinator getting bit by an overly protective canine.

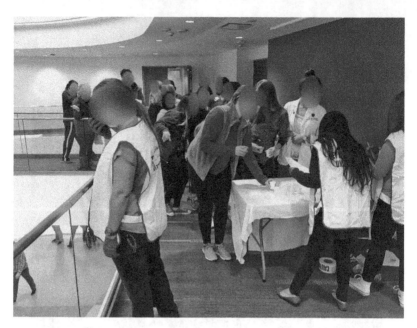

FIGURE 18.8 A POD exercise for Master of Public Health candidates in the University Population Health program. The "clients" were physician's assistant and nursing students who arrived at the POD expecting to receive prophylactic antibiotics for a meningitis outbreak.

BOX 18.2 **POD types**

Open: A POD that is unrestricted to anyone in need. *Example*: Distribution of potable water.

Closed: A POD that has been created to service a specific segment of the population for specific reasons. *Example*: COVID-19 vaccination program for the most vulnerable populations, like ICU healthcare providers.

Fixed: A POD that would function within an established edifice. This type of POD is easy to establish since it should have established amenities like communications, toilet facilities, entrances, exits, and parking. If the building is big enough, the public can be accommodated indoors. However, to wait on line outdoors could create a significant burden for vulnerable populations (e.g., geriatric, pregnant, special needs, functionally disabled).

Mobile: A transient POD; people would drive to the site to acquire the needed resource. Mobile PODs are best suited for individuals who have ambulatory/functional difficulties or who are responsible for accompanying individuals (e.g., children). When developing an improvisational POD, one should consider:

- Traffic patterns
- Terrain
- Weather vulnerabilities
- Flora and fauna threats
- Communication redundancy
- Vehicular requirements (cars, buses, etc.)
- Medical emergencies

With a mobile POD, there is less of a chance for interpersonal interaction that could spread infections or generate acts of mob displeasure.

ACFs

ACFs (also known as alternate care sites) are improvisational and transient venues in the community that have been created to provide care to a segment of the population while alleviating the increased burden of healthcare delivery on the traditional hospital network. This type of surge capacity is quite useful during complex and catastrophic disasters. In those situations, the healthcare system will have to meet the healthcare needs of the traditional baseline patient as well as those who have been victimized by the disaster itself either directly or indirectly (Figure 18.9).

ACFs have been around since the founding of this country. As you may remember, during the yellow fever epidemic in revolutionary Philadelphia the citizenry appropriated a mansion on top of an outlying hill and turned it into a hospital. During Hurricane Katrina, the New Orleans Convention Center became an ACF. In fact, 5 months after the that cyclone, the center was still caring for up to 5,000 individuals per month, and that included the uninsured poor.

Establishing an ACF requires coming up with a concept of operations: In other words, what will it be used for? One method of coming to grips with the development of the ACF is by using the time-honored 5W's and 1H system.

Who?

- For whom is the ACF intended? Ambulatory patients, acute care patients, subacute patients, chronic care patients?

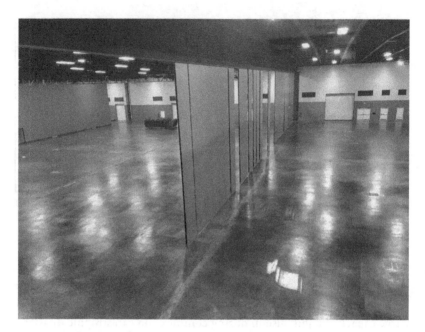

FIGURE 18.9 The convention center in the center of Toledo, Ohio, was scouted by local and state stakeholders as well as the U.S. Army Corps of Engineers and was approved by the governor as a possible ACF. The concept of operations changed from rendering care only to the Green patients in the region to housing recovering COVID-19 patients. Plans, personnel, and target activators were developed, but the building was never needed since the surge capacity of the hospitals in the region was sufficient to manage the COVID-19 numbers. This was quite fortunate. The cost to erect an ACF was $155.5 million in SUNY, Stony Brook, New York (number of beds: 1,000+; actual patients: 0); $118.5 million in SUNY, Westbrook, New York (number of beds: 1,000+; actual patients: 0); and $65.5 million in McCormick Place, Chicago (number of beds: 3,000; actual patients: 37).

- Who is in charge? An ICS structure for the ACF must be developed.
- Who are the caregivers? Medical specialists, nursing, physician's assistants, nurse practitioners, psychologists, respiratory therapists?
- Who will be needed as support staff? Aides, sanitation, maintenance, security, food workers, communications, mental health, social services, pastoral services, housekeeping, translators, transporters?

What?

- What is the concept of operations? What is the purpose of the ACF? Is it meant to care for people with minor problems (Green patients)? Major problems (Yellow and Red patients)? Trauma patients? Pediatric patients?
- To a certain extent, staffing personnel will be the same regardless of the concept of operations. On the other hand, the healthcare providers will be recruited based on the types of patients who have been selected to enter the ACF.
- What triggers will determine the activation of additional ACFs?

Where?

- The location to a large extent will be dictated by what is available in the community either in terms of a structure or in terms of acreage.
- Accessibility must also be considered.

When?

- There need to be clearly defined triggers that will determine when the ACF should activated. Examples of these triggers include:
  - A defined number of local hospitals that have reached a specific percentage increase in their surge capacity
  - A sustained increase (e.g., 7 days) in the percentage of pandemic patients per a given number of hospitals (e.g., 10%, 15%).
  - Modeling data predicting that the increase in future pandemic hospitalizations will reach a certain predetermined percentage within a specific period of time (e.g., 30 days).
- Some period of time will elapse between the decision to open the ACF and when it becomes operable. Therefore, trends must be followed assiduously so that the timing of the opening of the ACF is optimal.

Why?

- One or more of the triggers have been met.
- The Incident Commander has ordered it.
- Some state or federal power authority has requested the activation.

How?

- How will the ACF be activated?
- How will ACF policies and procedures be determined, developed, vetted, and instituted?
- How will the leadership of the ACF be determined?
- How will the activities of the ACF mesh with the established healthcare infrastructure?
- How will the personnel be specifically trained for the venue?
- How will the volunteers be coordinated?
- How will deactivation of the ACF be determined?
- How will the public be apprised of the ACF goals and objectives?
- How will the ACF appropriately accommodate the community's vulnerable populations?

Allocation of Scarce Resources

During complex and catastrophic disasters, resources may become so diminished that decisions will have to be made as to what victims are the best candidates to receive those resources. Reports indicate that this concept was implemented during the COVID-19 pandemic in resource-stressed sections of the United States and in other nations around the globe.

The problem is that these disasters have been so rare that policies and procedures surrounding allocation of scarce resources have not gone beyond the talking phase. The discussion began to bubble to the surface during the SARS-CoV-1 epidemic in Toronto. Peer-reviewed publications presented the problems associated with a scarcity of ventilators and the need to determine which patients should receive those ventilators and what parameters to employ to help with that decision. There was no true consensus in the literature. Sequential organ failure assessment (SOFA) scores, age criteria, and past medical history were all parameters under consideration. There were proponents and opponents to these concepts. Even the ethicists did not agree. However, nothing was ever truly decided. Consensus was never achieved. Meanwhile, the policymakers and legislators left well enough alone. They could not plead ignorance because national reports, white papers, and tabletop exercises were available for anyone who took an interest.

However, the COVID-19 pandemic made it clear that attention had to be paid not only to the ethical provision of scarce resources, but also what to do when that essential resource is not working with a particular patient but may be of use to a new patient (i.e., withdrawal of resources). With no legal guidelines and no ethical framework in place, arbitrary decisions about who gets what and who does not will contribute to communal fears and chaos. Box 18.4 shows an ethical framework to assist with the allocation of scarce resources and withdrawal of care.

Anecdotes nationally and globally underscore the need for ethical guidance and legislative specificities so that mistakes are not made, however inadvertent. These issues are rare but they do happen even now.

For example, in one country, in the event of a suicide bombing, the injured bomber would be triaged last regardless of that person's level of severity. In another country's disaster response, the powers that be insisted that foreign healthcare providers allocate units of blood to members of a particular religion first. In our own country during Hurricane Katrina, decisions regarding who had priority in terms of evacuation from a nonfunctional hospital were made based on living wills alone. It has also been reported that oxygen supplies were shipped to military hospitals primarily instead of civilian hospitals. Presumably, ill military personnel and their families had a higher status than the general public dying in civilian hospitals.

Fortunately, now, in the United States, legal considerations have been put in place to ensure that decision-making will not be based on race, gender, ethnic background, socioeconomic value, and current medical conditions. Through their publications and their communications with Congress, the U.S. Department of Health and Human Services Office for Civil Rights and the Consortium for Citizens with Disabilities have attempted to safeguard individuals with disabilities. Additionally, the Americans with Disabilities Act of 1990 and Section 504 of the Rehabilitation Act of 1973 state that decisions surrounding medical therapy provided to an individual should be based on one's current objective medical evidence and not on the patient's disability or past medical history.

With the COVID-19 pandemic we have gone from the theoretical to the actual. Therefore, there must be established an Allocation of Scarce Resource Advisory Body that can objectively and authoritatively establish guidelines to assist hospitals and other healthcare institutions. Their efforts may be superseded by state and federal authorities, but these external stakeholders usually will present a general framework. A local advisory body not only can provide deeper texture to those guidelines but can also add credibility to the community it serves.

KEY POINTS TO REMEMBER

- Determine your position in the local ICS.
- Determine your level of authority.
- Physicians have a different outlook regarding emergencies and disasters than public health authorities. Use that trait to the community's best advantage.
- PODs and ACFs are proven strategies to enhance the response to a complex and catastrophic disaster.
- Allocation of scarce resources is a medical, legal, and ethical issue, not only a public health one.

Further reading

Barry JM. *The Great Influenza: The Epic Story of the Deadliest Plague in History.* Viking Press; 2004.

Fenn EA. *Pox Americana: The Great Smallpox Epidemic of 1775–82.* Hill & Wang; 2001.

Influenza 1918. A Robert Kenner Films Production for The American Experience; 1998.

Leavitt JW. Public resistance or cooperation? A tale of smallpox in two cities. *Biosecur Bioterr.* 2003;1(3):185–192.

Markel H. Cholera, quarantines, and immigration restriction: The view from Johns Hopkins, 1892. *Bull Hist Med.* 1993;67:691–695.

Markel H. "Knocking out the cholera": Cholera, class and quarantines in New York City, 1892. *Bull Hist Med.* 1995;69:420–457.

Murphy J. *An American Plague: The True and Terrifying Story of the Yellow Fever Epidemic of 1793.* Clarion Books; 2003.

Rega P, Bork C, Chen Y, Woodson D, Hogue P, Batten S. Using an H1N1 vaccination drive-through to introduce healthcare students and their faculty to disaster medicine. *Am J Disaster Med.* 2010;5(2):129–136.

Reynolds G. Why were doctors afraid to treat Rebecca McLester? *NY Times Magazine,* April 18, 2004.

Risse GB. "A Long Pull, A Strong Pull, and All Together": San Francisco and bubonic plague, 1907–1908. *Bull Hist Med.* 1992;66:260–286.

Scheck A. Toronto's SARS epidemic reveals extraordinary human spirit. *Emerg Med News.* 2004;26(9):3.

The National Quarantine. Harper's Weekly, August 26, 1893.

Thompson WW, Shay DK, et al. Influenza-associated hospitalizations in the United States. *JAMA.* 2004;292:1333–1340.

19 My home, my castle—I hope!

You have just moved yourself and your family to the heartland of America along the Mississippi River. It is an opportunity for everyone to grow personally and for you to enhance your career. As you settle into the community you hear about the New Madrid Fault from your new friends and neighbors. You attend a lecture at the local university about the 1811–1812 New Madrid earthquakes. During the Q&A, you and your spouse are surprised to hear that a repeat seismic episode at a level of 6 magnitude or greater has a 25% to 40% chance of happening in the next 50 years. An area of 15,000 km² across five states would be impacted by ground liquefaction; flooding; impassable rivers; decimated roads, bridges, and highways; burst pipelines; and collapsed and quasi-collapsed buildings. Between 3,000 and 4,000 people would be dead and 86,000 would be injured. Economic losses would approach $300 billion. One hundred fifty hospitals in the region could be rendered inoperable. In the high-impact zones, 50% of residents would not have potable water and it would take weeks to restore it. An estimated 2.6 million people would also be without power. It suddenly dawns on both of you that you are more vulnerable than you previously thought.

What do I do now?

Here are some basic assumptions you should not forget:

- No one will be able to help you initially, so plan to rely on yourself and your family.
- There is no guarantee that your family members will be together when the Big One arrives. Kids go to school. Spouse goes to work. You go shopping. So what are your children's school emergency plans? Shelter? Food? Water?
- You need to be prepared for 72-hour self-sufficiency. That may suffice for most parts of the country, but on the West Coast or along the South Atlantic/Gulf Coast shores, 1- to 2-week self-sufficiency plans may be more appropriate.

Hazard vulnerability analysis

What are the hazards in your area that might destroy your home and force you to evacuate? Consider the following:

- Past history of the types of emergencies in your community
- Geographic characteristics
- Community characteristics
- Distance from transportation routes, cities, industries, or military bases
- Climatic variabilities

External chemical/radioactive release

Lock windows and doors for a better seal. Turn off any device or equipment and seal off any space that may transport external air into the internal environment. Put duct tape around doors and windows. In case of radiation, go to lowest part of the house or in the middle of the building.

Avoid tap water. Instead, drink from your supply cache.

Open communication channels with authorities.

Earthquake

"Drop, cover, and hold on." Secure heavy objects for possible aftershocks.

Floods/flash floods

Floods are the most common natural disaster in the United States. Reach the highest floor of the house or the roof. Avoid closed-off areas to avoid being trapped. Don't consume foods and fluids that have been damaged by flood waters; they may be contaminated.

Most homeowners do not carry flood insurance. Remember that coverage usually becomes effective 30 days after purchase.

Evacuation plans and routes

Do you have printed maps? Which roads have amenities, fuel, and food? It is safer to adhere to the evacuation routes identified by the proper authorities. Don't rely on non-FEMA phone apps for information, as they may be out of date or unavailable during a disaster.

Check-in phone numbers

Is there a check-in contact number that everyone in your family knows to use in the event of an emergency? Do you have two contact numbers, one near and one far? The distant contact number may be more readily available if the contact is not within the disaster zone. Texting may be more successful than phoning.

Home escape routes

Does each member of your family know how to escape from the home and each of the rooms in the event the house is actively compromised? Everyone should learn two escape routes for each room of the house. Does everyone know where to gather after evacuating the house? The meeting place should be secure and somewhere close to the home.

Food and water

Make sure there is enough canned food and potable water for all members of the family to last at least 72 hours. Dry ice (25 pounds) will keep the contents of a 10-cubic-foot freezer space frozen for 3 to 4 days.

Documents

You should have two copies of the following, one in your home and one in your bank's safety deposit box or with a trusted friend or family member living outside of the stricken area. All such items should be kept in a water-proof and portable container:

Will, insurance policies, deeds, stocks, bonds

Passports, social security cards, immunization records

Bank account numbers, credit card account numbers

Inventory of household goods for insurance purposes (photo/video and written documentation)

Family records (birth certificates, death certificates, marriage licenses, etc.)

Vehicle

Your vehicle may become your alternative home. Make sure it is ready (see Chapter 20 for more information).

Utilities

Make sure you know where the gas, electric, and water turn-off and turn-on valves or switches are located. Specific tools may be required to shut off utilities. Locate the shut-off valve for the water supply outside the house.

Unplug electrical equipment if you are evacuating home. In the event of an early return back home, leave the refrigerator plugged in.

Gas leaks and explosions can be secondary disasters following the primary one. There are different procedures to shut off the gas supply to your home. Ask the gas company for assistance prior to the disaster. If you turn it off, have an expert from the gas company turn it back on.

To avoid electrical sparks, which can lead to an explosion, turn off the individual electrical circuits before shutting down the main circuit to your property.

Don't run a generator in the house. Power it up 20 feet outside the house and away from windows to avoid carbon monoxide toxicity.

Medical necessities

This is especially important for those with disabilities. Make sure you have:

Prescription medications

Copies of medical prescriptions

Mobility aids

Auditory aids

Extra eyeglasses

Extra dentures

Batteries and information for medical devices (pacemakers, implantable devices, monitoring equipment, etc.)

Copies of medical insurance and appropriate documentation

List of physicians, medical history, medications, procedures, allergies, etc.

Assistance animal necessities/documentation

Credit cards and cash

Remember that ATMs may not function in a disaster.

Phone apps

Download the FEMA app to your smartphone (in English and Spanish) via Google Play or Apple.

NOAA weather alerts

Family notifications

Preparedness tips and checklists

Emergency shelter locations: Text SHELTER and a ZIP code to 43362

Disaster recovery centers: Text DRC and a ZIP code to 43362

Disaster assistance registration

Disaster information

Wireless Emergency Alerts (WEA) provide short emergency messages from authorized local to federal authorities. The Emergency Alert System (EAS) is a national public warning system within 10 minutes of a national emergency. The NOAA Weather Radio All Hazards (NWR) is a nationwide network of radio stations advising the public on weather conditions from the closest National Weather Service to one's location.

First aid/CPR

Law enforcement and EMS may not be readily available to deal with lacerations or a cardiac arrest. Table 19.1 lists the contents of a disaster first-aid kit.

TABLE 19.1 **Disaster first-aid kit**

Sunscreen	Surgical gloves	Soap
Bandages	Gauze pads	Surgical tape
Scissors	Tweezers	Needle
Moist towelettes	Antiseptic solution	Anti-diarrheal medications
Flashlights/batteries	Thermometer	Tongue blades
Triangular bandages	ACE bandages	Band-Aids
Pins	Scalpel	Isopropyl alcohol
Lubricant	Hypothermia blankets	

TABLE 19.2 **Disaster kit: baby/child**

Formula (premixed)	Prescription medications
Bottled water	Diapers
Baby bottles/nipples	Eye dropper
Diaper wipes	Diaper rash ointment
Pediatric sunblock	Pediatric analgesics/antipyretics
Comfort toys, pacifiers	Protective clothes
Hygiene products/baby shampoo	Hypothermia blankets

Contact information for your family's physicians/pediatricians

Children and pets

Table 19.2 lists the contents of a pediatric disaster kit and Box 19.1 gives information about pet safety in disasters.

Water

Water sustenance is essential in disaster planning. Anecdotal stories of survival have documented people living for more than a week or two on water alone. Therefore, serious consideration must be given to obtaining and storing uncontaminated water first and then planning what to do when there is nothing to drink except contaminated water.

Do not store water in empty juice or milk containers, since they may not be properly cleaned and can allow the formation of harmful bacteria. When storing uncontaminated water, typical planning calls for 1 gallon of water per person per day (2 quarts for drinking, 2 quarts for additional necessities). The amount may be higher for children, nursing mothers, and the ill. Requirements will also increase with exertional activity and hot climates.

Alcohol and caffeinated products are not suitable hydration replacements.

Plan for at least a 3-day supply of water, but again, depending on your hazard vulnerability analysis, it may be more comforting to have a 2-week supply handy. Obviously, storage of such a large cache may be impractical for most people. Water supplies should be rotated every 6 months. One way of preserving the integrity of the water and to prevent contamination is to store each quart of water with 4 drops of household bleach.

Never ration water unless you hear otherwise from local authorities.

Drink uncontaminated water first. Box 19.2 lists some easy-to-forget sources of uncontaminated water.

Sometimes, however, there is no choice but to drink contaminated water. Box 19.3 outlines methods to correct or to minimize contamination.

Food
Box 19.4 lists general food considerations.

Toilets
Box 19.5 explains how to make your own potty.

Tools and supplies
Finally, Box 19.6 lists tools and supplies to have on hand in case of disaster.

BOX 19.2 **Easy-to-forget home sources of uncontaminated water**

- Ice cube trays
- Juice and fluids from canned food
- Toilet tanks, as long as the tank was not treated with antiseptic or coloring solutions. Do not consider the water from the toilet bowl as potable.
- Indoor water pipes: Turn the faucet to the "on" position at the highest point in the house, then open the faucet at the lowest point. Drain into receptacle.
- Water heater: Turn off the power first.
- Waterbed: Only if fresh water was infused. Treat with 2 oz of household bleach per 120 gallons of water.

BOX 19.3 **Water decontamination**

- Filter visible debris; allow to stand for 24 hours; strain through layers of cloth.
- Boiling: 1–2 minutes of a rolling boil; add salt and aerate to improve taste.
- Distillation: Better than chlorination and boiling in terms of removing most microorganisms. Also removes heavy metals and salts in the water, which are not removed by boiling or chlorination.
- Household bleach (5.25–6% sodium hypochlorite): Add 16 drops of bleach per gallon of water and let stand for 30 minutes. Repeat if no chlorine smell and let stand for 15 minutes. Discard water and use another source if there is still no chlorine scent.

BOX 19.4   **General food considerations**

· Store a 3-day supply of food at least. In some high-threat areas, a 7- or even a 14-day supply may be indicated.
· Canned goods
    – Usually last 1 year; rotate stock every 6 months.
    – If using a Sterno to heat a can of food, open the can, but remove the label first. The label could ignite.
· Avoid thirst-provoking foods (high in fat or protein, salty) if potable water availability is questionable.
· Do not eat food that normally requires refrigeration and that has been left at room temperature for more than 2 hours.
· Avoid rationing in children and in pregnancy.
· Bury all garbage deep and away from shelter and water sources. Garbage can be a food source for feral animals and other scavengers.
· Do not use powdered formulas with untreated water.
· Example of a 3-day menu for the average adult/adolescent:
    – 3 cans tuna, chicken
    – 3 cans of ready-to-eat soup
    – 6 cans of juice
    – 3 cans of fruit/vegetables
    – 1 box of dry milk
    – 1 box of crackers
    – 1 jar of peanuts
    – 1 jar of jam
    – Treats
    – 1 manual can opener

BOX 19.5   **Creating a DIY potty**

Supplies

· Toilet paper/towelettes
· Hand-washing supplies (alcohol-based)
· Feminine hygiene items
· Plastic storage bags/bucket
· Shovel
· Household bleach
· Disinfectant
· Sanitizer

Method

· Obtain a suitably sized bucket with snug cover.
· Place an old toilet seat on top of the bucket for comfort.
· Line the bucket with two plastic bags.
· Sprinkle the waste with bleach.
· Bury the waste deep and away from food and water sources.
· Avoid urinating in the DIY potty, as the plastic bags may disintegrate. Instead, create a latrine (2 feet long, 6 inches wide, 2 feet deep) located away from food and water sources.

BOX 19.6 Disaster kit: tools and supplies

Portable generator
ABC fire extinguisher
NOAA weather radio
Duct tape
Waterproof matches
Compass
Mess kit/eating utensils
Manual can opener
Swiss Army knife
Pliers
Hammer/nails
Battery-operated radio
Compass
Flares
Pencils/markers
Waterproof containers
Disinfectants
Rope (100 feet or more)
Sewing kit
Kerosene heater
Tarpaulin
Hatchet
Flashlight
Work gloves
Work boots
Crescent wrench
Screwdriver
Whistle
Maps
Shovel
Garbage bags
Household bleach
Raft
Life preservers
Mosquito netting
Candles
Crowbar
Chain saw
Rock salt
Toilet paper
Portable toilet

- Perform a hazard vulnerability assessment for your community and your home.
- Determine the individual needs of each member of the family.
- Prepare your home for survival in the event that evacuation is impossible.
- Prepare your vehicle for survival in the event of an evacuation or an accident.
- Train all members of your family in basic survival techniques.
- Maintain a redundancy of communications options.

Further reading

Federal Emergency Management Administration. Make a Plan; Build a Kit; Individuals with Disabilities; Prepare Your Pets for Disasters; Seniors; Evacuation; Emergency Alerts. All available at Ready.gov.

Federal Emergency Management Administration. National Flood Insurance Program. FloodSmart: The National Flood Insurance Program. https://www.fema.gov/flood-insurance

U.S. Geological Service. *Earthquake Hazard in the New Madrid Seismic Zone Remains a Concern.* Fact Sheet 2009-3071; 2009.

U.S. Geological Service. *Putting Down Roots in Earthquake Country: Your Handbook for the Central United States.* General Information Product 119; 2011.

20 A vehicle for all seasons

You just received an urgent summons from your healthcare system that it needs ED coverage in one of their hospitals 800 miles from where you normally work. They are offering four times what you usually receive for locum tenens work, but it is the dead of winter and you would need to travel on I-80, a stretch of highway notorious for its multi-vehicular accidents even in the best of times. On top of that, the weather forecast predicts several inches of snow over the route in rather isolated spots. For further emphasis, this morning the news services are reporting a 60-vehicle pile-up in Pennsylvania, resulting in at least one death. Scrolling a little bit lower on the news site, you see that a snowstorm in Japan resulted in a chain-reaction vehicular accident that kept travelers isolated, hungry, and cold for up to 48 hours.

What do I do now?

You decide that it is worth the risk since you have time to prepare yourself and your vehicle. The vehicle is new and sturdy and has been recently serviced. Let's examine what your vehicle should have (Table 20.1) and what you should have (Table 20.2).

Bear in mind that this scenario—a long winter drive—is an elective situation. It involves an event that is stable, predictable, and relatively safe. However, emergency evacuations do not fall in that category. Finding yourself in the path of a Category 5 hurricane that will be making landfall in 5 days can be considered an urgent evacuation. It is far from predictable, but it is safer than staying along a coastline that will be directly impacted by the storm surge. The longer you delay evacuation in this circumstance, the greater your

TABLE 20.1 **Vehicular preparation**

In no-threat conditions, keep your fuel tank halfway filled at all times; in questionable circumstances, keep the fuel tank three-quarters filled. Depending on the type and year of the vehicle, fluid levels also need to be checked at regular intervals (antifreeze, windshield fluid, brake fluid, etc.).

Extra set of car keys	Booster/jumper cables	Hand-cranked radio
Battery-powered radio	Batteries	ABC fire extinguisher
Flashlight/batteries	Water (1 gallon/person/day)	Tow chain
Maps (hard copies)	Shovel	Flares
Tire repair kit	Tire pump	Spare tire
Rock salt (traction)	Sand (traction)	Kitty litter (traction)
Ice scraper	Hypothermia blanket	Zip-lock bags
Gloves	Toilet paper/hygiene products	All-purpose multi-tool
First-aid kit	Blankets	Hammer
Wrench	Pliers	Traffic triangles (hazard signs)
Brushes	Spare car phone charger	Matches/lighter (waterproof)
Duct tape		

TABLE 20.2 **Personal protection while on the road**

Multiple layers of clothing: The key is layering to fend off cold and wind chill factors	Traffic vests to increase your visibility in darkness
Sleeping bag	Hypothermia blankets
Thermal gloves	Thermal hats and face coverings
Sturdy, waterproof boots	Knife/hatchet
Personal sanitation necessities (sanitizers, wipes, bags, ties, etc.)	Communication equipment: whistles, bullhorn, air horn
Medication refills	Extra set of glasses
Cash	

High-energy food (with a long shelf life): peanut butter, assorted nuts, energy bars, dried fruit, MREs (Meals-Ready-to-Eat). Warming and can openers are not required

vulnerability factor, as roads will be clogged, fuel stations will be closed, and places to shelter will be limited. Don't drive through flood waters: 6 inches of water could make a car go out of control and 12 inches of moving water can make a car float away. Fallen power lines can kill; if a line falls across your vehicle, stay in your car until someone can safely neutralize the line.

An interesting conundrum should now be considered as this country enters the electric vehicle (EV) era. Is an EV owner more vulnerable to the exigencies of a sudden evacuation compared to the owner of a traditional gas-fueled vehicle? During Hurricane Irma (2017), 58%, 40%, and 35% of gasoline stations in Gainesville, Miami, and Tampa ran out of gasoline, respectively. Having some (yet to be determined) ratio of both traditional vehicles and EVs in a community may reduce long lines at gas stations, but will the local power grid be able to "juice up" a mass efflux of electric cars from a danger area? Currently, a hybrid power vehicle may be the best answer. A typical hybrid vehicle can drive on electricity for about 50 miles before needing a recharge and approximately 350 miles on a full tank of gasoline. Conceivably, using one type of energy may allow a family to flee from ground zero expeditiously enough so that they can reach a more available source of energy well away from the disaster site. Obviously, more research is indicated.

Similarly, the vulnerabilities are logarithmically increased during an emergent situation when, for example, the winds have changed 180 degrees and the wildfire that was just over the horizon is suddenly coming toward your community. That is why it is important to perform your hazard vulnerability analysis. Prepare and train accordingly. That admonition is also directed toward your entire family and anyone else for whom you have responsibility. Preparing for an elective departure by vehicle will pay dividends when a quick evacuation may be lifesaving.

KEY POINTS TO REMEMBER

- Have as many of the disaster preparedness necessities stored in one backpack or container for easy access and for easy checking (a "go-bag").
- Check little-used equipment at least with the change of seasons.
- Service your vehicle as per its maintenance guidelines.
- Keep a mental note of mile markers or road signs in case you need to communicate your location.
- Becoming a ham radio operator will enhance your communication capabilities.

Further reading

Federal Emergency Management Administration. Car Safety. https://www.ready.gov/car

Feng K, Lin N, Xian S, Chester MV. Can we evacuate from hurricane with electric vehicles? *Transportation Research Part D*. 2020;86:102458.

National Weather Service. Prepare for Cold Weather. https://www.weather.gov/safety/cold-before

"OK, so now I have an idea of what to do, but what about my team?" Over the course of time, you have acquired a great deal of knowledge regarding disaster preparedness and response. That is true not only in a general sense but also in a more specific one— your knowledge is based on a hazard vulnerability analysis (HVA) of your community. Now, hospital and community leaders wish to have that knowledge disseminated, not only to ED staff but to everyone else in the hospital. Who knows? The hospital's public relations department is thinking that if you are good enough, they may want you to be the voice of disaster medicine in the community.

What do I do now?

et's break this down to the essentials. First, teach your people—your ED. Much of what you will want them to know will be managed by hospital's administrators and nursing. Sometimes, the leadership will have very progressive ideas about how much the staff should absorb about a disaster response and will make the most of the various educational platforms available to deliver the content. Other times, that won't be the case, due to limited time, expense, and interest, and the paucity of real threats, and the disaster education provided will be just enough to get by and meet the minimums established by the Joint Commission's Emergency Management Standards. The basic components set by the Joint Commission deal with communications, resources, safety, responsibilities, utilities, and clinical support. That will also include the mandate to conduct at least two disaster drills per year. The staff will receive training on the hospital disaster plan, its specific annexes, and the various codes that could be announced over the PA system. Check out the syllabus and you may realize that the education is basic, infrequent, and boring.

So, if you have the power to make changes, evaluate the current syllabus and reinforce it by adding topics based on your HVA. For example, your hospital's educational program may include triage, incident command, and a general disaster response, but if you live in a hurricane-prone region you may wish to add specific topics like near-drowning, blunt force trauma, environmental exposure, etc. This is similar to FEMA's "discussion-based exercise." It is a forum where tactical and strategic disaster preparedness and response are presented, discussed, and tested. Depending on time, interest, and funding, these sessions can be as minimal as a lunch-break topic-of-the-week presentation and or as extensive as seminars, workshops, tabletop exercises, and gaming.

In my experience, seminars and workshops require more time and planning, and a lot of assistance from the hospital's continuing education department. As an example, let us say that your HVA indicates the need for more in-depth hospital-wide education on the impact of tornadoes on hospitals and the community. A 4-hour seminar might include topics such as the risk of tornadoes in the region, injuries associated with tornadoes, the risk of tornadoes on your hospital, personal and family preparedness during tornado season, and mental health issues during the recovery process.

TABLETOP EXERCISES AND GAMING

Tabletop exercises and gaming disaster scenarios take less time, involve fewer resources, and create a more intense learning environment in a no-threat atmosphere. Besides, if done correctly, they can be a lot of fun. What is needed, however, is an expert facilitator to develop the exercise or the game and oversee and guide the activity as it occurs. You would be that facilitator.

Tabletop exercises

Box 21.1 outlines a tabletop exercise involving a 24-vehicle crash on the turnpike.

BOX 21.1 **Tabletop exercise: turnpike crash**

Example: A 24-vehicle accident on the turnpike

Players: The incident commander (IC), security, heads of emergency services, surgery, radiology, laboratory services, and blood bank

Facilitator: You, the reader

Facilitator to IC: "You have received word that your hospital may be receiving 20 to 30 casualties from a vehicular MCI 2 miles away. You are the closest. What are your first steps?"

[Answer]

Facilitator to IC: "At this table is your team, IC. Who is Operations? Finance and administration? Logistics? Planning?"

[Answer]

Facilitator to Operations: "Your ED is 85% filled with patients and boarders. What are you going to do?"

[Answer]

Facilitator to Operations and Logistics: "The ED has received word that a bus containing 20 to 30 non-English-speaking tourists from France is involved. Any ideas?"

[Answer]

Facilitator to Surgery: "Where will you be positioning your team?"

[Answer]

"Are you canceling elective surgeries?"

[Answer]

Facilitator to Planning: "What are your plans for surge capacity? How are you addressing shift changes over the next 24 hours?"

[Answer]

Facilitator to Public Information Officer: "How have you served the needs of the media?"

[Answer]

"How often do you plan to provide updates?"

[Answer]

The idea is for the players to understand that while there is a plan, they must also appreciate the need to put that plan into action. Having a facilitator who knows the plan and who can ask granular hypotheticals will demonstrate to the key players whether the plan works or if there are specific challenges that need to be addressed. It is important that the facilitator operates in a non-confrontational manner. It is also worthwhile to have a secretary present to take notes and document ideas, suggestions, and challenges that require further evaluation at subsequent meetings.

Box 21.2 describes a tabletop exercise involving a mass shooting.

BOX 21.2 **Tabletop exercise: mass shooting**

Preparation

1. Simulate the mass shooting event in San Bernardino, CA (12/2/2015) as it relates to the actions of the ED at Loma Linda University Medical Center and Children's Hospital. The objectives of the exercise will change depending on the players as well as other variables.
2. Set the scene first. There are x number of patients in the ED waiting room. There are y number of patients (add a number relevant to your ED) already being treated in the ED:
   - A patient with an acute CVA
   - A patient in acute respiratory failure requiring immediate intubation
   - A patient with an acute arterial occlusion of an upper extremity
   - A Level 2 motor vehicle trauma coming in by ambulance
3. EMS calls in to the ED. Present a synopsis of the shooting to the players.
4. Discuss pre-arrival objectives:
   - Activation of disaster code
   - Assign duties to ED staff
   - Disposition of ED patients
   - Disposition of waiting room patients
   - Communication with critical departments
5. With the setting established, the first four shooting victims will arrive within 11 minutes. Present the cases and discuss with the players management strategies.

Victims
VICTIM #1 (11:44 arrival time): GSW in the anterior chest. Victim is alert but tachypneic. He is hemodynamically stable. Ultrasound is negative for pericardial tamponade, but a pneumothorax is likely.

Victim #1 objectives:

- Initial management based on primary and secondary surveys
- Differentiate between simple and tension pneumothorax
- Discuss treatment strategies for simple and tension pneumothorax
- Reassessment of patient when he suddenly becomes hypotensive
- Emergency management of a suddenly hypotensive gunshot victim

VICTIM #2 (11:48 arrival time): Laceration to the chest and multiple wounds to face, arm, and leg. Victim is alert and hemodynamically stable. Initial FAST exam is negative. Standard X-rays are positive for multiple metallic fragments. Leg wounds continue to bleed profusely.
Victim #2 objective:

- Diagnosis and management of serious vascular trauma in the ED

VICTIM #3 (11:50 arrival time): The victim is in critical condition with multiple GSWs to the chest and elsewhere. The victim is hypotensive and has a decreased level of consciousness. The FAST exam revealed bilateral pneumothoraces and X-rays indicated multiple metallic fragments.
Victim #3 objective:

- Prioritize emergency care in a victim with altered mental status, hypotension, and bilateral pneumothoraces

VICTIM #4 (11:55 arrival time): The victim has sustained multiple GSWs to the pelvic region and one leg. Plain films reveal multiple pelvic fractures. The FAST exam suggests blood in the bladder. The patient received tranexamic acid (TXA), the massive transfusion protocol, and an expeditious transfer to the OR.
Victim #4 objectives:

- Indications for the use of TXA in the trauma patient
- Discussion on the logistics of administering TXA
- Indications for the mass transfusion protocol
- Discussion on the rationale for a massive transfusion protocol

Gaming

FEMA classifies "gaming" as another example of a discussion-based exercise. However, to lump classroom PowerPoint lectures with facilitated tabletop exercises and gaming into one category does a disservice to those platforms. Many of the initial educational activities are passive in nature:

Instructor talks, students listen. With tabletop exercises and gaming, the activities are much more interactive. The students are required to act and, with the assistance of expert facilitators, learn. Studies indicate that gaming, for example, improves retention of complex concepts, hones interactive communications, and explores depths of the educational content that are not attained by routine classroom education. Unfortunately, FEMA's approach to gaming is a limited one. It does not address the different types of gaming such as competitive versus non-competitive and web-based versus boardgames.

Emergency medicine and disaster medicine personnel should explore and experiment with diverse teaching modalities, including educational gaming. Over the course of years, we have employed card games and dice throws to quiz students on the properties and clinical manifestations of bioterrorism agents and emerging infectious diseases. The key is to develop an educational platform that is cheap, efficacious, easy to teach, easy to learn, and fun.

We also explored the concept of non-competitive gaming to teach about a sudden-impact, no-warning event like an active assailant. The components of the game consisted of a board upon which was laid the schematic or footprint of the ED, a deck of cards, dice, player and patient tokens, and patient scenario cards (Box 21.3, Figures 21.1 and 21.2). The patient scenario cards indicate the level of criticality by means of diagnosis, diagnostic tests, and vital signs.

We discovered that the game is easily transportable, easy to explain, simple to comprehend, and quick to perform. The game itself was over in a matter of minutes. Where the players received their education was from each other in terms of best places to hide, how to hide, and what items in a patient care room would be good weapons if needed. The discussions grew even more interesting when each player stated their reasons as to whether or not they tried to protect their patients in the process. All this allowed everyone to explore ethics, legalities, stigmatization, and more granular strategies. It's important that there is a facilitator or two who can address these issues competently. Believe it or not, the entire game lasted no longer than 30 to 40 minutes. Because of its length of time it took to play and its transportability, we were able to "game" even in the ED during breaks and in the middle of the night, when personnel are not typically in the educator's sights for training.

BOX 21.3 **Active assailant board game (aka "52 Bang-Bang")**

Game components

- The board: A floor plan (with grids) of the ED
- Deck of conventional 52 playing cards + two jokers
- A pair of dice
- Player tokens
- Patient tokens
- Patient scenario cards: demographics, chief complaint/diagnosis, vital signs, stage of care
- Player demographic cards
- Writing instruments
- Commercial/improvisational tourniquets

Procedure

- The facilitator reviews the rules of play.
- The facilitator presents the floorplan (entrances, exits, patient care rooms, supply rooms, bathrooms, etc.). Areas and doors that can be locked are highlighted.
- By a roll of dice, one player becomes the charge nurse.
- Players randomly select a patient from the deck of patient scenario cards, one player per patient. The demographics of the patient are made known to everyone.
- Depending on the rules, the players can act as themselves or simulate another caregiver with a different set of demographics (e.g., age, disabilities, gender).
- The "charge nurse" places each player/patient duo in a specific patient care room that is appropriate to that patient's triage level.
- Once players and patients are in position, gunshot sound effects are heard ("bang, bang").
- With that alarum, each player simultaneously makes the decision to run to safety, barricade in place, and be prepared to fight with improvisational weapons if confronted.
- They have 20 seconds to write down their actions—(1) RUN, (2) HIDE, or (3) FIGHT—and HOW (i.e., list the barricade equipment, any improvisational weapons, and whether they are including the patient and/or families in their actions). The abbreviated amount of time allotted to write intentionally serves as a minor stressor for the players.
- The players move their tokens on the board based on the actions they described.
- Each player explains their actions to the group.

Continued

BOX 21.3 **Continued**

- Each action has a certain degree of difficulty based on the amount of time required to complete it. That degree of difficulty is exemplified by the number of playing cards that have to be turned over to complete the action. For example, a player who is running out of the room and through the ambulance entrance a short distance away will take little time. The brevity of that action is arbitrarily commensurate to turning over 3 playing cards. If the player decides to run with their patient, it will take longer to complete (4 cards) and even longer if that patient is comatose and on a ventilator (6 cards).
- The more cards that are turned over, the more likely it is that one or two of the jokers will be revealed. If no jokers are revealed, then the player has accomplished their objective successfully. If one joker is revealed, that signifies that the player has been shot in an extremity. If two jokers are revealed, that signifies that the player has been shot twice. (More jokers can be added to represent additional conditions that need to be corrected emergently. This depends on the objectives of the facilitator and the type of players.)
- Whether the stricken player survives their wounds will depend on the fellow player they select to apply the tourniquet or the needle thoracostomy or the IO infusion on simulation models. What happens at this stage is a refresher course or just-in-time training on certain emergency skills.
- Finally comes the debriefing, which is led by the facilitator. At this stage, all the players have an opportunity to discuss each other's actions and identify challenges and solutions.

Uniformly, in our trials with a variety of ED personnel and students, the reviews were extremely positive, in terms of interest and learning objectives, even among those who had already taken formal active shooter courses. The most tangible objective that was always met was that the players received training in applying both commercial and improvisational tourniquets.

This type of game can be expanded to include hospital security and external responding law enforcement agencies as players. It would be very educational and possibly even an eye-opening experience to have the healthcare personnel appreciate what law enforcement would need to do to neutralize the perpetrator before any search-and-rescue efforts.

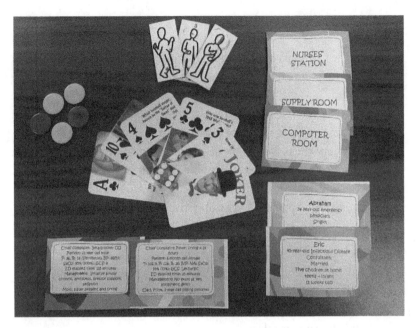

FIGURE 21.1 Components used in the "active assailant" exercise.

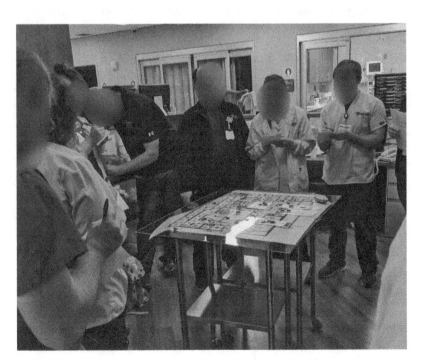

FIGURE 21.2 From presenting the rules to "52 Bang-Bang" to the players' final debriefing, the game can play out as quickly as 30 minutes. The photo demonstrates the simple fact that it can be played virtually anywhere at any time. In this instance, with administration's approval, we were able to play the game at 5 a.m. in a functioning ED. Trying to provide education to the night shift crew is always problematic.

Another set of players could be introduced into this gaming concept by inviting functionally disabled individuals (i.e., wheelchair-bound, the blind, the deaf, and their service animals or their equipment) to serve as the patients in the game. In this variation, there would be two types of players: the healthcare team and the functionally disabled persons.

An analysis of the players' subjective and objective measures was positive and it led to exploring the use of the same platform to teach other topics. One was a similar game, "Botulopoly," dealing with a botulism mass casualty incident (see Chapter 10). The objectives were as follows:

- Evacuating ED patients safely to make room for the prisoners with botulism who consumed tainted Pruno
- Developing management schemes to detect the patients' respiratory compromise as early as possible
- Allocating scarce resources (e.g., ventilators) to manage multiple botulism patients safely
- Identifying the pathway to access botulism antitoxin
- Triaging patients safely when the local hospital was overwhelmed.

DRILLS, FUNCTIONAL EXERCISES, AND FULL-SCALE EXERCISES

The discussion-based educational platforms we have just discussed are a prelude to operations-based exercises. According to FEMA, there are three basic types: drills, functional exercises (FEs), and full-scale exercises (FSEs). With these, the students get to move around and put didactics into play.

Drills serve to teach and/or maintain certain skills and procedures or work through a new policy or protocol. An FE is the next step up. Using real-time simulated scenarios and environments, this type of exercise evaluates policies, procedures, and capabilities. There is a great deal of dependence on facilitators, controllers, and evaluators. To be successful significant preparatory work is needed by a number of individuals to identify the objectives, educate the players beforehand on the means to achieve those objectives, and develop the exercise to meet those objectives.

The FSE remains the "gold standard" in disaster planning and mitigation efforts. To plan and develop an FSE requires time, dedication, facilitators, observers, subject matter experts, trusted agents, and money.

Multiple agencies and diverse stakeholders have agreed to come together to test plans, coordinate responses, enhance communications, and resolve unpredictable events. This is a goal to be valued and acted upon for the well-being of the community. Since this is a complicated endeavor, it will require an incident command hierarchy to identify key stakeholders and operatives (e.g., designers, controllers, safety officers, and facilitators), lay out the meeting schedules, develop a master scenario events list, create a Controller/Evaluator Handbook, and fix the exercise date. Obviously, this will take time and commitment. Human nature, as it is, may yield to the temptation of creating shortcuts that could destroy the very goals a full-scale exercise is meant to achieve. To counterbalance the foibles of human nature, recruiting the media and the public (especially those representing vulnerable populations) to serve as key stakeholders in the process is advisable.

Once the FSE is completed, a full-scale debriefing ("hot wash") should be initiated soon thereafter. The earlier the better; the same day, if possible. The final product of all this is an After-Action Report. This official document, which frequently is sent to state and federal authorities, presents the successes and the challenges of the exercise and serves as the fulcrum for further planning and testing.

Simulation Medical Education

Having access to a bona fide medical simulation center would be an excellent modality to enact operations-based exercises. Depending on the center's level of sophistication and commitment, the healthcare professionals in the ED can be exposed to various simulation models, simulated clinical settings, and even virtual immersive environments. For the past 10 years or so, on virtually a weekly basis, I have had the honor and privilege of teaching emergency medicine and skills to myriad numbers of students (medical, physician assistant, nursing, pharmacy, public health) and residents (emergency medicine and pharmacy) at the Lloyd A. Jacobs Interprofessional Immersive Simulation Center (IISC). In February–March 2020 we used the IISC for 2 weeks to train faculty, residents, and students on management strategies when attending to a possible COVID-19 patient in the ED (Figure 21.3).

Regarding disaster medical education, my team and I have used the IISC environment, human patient simulators, and other specialized resources to drill the classes on triage and tourniquets ("T-n-T"), active shooter, hospital

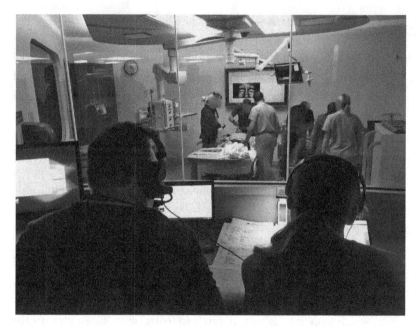

FIGURE 21.3 The management of a trauma patient by PGY 1 EM residents under the watchful eye of faculty in the IISC at the University of Toledo. Note the scenario script timeline beside the monitors. These are followed to advance or veer off the cases, depending on the residents' capabilities.

evacuation, blast injury, and other more specific disaster-related scenarios. Boxes 21.4, 21.5, 21.6, and 21.7 are examples of the various drills that we have created and conducted for multidisciplinary healthcare students, residents, faculty, and staff.

FULL-SCALE EXERCISE

Finally, we come to the FSE, the "gold standard." After receiving education from multiple discussion-based platforms and testing their mettle through drills and FEs, the players now experience a scenario from start to finish where they are on their own. Under the professional eyes of the evaluators, the players are displaying in real time, using actual resources, their actions to a critical incident. If the training was appropriate, the players will be

BOX 21.4 The active assailant blitz for healthcare students, residents, and staff

Pre-drill preparations

Players receive Run/Hide/Fight education prior to drill day or just-in-time education on drill day.

Notify security personnel regarding drill.

Seal off drill area from non-participants.

Brief players about rules, venue set-up, objectives, strictly voluntary participation, no-touch, no-harm environment.

- Have multidisciplinary players, if possible, in each room.
- Each participant team would evaluate each case scenario and begin management prior to the active shooter drill.

Random dispersal of participants in the simulated ED patient care rooms or multiple patients in the waiting room

"Patients": High-fidelity simulators or volunteer faculty as hybrid simulators

Patient scenarios are placed on the simulators for the players or given to live "patients" serving as standardized patients (see below).

Participants and faculty/staff/law enforcement are in place.

Patient scenarios

Patient Scenario #1

- Chief complaint: Weak left arm and droopy eyelids
- History: On June 29, 2014, Horatio P., a previously healthy male, aged 19 years, from Michoacán, Mexico, began working at a tomato farm in rural Indiana. After 1 day of work, the patient sought medical attention for generalized fatigue, left shoulder pain, left hand numbness, and blurry vision. No meds, no allergies, no significant PMH.
- Vital signs: T: 39.6°C; P: 124; R: 22; B/P: 116/56; SaO2: 97%
- Physical examination: Hyperesthesia of the left shoulder, weakness of the left hand, generalized areflexia, and drooping of the left upper eyelid. Additional findings: nuchal rigidity and disjointed answers.

Patient Scenario #2

- Chief complaint: A 7-day history of throat pain, difficulty swallowing, muffled voice, and subjective fevers

Continued

- History: A previously healthy 35-year-old woman, Melodie T., presents to the ED with a strep throat. Despite pain medications + antibiotics for 5 days, the pain is getting worse and it's getting harder to eat, talk, and swallow. Meds: penicillin & ibuprofen. Allergies: Eggs. PMH: PID 10 years ago.
- Vital signs: T: 36.6°C; P: 94; R: 18; B/P: 96/56; SaO2: 95%; Pain: 7/10
- Physical exam: Mild tenderness and swelling in the anterior neck; no cervical lymphadenopathy; no drooling

Patient Scenario #3

- Chief complaint: Fever and altered mental status in a child
- History: A 5-year-old boy was admitted to the general pediatrics inpatient service with fever, headache, fatigue, neck stiffness, buttock pain, and bilateral leg pain for the past 2 days, according to mother and father.

Meds: Ibuprofen & acetaminophen. Allergies: None. PMH: Bilateral myringotomies 4 years ago (multiple otitis media).

- Vital signs: T: 38.8°C; P: 157; R: 28; B/P: 100/56; SaO2: 95%; Pain: 7/10; LOC: Sleepy but rousable.
- Physical exam: Ill-appearing. His movements are restricted by pain, primarily in his neck. Pronounced nuchal rigidity.

Mucus membranes are moderately dry. Petechiae noted on both lower legs. Heart, lung, and abdominal exams are normal.

Patient Scenario #4

- Chief complaint: MCI. Right leg pain. Cannot walk.
- History: Ulisse B. is a 19-year-old sophomore from Wisconsin. He was in an MCI where he was driving a car that was in a 25-car chain reaction incident due to foggy conditions. He was not wearing a seatbelt and was thrown from the car, but another car part fell on his right thigh, trapping him in place for 6 hours. Rescuers found him eventually and brought him to ED by ambulance.
- Vital signs: T: 36.8°C; P: 127; R: 22; B/P: 90/76; SaO2: 93%; Pain: 10/10; LOC: Awake & alert.
- Physical exam: In pain; grimacing. Severely bruised right thigh and perineal hematoma. Pain with pelvic rocking.

Chest, abdomen exams are unremarkable. Positive Battle's sign behind left ear.

BOX 21.4 **Continued**

Patient Scenario #5

- Chief complaint: Lower abdominal pain
- History: Tallulah is an 18-year-old. For the past 12 hours (mostly overnight) she has been having worsening abdominal pain in the lower area diffusely. No history of trauma. She has had nausea and when the pain gets really bad she'll vomit. She has vomited three times. Some diarrhea. Periods always erratic. LMP: ~ 3 weeks ago; 1 day duration and heavier flow than unusual. PMH: Cholecystitis at 15 years of age. Recurrence when she was 17 years of age. G:0. P:0; Ab:0. Allergies: Tylenol, codeine. Meds: OCs, ibuprofen. Weight: 213.8 lbs. Height: 5-foot-11.
- Vital signs: T: 38.8°C; P: 117; R: 24; B/P: 102/86; SaO2: 96%; Pain: 7/10; LOC: Awake & alert.
- Physical exam: Diaphoretic, pale, sweaty patient who is in severe pain when they palpate her abdomen. Guarding, rebound. Pelvic exam: +++ cervical motion tenderness & ++ foul discharge.

Patient Scenario #6

- Chief complaint: Painful hemorrhoids.
- History: 55-year-old female, Esmeralda F. History of hemorrhoids. After a period of constipation, one of the hemorrhoids became swollen and tender.
- Vital signs: T: 36.4°C; P: 117; R: 16; B/P: 112/76; SaO2: 98%; Pain: 9/10; LOC: Awake & alert.
- Physical exam: Thrombosed hemorrhoid. Incision and drainage pending.
- Complicating factor: Mother (86 years old) ambulating with a cane has accompanied the patient.

Patient Scenario #7

- Chief complaint: Sudden back pain x 2 hours
- History: Howie P., a 75-year-old male; Full code. Patient has been having some increasing mid-back pain for the past couple of days. Then tonight, all of a sudden, he developed intense abdominal pain in association with the back pain.
- Vital signs: T: 37.4°C; P: 127 (AF); R: 26; B/P: 86/46; SaO2: 91%; Pain: 10/10; LOC: Awake & alert; GCS 14. Extremely diaphoretic.
- Physical exam: Periumbilical pulsatile mass.
- Imaging: US reveals an abdominal aortic aneurysm (AAA).

Continued

BOX 21.4 **Continued**

- Stat orders: 2 IVs, relevant labs, vascular surgery consultation and blood bank notification.
- Complication: 84-year-old ambulatory spouse is with the patient.

Active assailant drill begins
Observers are positioned to review and document player actions in all the rooms.
Players are escorted to patient care rooms to begin assessing and managing their patients. Time limit: Arbitrary.
General announcement: Bang-Bang-Bang (automatic gunfire heard over the public address system. "Active shooter, active shooter." Depending on the objectives, the PA announcer could state that the assailant is located on a separate floor in order to encourage players to escape from the ED. On the other hand, the announcement could indicate that the shooter is near the ED, which might encourage players to barricade the patient care room.

Official observers document the following:

- Initial reactions: Turn off lights, silence phones, etc.
- Players elect to either escape (by themselves or with their patients) or barricade in place (choose their barricade resources, arm themselves, and select their improvised weapons).

End of exercise is based on observers and lead facilitator.
Debriefing
Players with their official observers present their "patients" and discuss their actions.
Multidisciplinary faculty enhance discussion.
The ethics of Run/Hide/Fight versus Secure/Preserve/Fight strategies are presented and discussed.
Player evaluations
Faculty debriefing

displaying crisis leadership, critical decision-making, and competent interagency communications under high-stress conditions.

Developing an FSE will require time, expertise, and expense. It is no wonder that this ultimate educational experience may only occur annually, at best, if you're lucky. That is why there should be greater emphasis on tabletop exercises, gaming, and drills. They are a step higher than PowerPoint

BOX 21.5 **Hydrofluoric acid (HFA) scenario**

Targeted objectives
The learner will (Figure 21.4):
Discuss initial decontamination procedures at the scene and in the ED.
Demonstrate initial medical management measures.
Identify EKG abnormalities associated with HFA.
Order the necessary labs that are specific to HFA management.
Order the appropriate antidotal therapy.
Discuss the diverse methods of delivering the antidotes.
Contact the appropriate consultants.
Patient scenario stages

• Patient Scenario Stage 1

EMS calls into the ED: A male patient, Hondo K., is accidentally exposed to HFA. He is complaining of chest pain and shoulder pain on the right side where there is evidence of severe burns. Prior to the EMS transport, he was decontaminated at the glass plant's shower area for 10 minutes. He was then placed in the ambulance and is now being transported to your facility.

Hondo has been deposited in the decontamination room of the ER. He has undergone further washdown by the decontamination team. He is in severe pain. Treatment team awaits him in the "cold zone" of the ER (Room 10).

Vital signs in the decontamination zone: Temp: NA, HR: 122, BP: 164/87, ECG (rhythm): ST, RR: 28, SpO2: 95%, Breath Sounds: Full, Bowel Sounds: NA, Skin: diaphoretic, LOC: GCS 15, Pain: 10/10, Weight: ~85 kg, Height: 55 inches.

• Patient Scenario Stage 2

Upon arrival in Room 10, Hondo is screaming in pain despite adequate decontamination. Healthcare team in attendance. Hondo yells that his arm and right side of his chest are burning still and he cannot get comfortable. Pain remains at 10/10. His breathing is labored. PMH: History of untreated hypertension. He has no allergies. Surgical history: Appendectomy 20 years ago. He smokes 2 packs per day, drinks 2 or 3 beers on weekends, and does not use illicit drugs.

Repeat vital signs in the ED: Temp 98.3, HR: 118, BP: 160/98, ECG (rhythm): ST, RR: 24, SpO2: 96, Breath Sounds: Full, Bowel Sounds: NA, Skin: Diaphoretic, LOC: GCS 15, Pain: 10/10.

Continued

Physical examination: ABCs: Intact, Neuro exam: Normal (GCS 15), HEENT: Normal, Lungs: Clear; CVS: Tachycardia, no murmurs; Abdomen: Soft, non-tender, non-distended, bowel sounds present, Skin: Large reddish discoloration across the right side of his chest and on his arm. The overlying skin is partially burned away. Body surface area exposed is roughly 2.5% of his total BSA.

- Patient Scenario Stage 3

Treatment begins with initial assessment and therapy (e.g., ABCs, primary survey, antidotes, analgesia).
Vital signs: HR: 97, BP: 138/85, ECG (rhythm): NSR, RR: 20, SpO2: 98%, Breath Sounds: Full, Bowel Sounds: NA, Skin: Warm, LOC: GCS 15, Pain: 7/10.
Labs: CBC: normal, BMP: normal except K+ of 6.5, Calcium 7.3, Magnesium 1.4, EKG shows peaked T waves

- Patient Scenario Stage 4

More aggressive therapy is indicated.
Vital signs: HR: 97, BP: 138/85, ECG (rhythm): NSR, RR: 18, SpO2: 96%, Breath Sounds: Full, Bowel Sounds: NA, Skin: Warm, LOC: GCS 15; Pain: 7/10 down to 5/10 with appropriate therapy.

- Patient Scenario Stage 5

Vital signs: HR: 89, BP: 135/83, HR: Normal sinus rhythm, BP: Borderline hypertension, ECG (rhythm): NSR, RR: 20, SpO2: High 90s, Breath Sounds: Full, Bowel Sounds: NA, Skin: Warm, LOC: GCS 15, Pain: 5/10. Ca: 8.9, Mg: 1.9.

- Patient Scenario Stage 6

Admission to ICU
HR: 89, BP: 135/83, ECG (rhythm): NSR, RR: Low tachypnea, SpO2: 98%, Breath Sounds: Full, Bowel Sounds: NA, Skin: Warm, LOC: GCS 15, Pain: 1/10.

lectures and can effectively direct students to the correct way to function in an FSE.

Unless you have an enlightened hospital administration that will spend the time and the money to develop more frequent FSEs, concentrate on mini-drills. Do not worry about teaching the complete disaster. Drill the

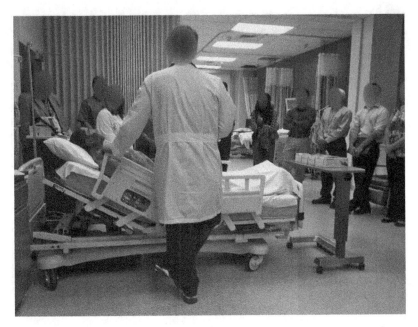

FIGURE 21.4 An HFA scenario class. These students are earning a degree in occupational health and safety.

BOX 21.6   **Primary blast injury: tension pneumothoraces and pericardial tamponade**

Learning objectives
1. Primary survey
2. Communication with patient, family, team
3. Emergency management of ABCs
4. Secondary survey
5. Disposition
6. Discuss all types of blast injuries

History
19-year-old female brought in by father after a grain silo explosion. Has soot, puncture wounds (PWs), and massive bruising and pain across chest. Bruised face. Whispers: "Can't . . . breathe." Parent provides history: Healthy, LMP 2 weeks ago, smokes 1 ppd, drinks EtOH occasionally, uses THC occasionally, employed at Subway, and lives with Mom and Dad. PMH: Broken leg 5 years ago. Allergies: None. Meds: OCs.

Continued

Treatment stages

- Stage 1: ED arrival of patient

Face sooty; shrapnel arms, legs, and face.
Blood from both ears.
Vital signs: HR: 150; BP: 60/30; RR: 36; SaO2: 71% (21% FiO2); LOC: GCS 10; Airway: Patent; Breathing: Shallow, grunting; Skin: Diaphoretic.
Assess team actions: Primary survey, communications, patient management.

- Stage 2: After needle decompression and evacuation of pericardial tamponade

"I'm breathing better."
Assessment: HR: 110; BP: 90/62; RR: 28; LOC: GCS 14; SaO2: 91% (100%); Airway: Patent; Breathing: 22; Skin: Less diaphoretic
Assess additional team actions: labs, imaging, etc.

- Stage 3

HR: 110; BP: 100/62; RR: 28; LOC: GCS 14; SaO2: 94% (100%); Airway: Patent; Breathing: 22; Skin: Less diaphoretic.
Lab, imaging results (e.g., +HCG).
Assess additional interventions and actions: antibiotics, tetanus prophylaxis, trauma center transfer.

BOX 21.7 **Quaternary blast injury: crush syndrome**

Background
Mikhail O. is a 19-year-old sophomore from Wisconsin. He was in his university classroom when a massive explosion in the chemistry department rocked the building (Figure 21.5). The building was partially destroyed. A major piece of artistic masonry fell and pinned his right thigh, trapping him in place for 6 hours. Rescuers were attending to others first. They found him and brought him to the ED. He is placed in a cervical collar and on a backboard.
PMH: Broken leg 5 years ago; no surgery. FH: Parents and sibling alive and well. Allergies: Sulfa. Meds: Vitamins.
Treatment stages
Stage 1: Mikhail is transported to the ED as a "load and go."

BOX 21.7 **Continued**

T: 98.4°F; P: 127; BP: 118/54; RR: 16; SpO2: 95. ST segments are unremarkable, but T waves are peaked. Breath Sounds: Clear. Bowel Sounds: Quiet. Skin: Severely bruised right thigh; LOC: 15; Pain: 9/10. Weight: 86 kg. Height: 71 inches.

Stage 2: Significance of peaked T waves not recognized immediately.

HR: 116; BP: 102/60; ECG (rhythm): ST; RR: 26; SpO2: 98; Breath Sounds: Clear. Bowel Sounds: Quiet. Skin: Clammy. LOC: Same. Pain: Same. Cardiac monitor: QRS complexes widen.

Stage 3: QRS complexes widen into sine waves.

P: 86; BP: 82/60; RR: 26; SpO2: 98. Breath Sounds: Clear. Bowel Sounds: Quiet. Skin: Diaphoretic. LOC: Decreased. ECG (rhythm): Sine waves.

Stage 4: Flat line on cardiac monitor: Peaked T waves not recognized on EKG.

P: 0; BP: 0; RR: 0; SpO2: 0; GCS: 3. Breath Sounds: None. ECG: Asystole. Successful resuscitation: Hyperkalemia recognized and treated.

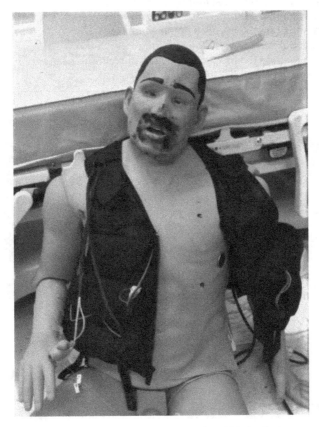

FIGURE 21.5 During blast injury exercises, we have introduced "victims" who are wearing suspicious attire. In this case, the victim is injured—or is he? No, he is one of the perpetrators. He is wearing a vest loaded with explosives and has a detonator in his hand. If the players do not address the situation or choose to ignore what is directly in front of them, there will be sound effects mimicking an actual explosion, and they are all casualties. If they do address the vest, the wires, and the detonator, then we evaluate the players' response to the discovery. Then comes the debriefing.

BOX 21.8 Hand-held radio education

The learner will:

- Activate the radio.
- Demonstrate proper radio etiquette.
- Explain the purpose of channels.
- Change the battery.
- Communicate via radios with partner.

BOX 21.9 Tourniquet education

The learner will:

- Apply the commercial tourniquet (CAT) properly.
- Demonstrate the proper locations at which to apply the CAT.
- Demonstrate the purpose of the windlass.
- List types of improvisational tourniquets.
- Demonstrate the proper application of an improvisational tourniquet (Figures 21.6 and 21.7).

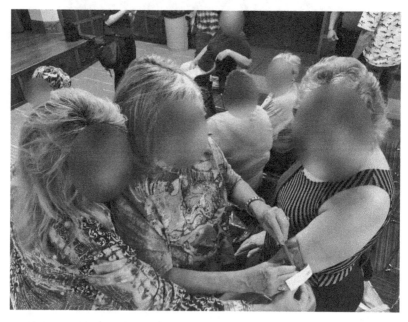

FIGURE 21.6 A tourniquet class for the general public.

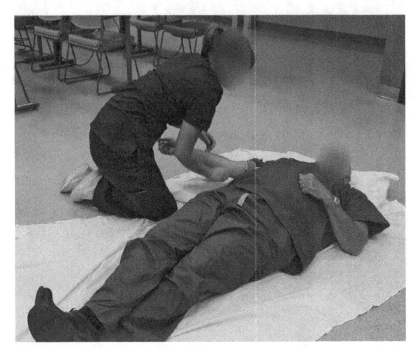

FIGURE 21.7 Tourniquet application drill. The scenario deals with an arterial hemorrhage in the upper arm, and the nursing student was timed in applying a commercial tourniquet properly.

BOX 21.10 **Emergency patient evacuation**

The learner will:

- Identify which patient impedimenta (catheters, tubing, etc.) must be secured with the "patient" for transport and which can be discontinued safely.
- Logroll, cocoon, and secure the "patient" using two bedsheets.
- Slide the "patient" off the bed using the patient's mattress.
- Slide the "patient" down the hall.
- Place mattresses down the stairs.
- Demonstrate how to use the Ambu safely while sliding an intubated "patient" down the stairs on the mattresses (Figures 21.8 and 21.9).
- Debrief.

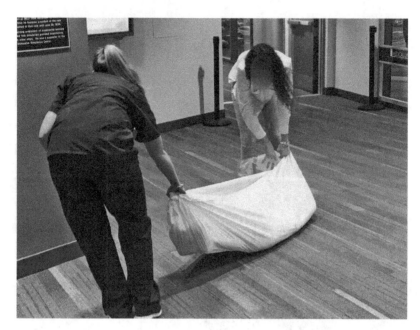

FIGURE 21.8 This non-ambulatory ICU patient has been placed in a double-sheeted cocoon and is being transported to the top of the stairs and will be slid down several flights on mattresses that are covering the steps.

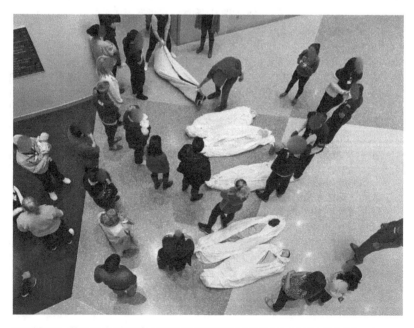

FIGURE 21.9 The termination of an emergency hospital evacuation exercise. The victims have been safely delivered outside of the hospital and are now being triaged for transportation to another hospital.

BOX 21.11 **Active shooter barricade options**

While being timed, the learner will:

- Enter a patient care room and prioritize silencing personal phones and turning off lights.
- Identify which items in the patient care room would serve as good barricade options against the entry of the active assailant.
- Place the most appropriate equipment/furniture against the entrance to the room to prevent entry.
- Debrief.

BOX 21.12 **Active shooter improvisational weapons**

While being timed, the learner will enter a patient care room and identify the types of equipment and other resources in that room or on their person that can be used as offensive and defensive weapons should an assailant invade that room. Debrief.

BOX 21.13 **START/SALT triage drill**

Learning objectives

The learner will:

- Triage Drill: An Explosive Event is an example of an exercise to teach and/or semonstrate proficiency in using START and/or SALT triage techniques.
- Explain the significance of RED, YELLOW, GREEN, (GRAY), and BLACK tags.

Triage Drill: An Explosive Event

Victims

Victim #1

- 43 y/o male, being carried in by family. Pumping right brachial artery. Shrapnel wounds on face, arms, legs.
- Respirations: 28. Radial pulse: Absent. Mentation: Only to intense verbal stimuli.
- Interventions?
- Triage Color: RED, YELLOW, GREEN, (GRAY) and BLACK?

Continued

BOX 21.13   **Continued**

Victim #2

- 63 y/o male, unresponsive. Burns on face/hands (2° & 3°): 25% TBSA; shrapnel wounds to face.
- Respirations: 24, noisy, partially obstructed by debris. Radial pulse: Present. Mentation: Unresponsive to pain.
- Interventions?
- Triage Color: RED, YELLOW, GREEN, (GRAY) and BLACK?

Victim #3

- 42-year-old female. No physical complaints; simply scared and crying. No bleeding, normal pulses, fast breathing.
- Respirations: 30. Pulse: Present. Mentation: Alert.
- Interventions?
- Triage Color: RED, YELLOW, GREEN, (GRAY) and BLACK?

Victim #4

- 26-year-old male. Contusions on head, bleeding from left ear; raccoon eyes; Battle's sign; one arm blown off (minimal active bleeding).
- Respirations: 8. Pulse: Present. Mentation: Unresponsive
- Interventions?
- Triage Color: RED, YELLOW, GREEN, (GRAY) and BLACK?

Victim #5

- 52-year-old female. Bleeding heavily: gaping abdominal wound; soaking clothes.
- Respirations: 10. Pulse: Absent. Mentation: Responsive to verbal stimuli.
- Interventions?
- Triage Color: RED, YELLOW, GREEN, (GRAY) and BLACK?

Victim #6

- 20-year-old male running around. Torn clothes. Yelling, "Help, help, help." Interfering with rescue operations. No obvious injuries.
- Prevents getting his vitals.
- Interventions?
- Triage Color: RED, YELLOW, GREEN, (GRAY) and BLACK?

Victim #7

- 18-year-old boy clutching left chest. Complains of severe pain and dyspnea: screaming and crying. Bruise along lower left chest and LUQ noted; crepitus noted over L chest wall; flail chest (L). Asymmetrical chest rise.

BOX 21.13 **Continued**

- Respirations: 28. Pulse: Present. Mentation: Alert
- Interventions?
- Triage Color: RED, YELLOW, GREEN, (GRAY) and BLACK?

Victim #8

- 27-year-old female, 8 months pregnant. Obvious open fracture at R ankle. Facial/hand: shrapnel injuries.
- Respirations: 26. Pulse: Present in wrists (Absent in R foot). Mentation: Alert.
- Interventions?
- Triage Color: RED, YELLOW, GREEN, (GRAY) and BLACK?

Victim #9

- 60-year-old male, brittle diabetic. Assorted shrapnel injuries to face, arms, and legs. Limps; no torso complaints. Just took his insulin 1 hour ago. Has not eaten since.
- Respirations: 24. Pulse: Present. Mentation: Alert.
- Interventions?
- Triage Color: RED, YELLOW, GREEN, (GRAY) and BLACK?

Victim #10

- 50-year-old male with tree branch embedded in right chest wall. "I can't breathe." Distant lung sounds on right; crepitus noted.
- Respirations: 38. Pulse: Present. Mentation: Alert
- Interventions?
- Triage Color: RED, YELLOW, GREEN, (GRAY) and BLACK?

Victim #11

- 30-year-old female whimpering. C/O LUQ pain; bruising and shrapnel wounds noted in LUQ.
- Respirations: 24. Pulse: Absent. Mentation: Alert
- Interventions?
- Triage Color: RED, YELLOW, GREEN, (GRAY) and BLACK?

Victim #12

- 23-year-old female. Partial amputated left hand. Father is carrying her mangled fingers separately.
- Respirations: 32. Pulse: Present. Mentation: Alert.
- Interventions?
- Triage Color: RED, YELLOW, GREEN, (GRAY) and BLACK?

Continued

BOX 21.13 **Continued**

Victim #13

- 33-year-old male. 95% amputation at R elbow; limb dangling and active bleeding.
- Respirations: 28. Pulse: Present (left radial artery), Absent (right radial artery). Mentation: Alert.
- Interventions?
- Triage Color: RED, YELLOW, GREEN, (GRAY) and BLACK?

Victim #14

- 43-year-old male. His partner just died in his arms. No injuries; heavy chest pain into shoulders; weeping. Sweaty; clutching chest. Pale appearance. PMH: 3 MIs in past.
- Respirations: 24. Pulse: Present. Mentation: Alert.
- Interventions?
- Triage Color: RED, YELLOW, GREEN, (GRAY) and BLACK?

Victim #15

- 73-year-old female. No injuries; difficulty breathing due to smoke. Sweaty; pale. PMH: Asthma; lost her asthma inhaler.
- Respirations: 34 wheezing. Pulse: Present. Mentation: Verbal.
- Interventions?
- Triage Color: RED, YELLOW, GREEN, (GRAY) and BLACK?

Victim #16

- 33-year-old female. Right eye (OD) totally avulsed; hanging by optic nerve; cannot see. 5-cm laceration and deformity along paralyzed right side of face.
- Respirations: 14. Pulse: Present. Mentation: Alert; Pain level: 9/10.
- Interventions?
- Triage Color: RED, YELLOW, GREEN, (GRAY) and BLACK?

Victim #17

- 3-year-old girl. Holding right side of abdomen (15-cm laceration). Bowel protrusion.
- Respirations: 34. Pulse: Absent. Mentation: Verbal, whimpering.
- Interventions?
- Triage Color: RED, YELLOW, GREEN, (GRAY) and BLACK?

BOX 21.13 **Continued**

Victim #18

- 53-year-old male. Trapped in vehicle on fire from burning, fiery debris. Major burns, soot, charred skin to face and hands; 12% TBSA.

BOX 21.13 **Continued**

- Respirations: 44; stridor. Pulse: Present. Mentation: Verbal.
- Interventions?
- Triage Color: RED, YELLOW, GREEN, (GRAY) and BLACK?

Victim #19

- 19-year-old disabled male (wheelchair-bound). Was trampled by fleeing crowd; left side of chest crushed; flail. "Can't breathe!"
- Respirations: 8. Pulse: Present. Mentation: Verbal.
- Interventions?
- Triage Color: RED, YELLOW, GREEN, (GRAY) and BLACK?

Victim #20

- 29-year-old female. Hobbling on makeshift crutch. Left proximal fibula protruding through pants. No other obvious injuries.
- Respirations: 24. Pulse: Present (left leg also). Mentation: Alert.
- Interventions?
- Triage Color: RED, YELLOW, GREEN, (GRAY) and BLACK?

Victim #21

- 43-year-old female. Dislocated R elbow; 3–5-cm lacerations: chin, left arm, lower lip.
- Respirations: 22. Pulse: Present (left wrist); Absent (right wrist). Mentation: Alert.
- Interventions?
- Triage Color: RED, YELLOW, GREEN, (GRAY) and BLACK?

Victim #22

- 83-year-old female. Wheezing due to smoke inhalation. Minor facial lacerations. Sweaty; pale. PMH: COPD.
- Respirations: 38 (barely audible wheeze; mild stridor). Pulse: Present. Mentation: Semi-responsive.

Continued

BOX 21.13 **Continued**

- Interventions?
- Triage Color: RED, YELLOW, GREEN, (GRAY) and BLACK?
- *SUDDEN STATUS CHANGE*: Respirations: 0. Pulse: 0. Mentation: Unresponsive.
- Interventions?
- Triage Color: RED, YELLOW, GREEN, (GRAY) and BLACK?

Victim #23

- 3-year-old male. Down's syndrome; 3-cm laceration on left leg below knee down to tendons. Sweaty; pale; whimpering. PMH: Deaf after infantile meningitis (from 18-year-old consoling brother).
- Respirations: 34; audible wheeze. Pulse: Present. Mentation: Verbal.
- Interventions?
- Triage Color: RED, YELLOW, GREEN, (GRAY) and BLACK?

Victim #24

- 6-year-old girl consoled by bystander. Dislocated hip after blown out of window; crying in pain.
- Respirations: 26. Pulse: Present x 4. Mentation: Verbal.
- Interventions?
- Triage Color: RED, YELLOW, GREEN, (GRAY) and BLACK?

Victim #25

- 12-year-old male. 10-cm laceration of abdominal wall; metal protruding from it.
- Respirations: 16. Pulse: Absent. Mentation: Verbal.
- Interventions?
- Triage Color: RED, YELLOW, GREEN, (GRAY) and BLACK?

Victim #26

- 30-year-old ambulatory male. Left shoulder pain. Dislocated left shoulder. Pain level: 8/10.
- Respirations: 24. Pulse: Present. Mentation: Alert.
- Interventions?
- Triage Color: RED, YELLOW, GREEN, (GRAY) and BLACK?

Victim #27

- 15-year-old male with 3 fingers of left hand amputated; father has two of the fingers.
- Respirations: 26. Pulse: Present. Mentation: Alert.

BOX 21.13 **Continued**

- Interventions?
- Triage Color: RED, YELLOW, GREEN, (GRAY) and BLACK?

Victim #28

- 62-year-old male on warfarin (chronic atrial fibrillation). Dirt in both eyes (painful); broken nose with major bleeding.
- Respirations: 26. Pulse: Present. Mentation: Alert.
- Interventions?
- Triage Color: RED, YELLOW, GREEN, (GRAY) and BLACK?

Victim #29

- 23-year-old male. Blind since birth; uninjured assistance dog on lap. No injuries; wheezing; minor lacerations on face and arms.
- Respirations: 34. Pulse: Present. Mentation: Alert.
- Interventions?
- Triage Color: RED, YELLOW, GREEN, (GRAY) and BLACK?

Victim #30

- 33-year-old male. Chest/abdominal discomfort after crushed by other victims.
- Respirations: 28. Pulse: Present. Mentation: Alert.
- Interventions?
- Triage Color: RED, YELLOW, GREEN, (GRAY) and BLACK?

Victim #31

- 11-year-old female. Obvious head, chest, and abdominal injuries. Carried by an uninjured parent.
- Respirations: 0. Pulse: 0. Mentation: Unresponsive.
- Interventions?
- Triage Color: RED, YELLOW, GREEN, (GRAY) and BLACK?

BOX 21.14 **PPE drill**

The learner will:

- Don an N-95 respirator.
- Don a PAPR (powered air-purifying respirator).
- Don and doff all PPE established for contagious infectious diseases.
- Success or failure based on the presence of fluorescent powder visible with a black light after doffing PPE.
- Debrief.

little concepts more diligently and more frequently. Boxes 21.8, 21.9, 21.10, 21.11, 21.12, 21.13, and 21.14 offer examples of mini-drills.

Further reading

American College of Emergency Physicians. Hospital Disaster Preparedness Self-Assessment Tool. http://cdphready.org/hospital-disaster-preparedness-self-assessment-tool/

Centers for Disease Control and Prevention. Explosions and Blast Injuries. https://www.cdc.gov/masstrauma/preparedness/primer.pdf

Federal Emergency Management Administration. IS-120.C: An Introduction to Exercises. https://training.fema.gov/is/courseoverview.aspx?code=IS-120.c

Lee C, Walters E, Borger R, Clem K, Fenati G, Kiemeney M, Seng S, Yuen HW, Neeki M, Smith D. The San Bernardino, California, terror attack: Two emergency departments' response. *West J Emerg Med.* 2016;17(1):1–7.

Pennardt A. Blast Injuries. https://emedicine.medscape.com/article/822587-overview

Rega P. Utilizing medical gaming principles to teach emergency management strategies and crisis leadership during a botulism mass casualty incident. *EC Nursing and Healthcare.* 2020;2(1):39–45.

The Joint Commission. Emergency Management. https://www.jointcommission.org/resources/patient-safety-topics/emergency-management/

Appendix A

Select hazardous materials: intentional and accidental

VESICANTS

VESICANTS - MUSTARD AGENTS (H, HD)

ONSET OF SYMPTOMS: DELAYED (2–24H)

Management Overview
Don PPE
Remove from source
Decon immediately despite
lack of symptoms

NASOPHARYNGEAL
Rhinorrhea, irritation,
epistaxis, ulcers, edema,
necrosis

RESPIRATORY
(usually occur after
cutaneous symptoms)
Laryngospasm,
hoarseness, cough,
dyspnea
Pneumonia
Pulmonary edema (rate)

Usually
occur with
prolonged
exposure

CARDIOVASCULAR
(Severe exposure)
Arrhythmias, shock

HEMATOPIETIC
Bone marrow suppression
(severe exposure: poor
prognosis)

OCCULAR (most sensitive)
Conjunctival irritation, lacrimation,
Miosis
Blepharospasm ⎫
Corneal damage ⎬ Severe
Temporary blindness ⎭ Exposure

CUTANEOUS (Latent period
shortened with heat/humidity)
Erythema, Intense pruritus, Pain
(within 4–8h)
Vesicles (within 2–18h)
Bullae
Central
necrosis
GI
Nausea, vomiting, diarrhea
(severre exposure)

™

Malaise, Prostration, Fever (Severe Exposure)

Topical Contact
Systemic Absorption
Major Affected Areas

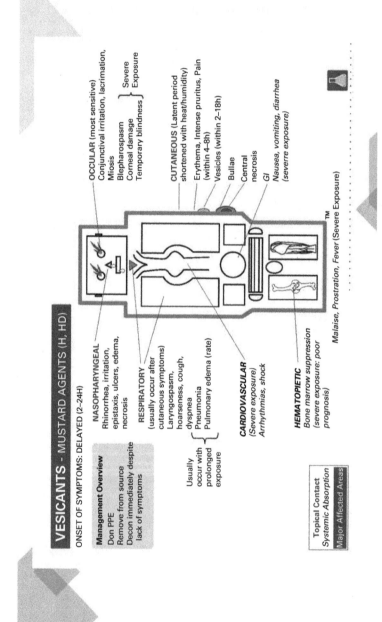

FIGURE A.1 Mustard agents. First and foremost is appreciating that the clinical effects of mustard agents are delayed even though the cellular damage can be immediate. Secondarily, these agents are persistent when released and are heavier than air. This means that children and those of short stature may be the most vulnerable. There is no antidote. Prolonged exposure will cause systemic effects that can be lethal.

VESICANTS - LEWISITE (L)

ONSET OF SYMPTOMS: IMMEDIATE

Management Overview
Don PPE
Remove from source
Decon immediately
Consider BAL

RESPIRATORY
Cough, dyspnea,
laryngospasm
Pseudomembrane formation
Local airway obstruction
Severe Exposure { Pneumonia (3-5d later)
Pulmonary edema

VASCULAR
(Prolonged exposure)
Capillary leak
Third spacing
Hypotension ("Lewisite Shock")

MULTI-ORGAN DAMAGE
(Severe exposure)
Encephalopathy
Hepatic necrosis
Renal necrosis
GI effects

OCULAR
Conjunctival irritation/pain,
blepharospasm, lacrimation,
photophobia, {corneal damage/
blindness (severe exposure)}

NASOPHARYNGEAL
Pain, irritation, sneezing,
rhinorrhea, epistaxis

GI: Vomiting

CUTANEOUS (immediate pain)
Rash
Vesicles
Bullae
(Maximum size usually occurs by 4th day)
Necrosis (Severe exposure)

HEMATOLOGICAL
(Severe exposure)
Hemolytic anemia

Topical Contact
Systemic Absorption
Major Affected Areas

TM

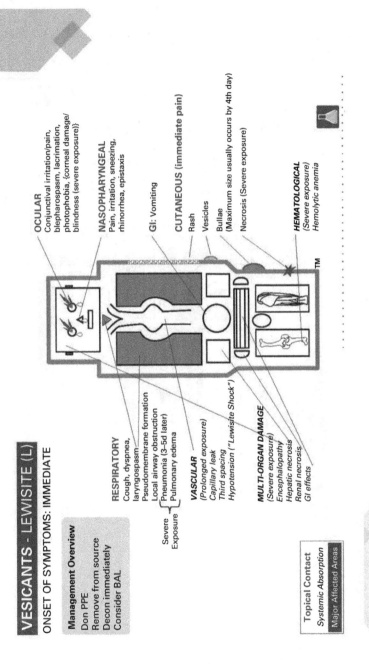

FIGURE A.2 Lewisite. This chemical warfare agent was developed by Allied researchers during World War I in response to the chemical agents developed by Germany. British Anti-Lewisite (BAL) was developed as an antidote. In contrast to the mustard agents, the clinical effects of a Lewisite exposure are immediate.

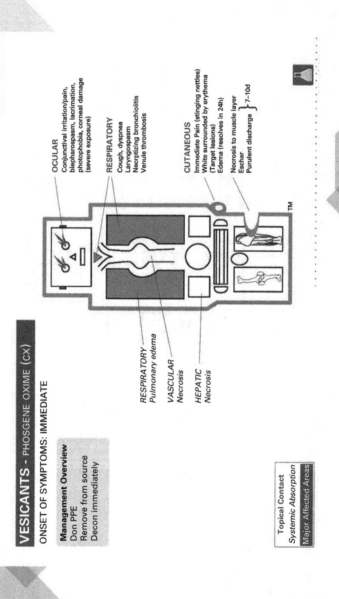

VESICANTS - PHOSGENE OXIME (CX)

ONSET OF SYMPTOMS: IMMEDIATE

Management Overview
Don PPE
Remove from source
Decon immediately

OCULAR
Conjunctival irritation/pain, blepharospasm, lacrimation, photophobia, corneal damage (severe exposure)

RESPIRATORY
Cough, dyspnea
Laryngospasm
Necrptizing bronchiolitis
Venule thrombosis

CUTANEOUS
Immediate Pain (stinging nettles)
White surrounded by erythema (Target lesions)
Edema (resolves in 24h)
Necrosis to muscle layer
Eschar
Purulent discharge } 7–10d

RESPIRATORY
Pulmonary edema

VASCULAR
Necrosis

HEPATIC
Necrosis

TM

Topical Contact
Systemic Absorption
Major Affected Areas

FIGURE A.3 Phosgene oxime. This agent does not blister like a true vesicant, but it does destroy tissue immediately. Like mustard agents and Lewisite, it is heavier than air, making children and people of short stature more vulnerable.

NERVE AGENTS

NERVE AGENTS

LOW VAPOR EXPOSURE

Management Overview
Don PPE
Remove from source
Decon immediately
Atropine
2-PAMCl
Diazepam

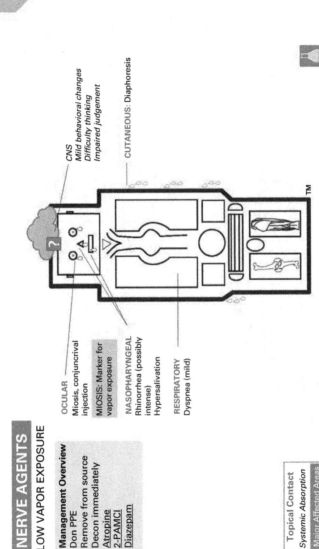

OCULAR
Miosis, conjunctival injection

MIOSIS: Marker for vapor exposure

NASOPHARYNGEAL
Rhinorrhea (possibly intense)
Hypersalivation

RESPIRATORY
Dyspnea (mild)

CNS
Mild behavioral changes
Difficulty thinking
Impaired judgement

CUTANEOUS: Diaphoresis

Topical Contact
Systemic Absorption
Major Affected Areas

FIGURE A.4 The effects of a low vapor exposure to a nerve agent. Nerve agents inhibit cholinesterase enzyme activity at synaptic sites and create an abnormal accumulation of acetylcholine at the nicotinic and muscarinic receptors. A mnemonic for the manifestations associated with nerve agents is SLUDGEBAM: salivation, lacrimation, urination, defecation, gastric secretions, emesis, bronchorrhea, abdominal distress, and miosis.

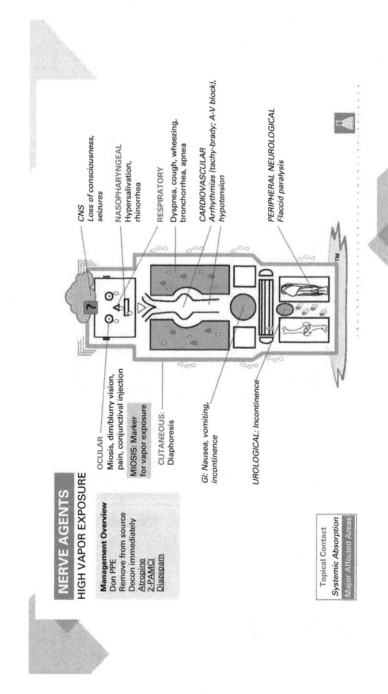

NERVE AGENTS
HIGH VAPOR EXPOSURE

Management Overview
Don PPE
Remove from source
Decon immediately
Atropine
2-PAMCl
Diazepam

OCULAR
Miosis, dim/blurry vision,
pain, conjunctival injection

MIOSIS: Marker
for vapor exposure

CUTANEOUS:
Diaphoresis

GI: Nausea, vomiting,
incontinence

UROLOGICAL: Incontinence

CNS
*Loss of consciousness,
seizures*

NASOPHARYNGEAL
Hypersalivation,
rhinorrhea

RESPIRATORY
Dyspnea, cough, wheezing,
bronchorrhea, apnea

*CARDIOVASCULAR
Arrhythmias (tachy-brady; A-V block),
hypotension*

*PERIPHERAL NEUROLOGICAL
Flaccid paralysis*

Topical Contact
Systemic Absorption
Major Affected Areas

FIGURE A.5 The effects of a high vapor exposure to a nerve agent. There are multiple versions of nerve agents: VX, GA (Tabun), GB (Sarin), GD (Soman), and GF: VX has the highest incapacitation and mortality potential. All the common varieties of nerve agents are heavier than air, making them most perilous to children and those of short stature.

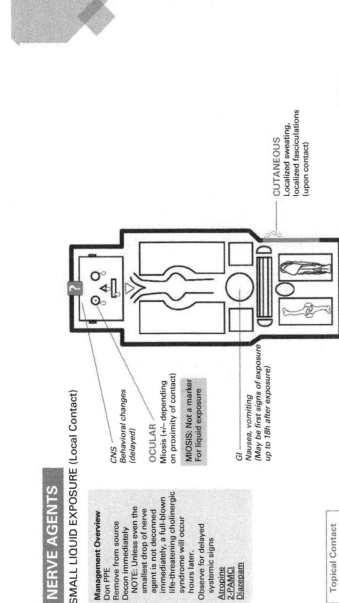

NERVE AGENTS

SMALL LIQUID EXPOSURE (Local Contact)

Management Overview
Don PPE
Remove from source
Decon immediately
NOTE: Unless even the smallest drop of nerve agent is not deconned immediately, a full-blown life-threatening cholinergic syndrome will occur hours later.
Observe for delayed systemic signs
Atropine
2-PAMCl
Diazepam

CNS
Behavioral changes
(delayed)

OCULAR
Miosis (+/– depending on proximity of contact)

MIOSIS: Not a marker
For liquid exposure

GI
Nausea, vomiting
(May be first signs of exposure
up to 18h after exposure)

CUTANEOUS
Localized sweating,
localized fasciculations
(upon contact)

Topical Contact
Systemic Absorption
Major Affected Areas

FIGURE A.6 The effects of a small liquid exposure to a nerve agent. A droplet, the size of a pinhead, can be lethal if it is not removed by blotting and then by washing. The initial manifestations will be noted only at the site of contact, but in time, as the nerve agent is absorbed, the systemic signs and symptoms will develop.

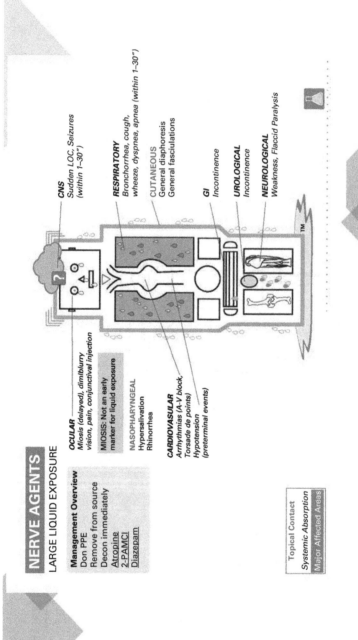

NERVE AGENTS

LARGE LIQUID EXPOSURE

Management Overview
Don PPE
Remove from source
Decon immediately
Atropine
2-PAMCl
Diazepam

OCULAR
*Miosis (delayed), dim/blurry
vision, pain, conjunctival injection*

MIOSIS: Not an early
marker for liquid exposure

NASOPHARYNGEAL
Hypersalivation
Rhinorrhea

CARDIOVASULAR
*Arrhythmias (A-V block,
Torsade de points)
Hypotension
(preterminal events)*

CNS
*Sudden LOC, Seizures
(within 1–30")*

RESPIRATORY
*Bronchorrhea, cough,
wheeze, dyspnea, apnea (within 1–30")*

CUTANEOUS
General diaphoresis
General fasciulations

GI
Incontinence

UROLOGICAL
Incontinence

NEUROLOGICAL
Weakness, Flaccid Paralysis

Topical Contact
Systemic Absorption
Major Affected Areas

FIGURE A.7 The effects of a significant liquid exposure to a nerve agent. There is a bonding that develops between the agent and acetylcholinesterase. The longer it persists or "ages," the greater the likelihood that the bond will be irreversible. The aging half-life for VX is 48 hours, while it is only 2 minutes for GD.

BLOOD AGENTS

BLOOD AGENTS - CYANIDES (AC)

LOW CONCENTRATION

Management Overview
Don PPE
Remove from hazard
Decon as needed

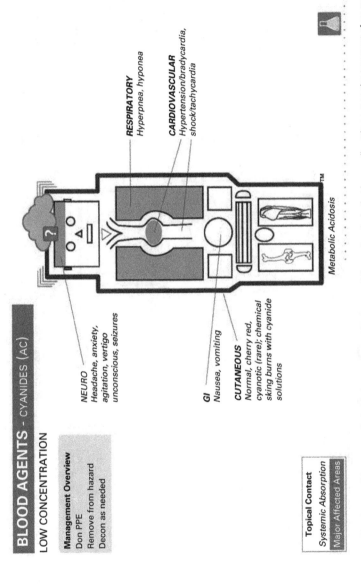

NEURO
Headache, anxiety, agitation, vertigo unconscious, seizures

GI
Nausea, vomiting

CUTANEOUS
Normal, cherry red, cyanotic (rare); chemical sking burns with cyanide solutions

RESPIRATORY
Hyperpnea, hyponea

CARDIOVASCULAR
Hypertension/bradycardia, shock/tachycardia

Metabolic Acidosis

Topical Contact
Systemic Absorption
Major Affected Areas

FIGURE A.8 "Blood agents" is a somewhat archaic term meant to represent those chemicals that have a direct impact on the transport of oxygen to the tissues. As the cyanides attach themselves to the cells' cytochrome oxidase system, a cascade effect will occur starting with an anaerobic metabolism, lactic acidosis, cell hypoxia, and cell death.

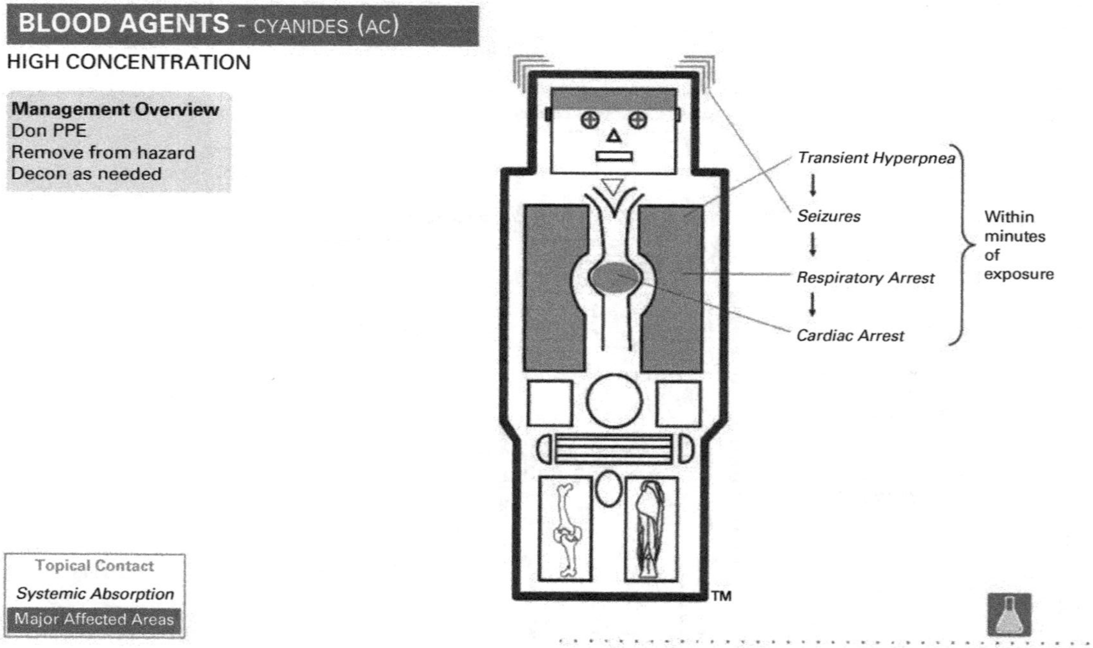

BLOOD AGENTS - CYANIDES (AC)

HIGH CONCENTRATION

Management Overview
Don PPE
Remove from hazard
Decon as needed

Transient Hyperpnea → Seizures → Respiratory Arrest → Cardiac Arrest

Within minutes of exposure

Topical Contact
Systemic Absorption
Major Affected Areas

TM

FIGURE A.9 There are two major types of cyanide: cyanogen chloride (CK) and hydrogen cyanide (AC). In the past, antidotal therapy consisted of amyl nitrite, sodium nitrite, and sodium thiosulfate. Currently, the principal antidote of choice is hydroxocobalamin. Unlike the nitrite antidotes, hydroxocobalamin has virtually no clinical adverse reactions.

BLOOD AGENTS - ARSINE (SA)

LOW CONCENTRATION

Management Overview
Don PPE
Remove from source
Consider Decon
Supportive therapy

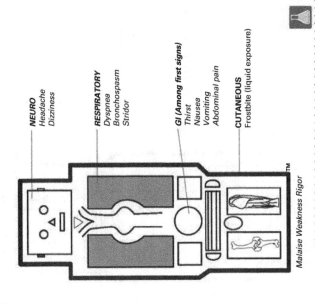

NEURO
Headache
Dizziness

RESPIRATORY
Dyspnea
Bronchospasm
Stridor

GI (Among first signs)
Thirst
Nausea
Vomiting
Abdominal pain

CUTANEOUS
Frostbite (liquid exposure)

Malaise Weakness Rigor

Topical Contact
Systemic Absorption
Major Affected Areas

FIGURE A.10 Arsine binds to hemoglobin, thereby inhibiting oxygen exchange. It also can induce intravascular hemolysis.

BLOOD AGENTS - ARSINE (SA)

MODERATE-HIGH CONCENTRATION

Management Overview
Don PPE
Remove from source
Consider Decon
Supportive therapy

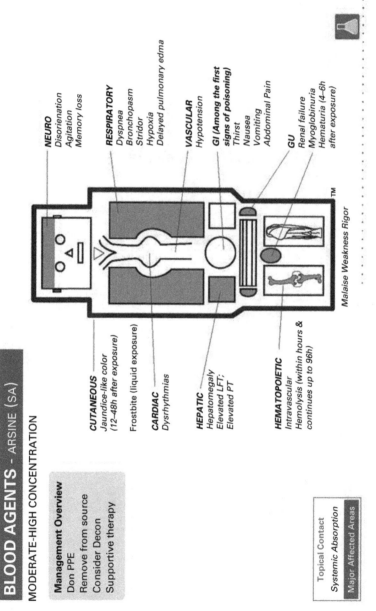

NEURO
Disorienation
Agitation
Memory loss

RESPIRATORY
Dyspnea
Bronchopasm
Stridor
Hypoxia
Delayed pulmonary edma

VASCULAR
Hypotension

GI (Among the first signs of poisoning)
Thirst
Nausea
Vomiting
Abdominal Pain

GU
Renal failure
Myoglobinuria
Hematuria (4-6h after exposure)

CUTANEOUS
Jaundice-like color (12-48h after exposure)
Frostbite (liquid exposure)

CARDIAC
Dysrhythmias

HEPATIC
Hepatomegaly
Elevated LFT;
Elevated PT

HEMATOPOIETIC
Intravascular
Hemolysis (within hours & continues up to 96h)

Malaise Weakness Rigor

Topical Contact
Systemic Absorption
Major Affected Areas

FIGURE A.11 Arsine is extremely flammable. Its manifestations are delayed from 1 up to 24 hours post-exposure. Mortality potential is moderate to high. There is no antidote. Survivors need to be monitored for up to 72 hours to check for hemolysis and renal compromise.

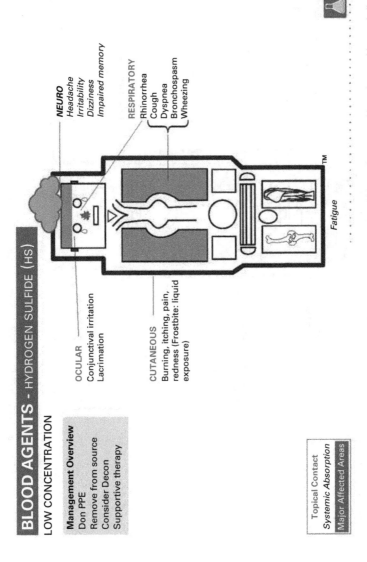

BLOOD AGENTS - HYDROGEN SULFIDE (HS)

LOW CONCENTRATION

Management Overview
Don PPE
Remove from source
Consider Decon
Supportive therapy

NEURO
Headache
Irritability
Dizziness
Impaired memory

RESPIRATORY
Rhinorrhea
Cough
Dyspnea
Bronchospasm
Wheezing

OCULAR
Conjunctival irritation
Lacrimation

CUTANEOUS
Burning, itching, pain, redness (Frostbite: liquid exposure)

Fatigue

TM

Topical Contact
Systemic Absorption
Major Affected Areas

FIGURE A.12 Hydrogen sulfide, besides being a local irritant, binds to iron in the mitochondrial cytochromes and impedes aerobic metabolism. It is a flammable explosive.

BLOOD AGENTS - HYDROGEN SULFIDE (HS)

HIGH CONCENTRATION

Management Overview
Don PPE
Remove from source
Consider Decon
Supportive therapy

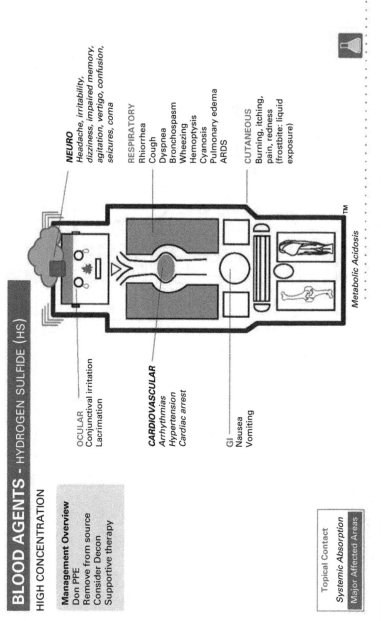

OCULAR
Conjunctival irritation
Lacrimation

CARDIOVASCULAR
Arrhythmias
Hypertension
Cardiac arrest

GI
Nausea
Vomiting

NEURO
Headache, irritability,
dizziness, impaired memory,
agitation, vertigo, confusion,
seizures, coma

RESPIRATORY
Rhiorrhea
Cough
Dyspnea
Bronchospasm
Wheezing
Hemoptysis
Cyanosis
Pulmonary edema
ARDS

CUTANEOUS
Burning, itching,
pain, redness
(frostbite: liquid
exposure)

Metabolic Acidosis

Topical Contact
Systemic Absorption
Major Affected Areas

FIGURE A.13 The potential for incapacitation and death is high once an individual has been exposed to a significant concentration of the chemical. Once in contact with water, H_2S can be converted to sulfuric acid.

PULMONARY (CHOKING) AGENTS

PULMONARY (CHOKING) AGENTS - CHLORINE (CL)

Management Overview
Don PPE
Remove from source
Decon as needed
Supportive therapy
Respiratory management

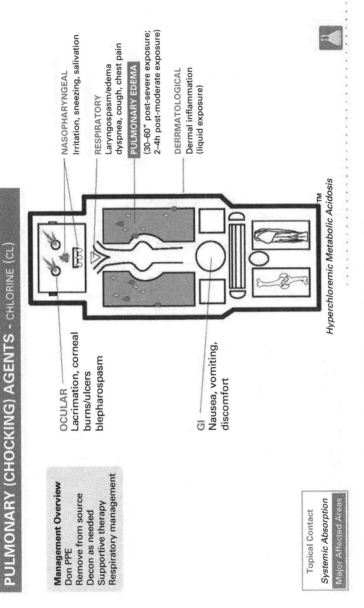

OCULAR
Lacrimation, corneal burns/ulcers blepharospasm

GI
Nausea, vomiting, discomfort

NASOPHARYNGEAL
Irritation, sneezing, salivation

RESPIRATORY
Laryngospasm/edema dyspnea, cough, chest pain

PULMONARY EDEMA
(30–60" post-severe exposure; 2–4h post-moderate exposure)

DERRMATOLOGICAL
Dermal inflammation (liquid exposure)

Hyperchloremic Metabolic Acidosis

Topical Contact
Systemic Absorption
Major Affected Areas

FIGURE A.14 Chlorine, upon contact with water, forms hydrochloric acid and oxygen free radicals.

PULMONARY (CHOKING) AGENTS - PHOSGENE (CG), DIPHOSGENE (DP)

EARLY SYMPTOMS

Management Overview
Don PPE
Remove from hazard
Decon as needed
Supportive therapy
Enforce rest
Caution during relatively
asymptomatic latent period
Observe for delayed
pulmonary effects

OCULAR
Irritation, burning,
lacrimation

RESPIRATORY
Oropharyngeal irritation,
Laryngospasm
Dry cough, chest rightness

DERMATOLOGICAL
Burns/frostbite
(liquid phosgene)

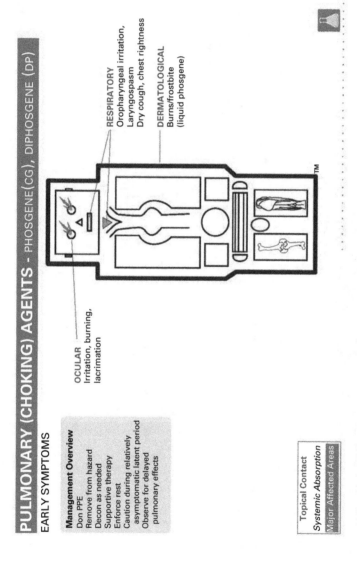

Topical Contact
Systemic Absorption
Major Affected Areas

FIGURE A.15 Unlike chlorine, CG and DP have high incapacitation and mortality potentials. A unique feature of these chemicals is their latency: It may take a couple of days before severe respiratory symptoms develop.

PULMONARY (CHOKING) AGENTS - PHOSGENE (CG), DIPHOSGENE (DP)

LATE SYMPTOMS (2–72 HOURS POST-EXPOSURE)

Management Overview
Supportive therapy
Enforce rest
Aggressive respiratory management

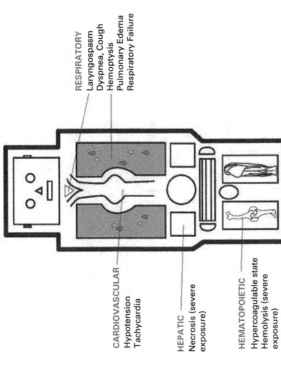

RESPIRATORY
Laryngospasm
Dyspnea, Cough
Hemoptysis
Pulmonary Edema
Respiratory Failure

CARDIOVASCULAR
Hypotension
Tachycardia

HEPATIC
Necrosis (severe exposure)

HEMATOPOIETIC
Hypercoagulable state
Hemolysis (severe exposure)

Topical Contact
Systemic Absorption
Major Affected Areas

FIGURE A.16 Asymptomatic victims should be observed for at least 6 hours for signs of latent manifestations. Those with mild respiratory symptoms may need to be observed for up to 48 hours.

INCAPACITATING AGENTS

INCAPACITATING AGENTS - QUINUCLIDIMYL BENZILATE (BZ)

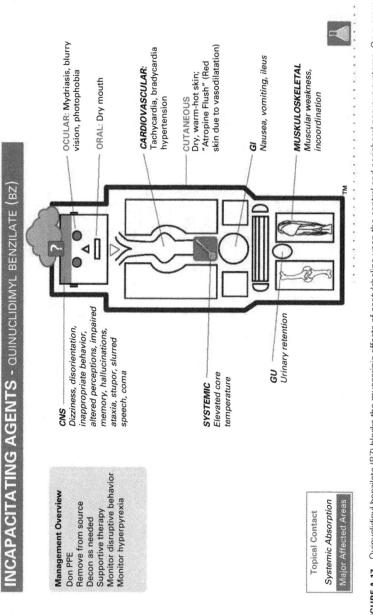

Management Overview
Don PPE
Remove from source
Decon as needed
Supportive therapy
Monitor disruptive behavior
Monitor hyperpyrexia

CNS
Dizziness, disorientation, inappropriate behavior, altered perceptions, impaired memory, hallucinations, ataxia, stupor, slurred speech, coma

SYSTEMIC
Elevated core temperature

GU
Urinary retention

OCULAR: Mydriasis, blurry vision, photophobia

ORAL: Dry mouth

CARDIOVASCULAR:
Tachycardia, bradycardia hypertension

CUTANEOUS
Dry, warm-hot skin; "Atropine Flush" (Red skin due to vasodilatation)

GI
Nausea, vomiting, ileus

MUSKULOSKELETAL
Muscular weakness, incoordination

Topical Contact
Systemic Absorption
Major Affected Areas

FIGURE A.17 Quinuclidinyl benzilate (BZ) blocks the muscarinic effects of acetylcholine upon the central and peripheral nervous systems. On average, clinical manifestations may be delayed for a couple of hours (range: 1 to 20 hours). "Dry as a bone. Blind as a bat. Red as a beet. Hot as a hen. Mad as a hatter." Its incapacitation potential is high but its mortality potential is low. Administering physostigmine as an antidote is controversial.

INCAPACITATING AGENTS - LYSERGIC ACID DIETHULAMIDE (LSD)

Management Overview
Don PPE
Remove from source
Decon as needed
Supportive therapy
Monitor distruptive behavior
Reassure
Sedate as needed

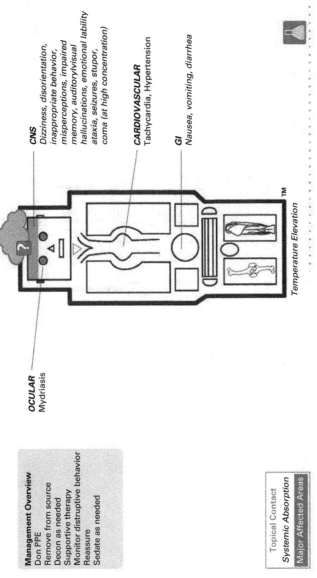

OCULAR
Mydriasis

CNS
Dizziness, disorientation, inappropriate behavior, misperceptions, impaired memory, auditory/visual hallucinations, emotional lability ataxia, seizures, stupor, coma (at high concentration)

CARDIOVASCULAR
Tachycardia, Hypertension

GI
Nausea, vomiting, diarrhea

™

Temperature Elevation

Topical Contact
Systemic Absorption
Major Affected Areas

FIGURE A.18 LSD, a sympathomimetic, releases serotonin within the cerebral cortex, causing mental and somatic excitatory symptoms. Manifestations will occur within minutes if inhaled and about an hour if ingested. One concern of an intentional mass casualty release is the possibility of a toxic psychosis that could last for months and flashbacks that could continue for years.

INCAPACITATION AGENTS - FENTANYL

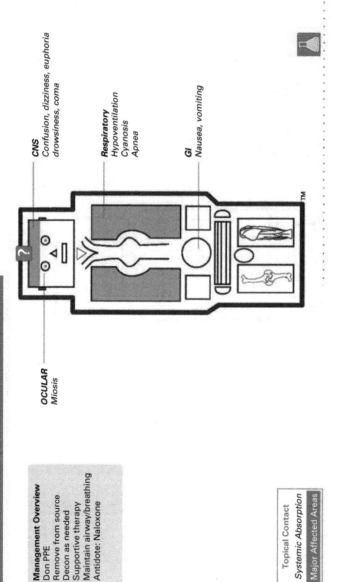

Management Overview
Don PPE
Remove from source
Decon as needed
Supportive therapy
Maintain airway/breathing
Antidote: Naloxone

OCULAR
Miosis

CNS
*Confusion, dizziness, euphoria
drowsiness, coma*

Respiratory
*Hypoventilation
Cyanosis
Apnea*

GI
Nausea, vomiting

Topical Contact
Systemic Absorption
Major Affected Areas

™

FIGURE A.19 In 2002, Russian troops launched a gas attack upon Chechen rebels and their hostages. The gas, thought to be carfentanil, overcame the rebels and also killed more than 120 hostages. A naloxone antidote was not available at the time of the counterattack.

RIOT CONTROL AGENTS

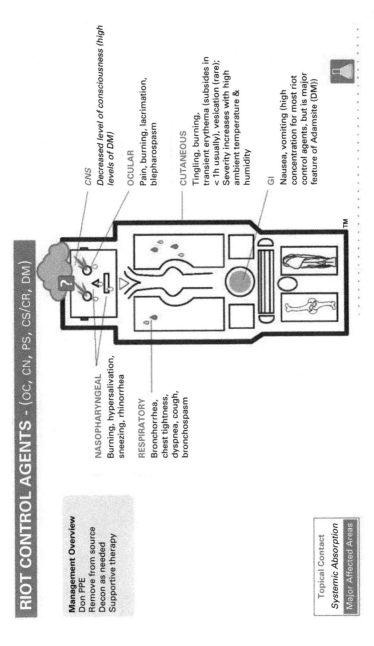

RIOT CONTROL AGENTS - (OC, CN, PS, CS/CR, DM)

Management Overview
Don PPE
Remove from source
Decon as needed
Supportive therapy

NASOPHARYNGEAL
Burning, hypersalivation, sneezing, rhinorrhea

RESPIRATORY
Bronchorrhea, chest tightness, dyspnea, cough, bronchospasm

CNS
Decreased level of consciousness (high levels of DM)

OCULAR
Pain, burning, lacrimation, blepharospasm

CUTANEOUS
Tingling, burning, transient erythema (subsides in < 1h usually), vesication (rare); Severity increases with high ambient temperature & humidity

GI
Nausea, vomiting (high concentration for most riot control agents, but is major feature of Adamsite (DM))

Topical Contact
Systemic Absorption
Major Affected Areas

FIGURE A.20 There are a number of riot control agents, many of which are against the law both for civilians and for law enforcement and the military. OC = Pepper spray; CN = Adamsite; CN = Mace; PS = Chloropicrin; CS/CR = Tear gas. Severe injury and even death can occur if these agents are released in a closed space.

Appendix B
Category A bioterror agents and beyond

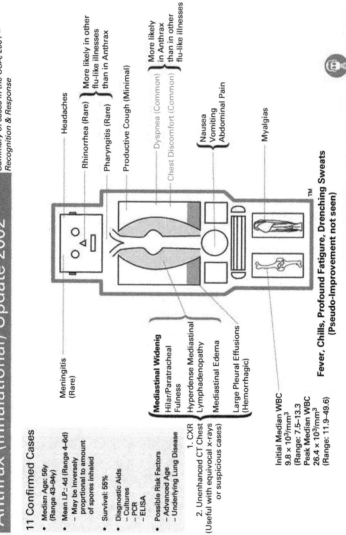

Anthrax (Inhalational) Update 2002

Summary of cases in the USA, 2001 –
Recognition & Response

11 Confirmed Cases

- Median Age: 56y (Range 43–94y)
- Mean I.P.: 4d (Range 4–6d)
  - May be inversely proportional to amount of spores inhaled
- Survival: 55%
- Diagnostic Aids
  - Cultures
  - PCR
  - ELISA
- Possible Risk Factors
  - Advanced Age
  - Underlying Lung Disease

1. CXR
2. Unenhanced CT Chest
(Useful with equivocal x-rays or suspicious cases)

Meningitis (Rare)

Headaches
Rhinorrhea (Rare) } More likely in other flu-like illnesses than in Anthrax
Pharyngitis (Rare)
Productive Cough (Minimal)

Dyspnea (Common) } More likely in Anthrax than in other flu-like illnesses
Chest Discomfort (Common)

Nausea
Vomiting
Abdominal Pain

Myalgias

Mediastinal Widenig
Hilar/Paratracheal Fulness
Hyperdense Mediastinal Lymphadenopathy
Mediastinal Edema
Large Pleural Effusions (Hemorrhagic)

Initial Median WBC
9.8 x 10³/mm³
(Range: 7.5–13.3
Peak Median WBC
26.4 x 10³/mm³
(Range: 11.9–49.6)

Fever, Chills, Profound Fatigue, Drenching Sweats
(Pseudo-Improvement not seen)

™

FIGURE B.1 Anthrax. This represents a visual summary of the 11 confirmed cases of inhalational anthrax that occurred in the United States in 2001. Key findings were the mediastinal lymphadenopathy, the significant hemorrhagic pleural effusions, and the high mortality rate.

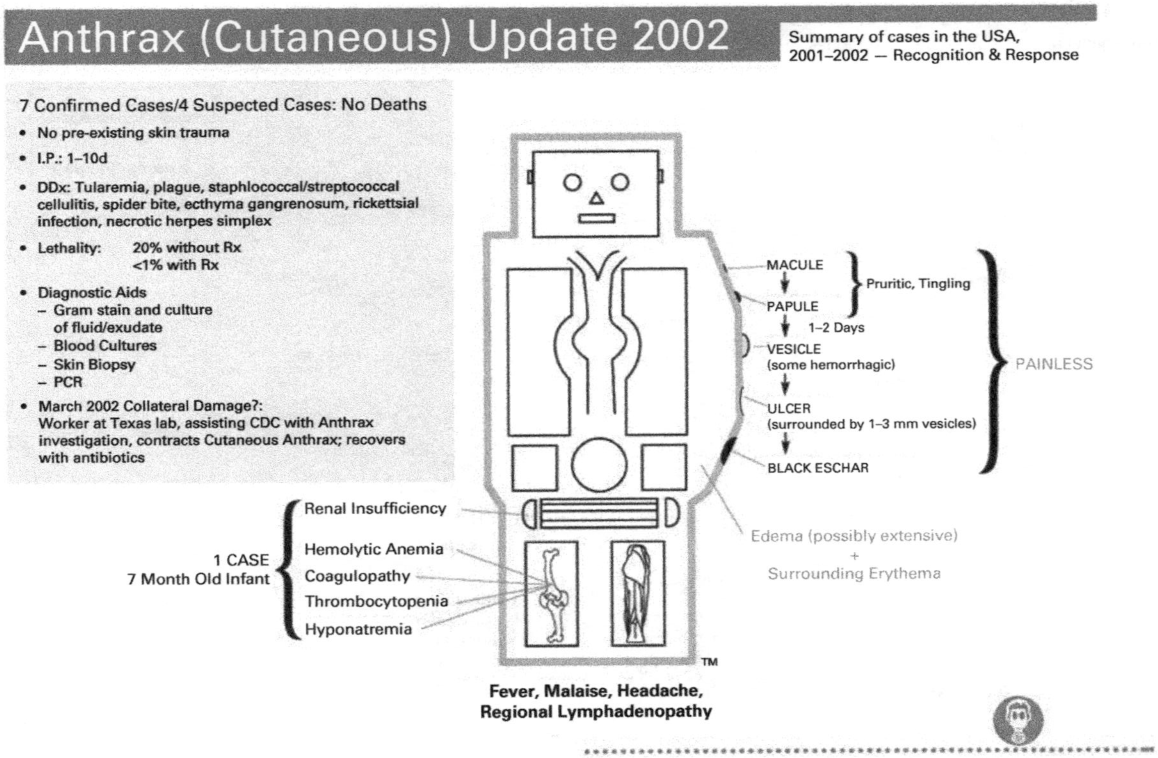

Anthrax (Cutaneous) Update 2002

Summary of cases in the USA,
2001–2002 — Recognition & Response

7 Confirmed Cases/4 Suspected Cases: No Deaths

- No pre-existing skin trauma
- I.P.: 1–10d
- DDx: Tularemia, plague, staphlococcal/streptococcal cellulitis, spider bite, ecthyma gangrenosum, rickettsial infection, necrotic herpes simplex
- Lethality: 20% without Rx
                      <1% with Rx
- Diagnostic Aids
    - Gram stain and culture of fluid/exudate
    - Blood Cultures
    - Skin Biopsy
    - PCR
- March 2002 Collateral Damage?: Worker at Texas lab, assisting CDC with Anthrax investigation, contracts Cutaneous Anthrax; recovers with antibiotics

MACULE
Pruritic, Tingling
PAPULE
1–2 Days
VESICLE
(some hemorrhagic)
ULCER
(surrounded by 1–3 mm vesicles)
BLACK ESCHAR

PAINLESS

Edema (possibly extensive)
+
Surrounding Erythema

Renal Insufficiency
Hemolytic Anemia
Coagulopathy
Thrombocytopenia
Hyponatremia

1 CASE
7 Month Old Infant

Fever, Malaise, Headache, Regional Lymphadenopathy

FIGURE B.2 Anthrax. In 2001–2002, there were seven confirmed and four suspected cases of intentional cutaneous anthrax. A black eschar is characteristic of cutaneous anthrax. A 7-month-old infant had unrecognized cutaneous anthrax that became systemic with renal compromise, hemolytic anemia, and thrombocytopenia. She recovered. Anthrax is a Category A agent.

Botulinum Toxin (Clostridium botulinum)

Syndromes
NEUROLOGICAL

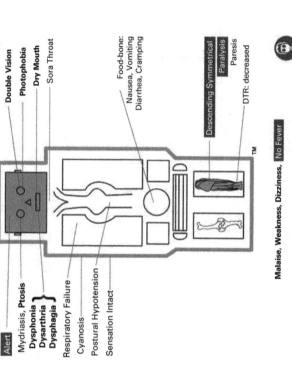

Double Vision

Photophobia

Dry Mouth

Sora Throat

Alert

Mydriasis, **Ptosis**

Dysphonia
Dysarthria
Dysphagia

Respiratory Failure

Cyanosis

Postural Hypotension

Sensation Intact

Food-bone:
Nausea, Vomiting
Diarrhea, Cramping

Descending Symmetrical
Paralysis

Paresis

DTR: decreased

Malaise, Weakness, Dizziness, No Fever

Early Symptoms
Delayed Symptoms
Classic Symptoms

FIGURE B.3 Botulism. Intentional botulism can develop through an aerosol attack over a populated area or sabotage of a food source. The incubation period is typically less than a week. It is characterized by a descending symmetrical paralysis from head to toe.

Pneumonic Plague Primary *(Yersinia pestis)*

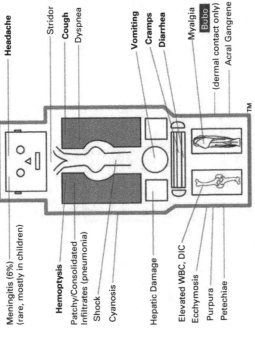

Syndromes

INFLUENZA

PULMONARY

DERMATOLOGICAL

Meningitis (6%)
(rare, mostly in children)

Headache

Stridor

Cough

Dyspnea

Hemoptysis

Patchy/Consolidated
Infiltrates (pneumonia)

Shock

Cyanosis

Hepatic Damage

Vomiting

Cramps

Diarrhea

Elevated WBC, DIC

Ecchymosis

Purpura

Petechiae

Myalgia

Bubo
(dermal contact only)

Acral Gangrene

Fever, Chills, Malaise

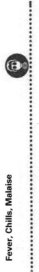

Early Symptoms
Delayed Symptoms
Classic Symptoms

FIGURE B.4 Plague, from *Yersinia pestis*, is a highly transmissible disease that can be highly lethal without prompt antibiotic therapy. This is a Tier 1 or Category A agent according to CDC. The incubation period is less than 1 week. Mortality rates are high even with early recognition and management. The WHO has estimated that intentionally spraying *Y. pestis* over a city with a population of 5 million could lead to 150,000 cases of pneumonic plague and 36,000 deaths. In the event that this is an act of bioterrorism, CDC's concern is that, due to an initial paucity of antibiotics for large numbers of victims, mild to moderate cases should be treated with oral antibiotics, leaving the parenteral antibiotics for the moderate to severe cases. Second, since it is always possible that the bacterium has been genetically altered, CDC recommends that the victims receive dual antibiotic therapy from different classes (e.g., fluoroquinolone + aminoglycoside) initially.

Ricin Toxin (Ricinus communis - Castor Bean)

Syndromes
INFLUENZA
PULMONARY

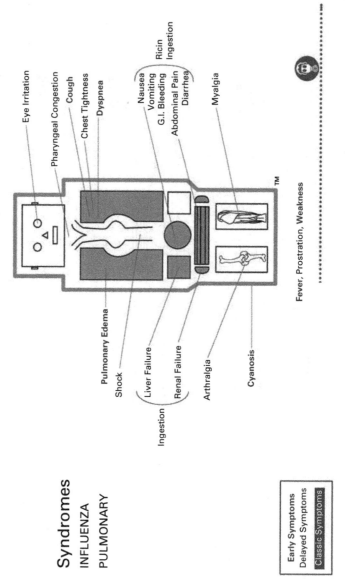

| Early Symptoms |
| Delayed Symptoms |
| Classic Symptoms |

FIGURE B.5 Ricin is a highly lethal toxin that is produced from castor beans (*Ricinus communis*). Each bean contains 1% to 5% ricin. Once absorbed, the toxin inhibits ribosomal function and protein synthesis. The incubation period can be as short as a couple of hours up to 24 hours. Mortality rate is elevated and is related to multiple-organ failure. It is estimated that the LD_{50} in humans is 1 to 20 µg/kg.

Smallpox

(Variola virus)

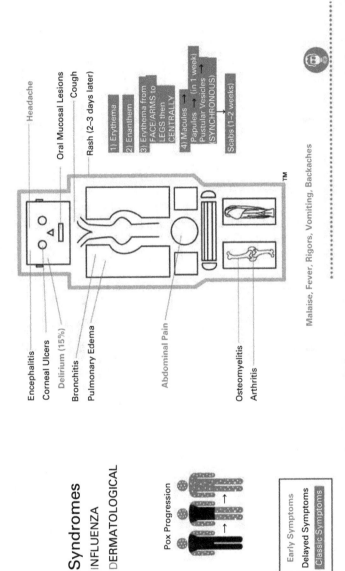

Syndromes

INFLUENZA

DERMATOLOGICAL

Pox Progression

Encephalitis
Corneal Ulcers
Delirium (15%)
Bronchitis
Pulmonary Edema

Abdominal Pain

Osteomyelitis
Arthritis

Headache
Oral Mucosal Lesions
Cough
Rash (2–3 days later)

1) Erythema
2) Enanthem
3) Erythema from FACE/ARMS to LEGS then CENTRALLY
4) Macules → Papules → (in 1 week) Pustular Vesicles (SYNCHRONOUS)
Scabs (1–2 weeks)

Malaise, Fever, Rigors, Vomiting, Backaches

Early Symptoms
Delayed Symptoms
Classic Symptoms

FIGURE B.6 This is a highly transmissible viral disease with a mortality rate of 30%. This is all based upon historical reviews since the disease was officially eradicated in 1979, but viral stocks are said to remain in certain U.S. and Russian labs for research purposes. The incubation period can be as long as 2.5 weeks.

Trichothecene (T2) Mycotoxin

Syndromes
DERMATOLOGICAL
PULMONARY

Coma←Seizures
Sneezing, Rhinorrhea,
Epistaxis
Wheezes

Pulmonary Edema
Tachycardia
Hypotension

Bone Marrow Suppression
→
Pancytopenia
→ Sepsis
Coagulopathy

Tearing, Blurry Vision
Irritation
Salivation
Sore Throat
Hoarseness

Cough, Hemoptysis
Dyspnea
Chest Pain

Nausea, Vomiting
Cramping,
Bloody Diarrhea
Red Burning Skin
→ Blisters→
Skin Necrosis →
Skin Sloughing
Yellow Fluid Droplets
(YELLOW RAIN)

™

Weakness, Prostration, Dizziness,
Ataxia, Loss of Coordination, Hypothermia

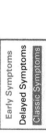

Early Symptoms
Delayed Symptoms
Classic Symptoms

FIGURE B.7 This is virtually the only acknowledged bioterrorism agent that has no incubation period. In an aerosol release, the droplets, "yellow rain," will cause immediate pain and dermatological changes. Rendering care to victims of a T2 mycotoxin attack without suitable PPE will expose the first responders to unnecessary contamination. The initial decontamination will begin with blotting the droplets instead of wiping them off so as to lessen the agent's contact with skin.

Tularemia (*Francisella tularensis*)

Syndromes

INFLUENZA

PULMONARY

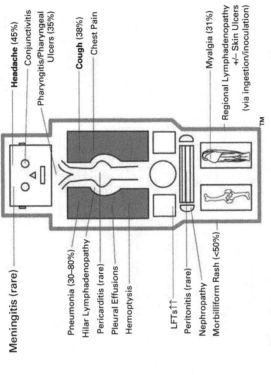

Meningitis (rare)

Headache (45%)
Conjunctivitis
Pharyngitis/Pharyngeal Ulcers (35%)

Cough (38%)
Chest Pain

Myalgia (31%)

Regional Lymphadenopathy +/– Skin Ulcers (via ingestion/inoculation)

Pneumonia (30–80%)
Hilar Lymphadenopathy
Pericarditis (rare)
Pleural Effusions
Hemoptysis

LFTs↑↑
Peritonitis (rare)
Nephropathy
Morbilliform Rash (<50%)

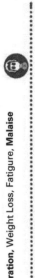

Fever (85%), Chills (52%), Prostration, Weight Loss, Fatigue, Malaise

Early Symptoms
Delayed Symptoms
Classic Symptoms

FIGURE B.8 Tularemia, while not transmissible from person to person, is still considered a Category A agent by CDC. The mean incubation period is from 3 to 5 days. Mortality is low with early recognition and treatment but otherwise could climb from less than 5% to 60%.

Viral Hemorrhagic Fever (VHF)

Syndromes

INFLUENZA
PULMONARY
HEPATIC
NEUROLOGICAL
DERMATOLOGICAL

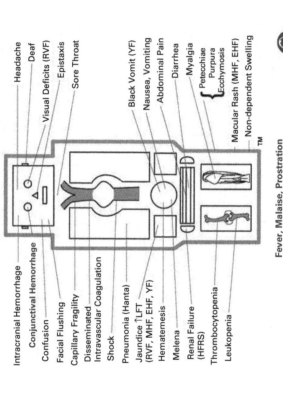

Intracranial Hemorrhage
Conjunctival Hemorrhage
Confusion
Facial Flushing
Capillary Fragility
Disseminated
Intravascular Coagulation
Shock
Pneumonia (Hanta)
Jaundice ↑LFT
(RVF, MHF, EHF, YF)
Hematemesis
Melena
Renal Failure
(HFRS)
Thrombocytopenia
Leukopenia

Headache
Deaf
Visual Deficits (RVF)
Epistaxis
Sore Throat

Black Vomit (YF)
Nausea, Vomiting
Abdominal Pain
Diarrhea
Myalgia
Petechiae
Purpura
Ecchymosis
Macular Rash (MHF, EHF)
Non-dependent Swelling
™

Fever, Malaise, Prostration

Early Symptoms
Delayed Symptoms
Classic Symptoms

FIGURE B.9 VHF, a Category A bioterror agent, as a group is transmissible from person to person. Bunyaviridae include Hantavirus, Rift Valley fever, and Congo-Crimean fever. The Arenaviridae include Lassa fever. Included among the Filoviridae are Marburg virus and Ebola virus. The Flaviviridae include yellow fever and dengue hemorrhagic fever. Transmission between individuals is highly possible, but the severity of disease manifestations will depend on the individual virus. Similarly, incubation periods, mortality rates, and duration of illness will also depend on the specific virus.

FURTHER READING

Nelson CA, Meaney-Delman D, Fleck-Derderian S, Cooley KM, Yu PA, Mead PS. Antimicrobial treatment and prophylaxis of plague: Recommendations for naturally acquired infections and bioterrorism response. *MMWR Recomm Rep.* 2021;70(3):1–27.

Appendix C

A calendar of major disasters in history

January 1, 2001: Shortly after midnight, a fire in a Volendam café in The Netherlands trapped over 300 revelers. Four died immediately in the fire. Mobile medical teams transported the survivors to surrounding hospitals and 182 required admission. Of the 112 who required ICU admission, 96 sustained inhalation injuries and 27 had TBSA burns that equaled or exceeded 40%. There was a high degree of secondary transfers to specialty centers. Ultimately, it was discovered that 27 hospitals in three countries rendered care to these patients. Amazingly, considering the severity of the trauma, only 10 of those hospitalized died.

January 2, 2006: A methane gas explosion occurred in the Sago mine in West Virginia. One miner died in the explosion. A dozen men were trapped underground. By the time they were rescued 41 hours later, 11 of the 12 had died from carbon monoxide poisoning.

January 10, 1977: The lava lake located atop Mount Nyiragongo in the Democratic Republic of Congo drained as its natural containment walls ruptured. Lava flowed down the mountain at a rate as high as 60 kmh, overwhelming villages and killing at least 70 inhabitants.

January 12, 2010: A 7.0M earthquake struck Haiti, killing more than 300,000 people and injuring another 300,000. More than 100,000 structures collapsed and another 200,000 were damaged. One million people were displaced.

January 13, 1982: An Air Florida Boeing 727 plunged into the Potomac River in Washington, DC, killing 78 people.

January 15, 1917: In the North End of Boston, a storage tank containing 12,000 tons of molasses burst. A tidal wave of molasses coursed through the streets of Boston, approaching speeds of 35 mph. The highest wave was 25 feet high and the sweet, sticky glop became a flood that was reported to be 2 to 3 feet deep. Twenty-one people died and 150 were injured.

January 17, 2002: The stratovolcano Nyiragongo in the Democratic Republic of Congo erupted. Lava flows were over 3,000 feet wide and 6 feet deep. Four hundred thousand people were evacuated from the city of

Goma. There were at least 245 deaths due to a variety of causes, such as asphyxiation and blunt force trauma.

January 23, 1556: An earthquake in Shaanxi, China, killed an estimated 830,000 people.

January 24, 2011: A bomb exploded in the International Arrivals Hall of Moscow's Domodedovo International Airport, killing 35 people and injuring 173.

January 27, 1982: A coal mine explosion occurred just outside of Glasgow. There were 40 casualties, mostly thermal trauma. One criticism of the response was that there was no communication between EMS and the hospitals. Most of the hospitalized required burn management; 18 patients suffered more than 15% TBSA burns. Average length of hospital stay was 24 days.

January 27, 2019: On the island of Jolo in the Philippines, two bombs were detonated in the Cathedral of Our Lady of Mount Carmel. At least 20 were killed and scores more were injured. The first bomb exploded in the Cathedral and the second was detonated in the parking lot as people were fleeing the chaos.

January 28, 1986: The *Challenger* explosion.

February 7, 1967: At Dale's Penthouse in Montgomery, Alabama, a cloakroom fire grew out of control and 26 people died.

February 8, 1947: In the British sector of Berlin, a fire erupted within Karlslust dance hall. It is believed that 81 people perished. Stovepipes from three active potbelly stoves were hot enough to ignite the overhead wooden beams. Escape was rendered nearly impossible due to barred windows and walled-up doors; the building had recently served as a jail. Of the 150 injured, 40 required hospitalization.

February 11, 2021: Outside of Ft. Worth, Texas, a massive traffic pile-up occurred on icy Interstate 35. More than 130 vehicles were entangled in the chain-reaction incident. At least six people died and 65 were injured, many of whom required transportation to hospitals. Buses were used at the scene to protect and warm victims.

February 14, 1981: Shortly after midnight on Valentine's Day, Dublin's Stardust nightclub was encased in fire. The city's disaster plan sent all available ambulance and fire engines to the scene and the six main local hospitals were immediately notified of the disaster. A total of 214 victims were transported to these hospitals, suffering from thermal and inhalation injuries. Of the 40 deaths, the majority died at the scene.

February 14, 2018: A 19-year-old expelled high school student entered the Marjory Stoneman Douglas High School in Parkland, Florida, and opened fire on students and faculty with an AR-15 semiautomatic rifle. Seventeen were killed and 17 more were wounded in an attack that lasted less than 4 minutes.

February 15, 1898: The USS *Maine* blew up in Havana harbor. Of the 400 crewmembers on board, 260 were killed. The cause of the explosion has been debated for more than a century, but it ignited a nationalistic sentiment that led to a declaration of war between the United States and Spain.

February 20, 2003: A pyrotechnic show during Great White's set at The Station nightclub in West Warwick, Rhode Island, accidentally ignited a conflagration that killed 100 and injured 200. Most of the Rhode Island hospitals received some sort of prenotification. Several received limited, incorrect, or no information at all. A perceived lack of central coordination among the receiving hospitals impeded their own ability to communicate, to deliver critical resources, and to surge additional personnel. Kent County Hospital received 82 patients, most within a span of 90 minutes. They treated and released 43, admitted 21, and transferred another 18 by ground and air. A 2014 study on 104 survivors revealed that 27% reported having pain for more than 2 years after the fire. Another 2014 study explored the psychological aftermath of the survivors. Whether the survivors were injured or not, there was significant evidence of posttraumatic stress—this was particularly evident in the survivors who did not sustain any injuries. Their rehabilitation was complicated by guilt, self-blame, helplessness, and bitterness.

February 22, 2011: At 12:51 p.m. local time, a 6.3M earthquake struck Christchurch, New Zealand (population. 400,000). Eighty percent of the city center was reduced to rubble and 185 people died.

March 1, 1910: In Wellington, Washington, an avalanche from the Cascade Mountains swept two trains off the rails into a gorge 150 feet deep. Ninety-six people perished.

March 2, 1944: During WWII in Italy, a freight train loaded with Italian troops was forced to stand idle in a tunnel near Salerno. Due to the fact that the train was using low-grade coal as fuel, the idling in an enclosed space caused volumes of carbon dioxide to fill the tunnel. Over 500 troops were asphyxiated.

March 3, 1974: A faulty rear-hatch door exploded open in midflight and severed the control cables. The DC-10's sudden decompression doomed the pilot's attempt to gain control, and it crashed into the woods outside Paris. Six passengers near the door were sucked out immediately and the remaining 340 souls died on impact 90 seconds later. The problem with the DC-10's door had been known in the aviation industry since 1972, when a similar event occurred that did not lead to a crash, but there had not been any universal recall to fix the system.

March 4, 1908: The Lakeview Elementary School in Collinwood, Ohio (outside Cleveland), was enveloped in flames. Within 30 minutes, 174 students and two teachers died. The fire, which had started in the basement, consumed the first floor and blocked everyone's principal escape route. Alternate routes of escape were narrow; children fell upon and crushed each other and soon perished from crush, flames, and smoke. It was later discovered that the children's bodies were piled up to 5 feet high in the vestibule as they were fighting to get out. Firefighters arrived late and did not have the aerial ladders to reach the upper floor. They also forgot their axes to crash through the wooden doors of the school. The water pressure for their hoses was also too weak to have any major impact. Because of this tragedy, Ohio and the nation's fire laws became stricter, including such measures as increasing the frequency of fire drills in schools and requiring "panic bars" on exit doors.

March 6, 1987: The *Herald of Free Enterprise* ferry capsized off the Belgian coast. It had left Zeebrugge harbor with 543 people, 84 cars, and 36 trucks on board, but the person responsible for closing the bow doors as the ferry got under way was asleep. As a consequence, water came in through the opening, shifting the cargo and tipping the boat to port. The ferry sank, costing the lives of 188 people. Safety regulations for ferries crossing the English Channel were reviewed and tightened as a result.

March 7, 2021: In Equatorial Guinea, a fire in a military barracks set off a series of explosions that killed at least 60 and wounded 600. The president of the country blamed negligence in the handling of dynamite as the cause of the disaster.

March 8, 2014: Malaysia Airlines Flight 370 took off from Kuala Lumpur, veered off course, and disappeared, along with 227 passengers and

12 crew. A massive search by many nations ensued over the plane's intended course and into the Indian Ocean. Periodically, over time, the plane's debris washed up on scattered shores, but the actual aircraft was never found. Theories were plentiful such as terrorism, pilot suicide, and sudden oxygen deprivation, but the mystery continues.

March 9, 1981: At the Japan Atomic Power Company plant in Tsuruga, Japan, a radioactive sludge tank overflowed due to human error. Efforts to contain the sludge were unsuccessful and 16 tons of radioactive waste contaminated Wakasa Bay. Fifty-nine workers were exposed to radiation. Despite the gravity of the mishap, news of the incident was concealed from the public. When the media got wind of the story, it led to a recall of all fish caught from the bay. It was said that over the next several years, the fish from the bay showed evidence of more mutations than previously noted. In May, the president and chairman of the company resigned.

March 10, 1906: At the Courrières Colliery in northern France, an underground fire that refused to be extinguished spawned a massive explosion that killed 1,060 miners. Hundreds of survivors sustained devastating burn injuries.

March 11, 2011: A 9M earthquake in the Pacific triggered a tsunami that inundated the northeast coastline of Japan. The cascade of destruction also spawned a meltdown at the Fukushima Daiichi nuclear power plant. Ultimately, this series of events devastated towns and villages, killed 18,000 people, and forced the evacuation of nearly half a million inhabitants. To this day, countries like China and South Korea have banned produce and fish from the Fukushima prefecture. The prolonged evacuation status of thousands underscored the myriad physical and mental health needs that would develop both acutely and chronically. Additionally, while the acute effects of this disaster cascade are well documented, experts debate the long-term public health consequences of low-dose radiation exposure.

March 11, 1669: Mount Etna in Sicily began belching noxious fumes, causing the asphyxiation of 3,000 people living along its fertile slopes. Ash and lava soon followed. Efforts to save Catania, 18 miles away, from the lava flood proved fruitless, and over the course of weeks, nearly 17,000 Catanians perished and 27,000 were rendered homeless.

March 11, 2004: During the Madrid rush hour, terrorists carrying backpacks detonated a series of improvised explosive devices on four crowded trains at three busy stations. The incidents left 193 dead and about 2,000 wounded.

March 11, 1888: The Great Blizzard of '88 maimed the east coast of the United States. In some places, up to 55 inches of snow fell. More than 400 people died, 200 in New York City alone.

March 12, 1988: A sudden hailstorm caused panic amid fans at a soccer stadium in Kathmandu, Nepal. As they rushed toward the exits, they discovered that the exit doors were closed and locked. This created a pile-up. Seventy died and hundreds were injured.

March 15, 2019: During Friday prayer, two mosques were attacked in Christchurch, New Zealand, by a lone gunman armed with a semiautomatic shotgun and a AR-15–style rifle. Fifty-one people were killed and 40 were wounded. Of the 37 patients who were admitted with gunshot wounds, the average amount of RBCs, FFP, cryoprecipitate, and platelets transfused was 4.0, 3.1, 1.2, and 0.4 units, respectively (https://doi.org/10.1111/vox.12907).

March 16, 2021: Three spas in Atlanta, Georgia, were targeted by a lone gunman who was known to have visited at least two of them in the past. Eight people were killed, six of them of Asian descent.

March 18, 1925: For 3 hours, the infamous "Tri-State Tornado" wreaked havoc across eastern Missouri, southern Illinois, and southern Indiana, a total of 219 miles. The tornado was more than a mile across and it topped speeds of 70 mph. It accounted for 695 deaths, and 13,000 people sustained injuries. It is still considered the worst tornado in U.S. history.

March 18, 1937: A natural gas explosion decimated the Consolidated School of New London, Texas. The explosion occurred at the end of the school day. Apparently there was a gas leak into a closed space in the school, but due to the odorless nature of natural gas, it was not detected. Of the more than 700 students and teachers present, nearly 300 were killed. It was because of this tragedy that a new Texas law was passed mandating that malodorants be added to natural gas in order to warn people of a possible natural gas leak. Mercaptan is now added because of its distinctive "rotten egg" odor. It is now an industry standard.

March 20, 1995: Packages of sarin gas were activated within the subway system of Tokyo. Over 1,300 EMTs and more than 130 ambulances were dispatched to 15 subway stations to render care. The chemical assault, conceived by the Aum Shinrikyo cult, killed 12 and sent more than 5,000 to hospitals for treatment.

March 21, 1960: Unarmed Black demonstrators, protesting South African travel restrictions, were mowed down by the submachine guns of the Afrikaner police in Sharpeville, South Africa. Sixty-nine were killed and 180 were wounded.

March 22, 2014: After weeks of rain, a wall of mud came crashing down on Oso, Washington, destroying homes and burying entire families. Forty-three people died. An investigation revealed that the mudslide, one of the most serious in American history, covered a 1-square-mile area and in some places was 80 feet deep.

March 22, 2021: A 21-year-old man wearing an armored vest and armed with a handgun and a military-style assault rifle began a deadly shooting rampage in the parking lot of King Soopers grocery store, Boulder, Colorado, and continued into the store. By the time the alleged assailant was apprehended, 10 people lay dead, including one police officer.

March 24, 2015: The co-pilot of a German airliner locked the cockpit door on the pilot and, based on the black box recordings, intentionally crashed the Airbus A320 into mountainous terrain in southern France. The suicidal flight claimed 150 lives.

March 24, 1989: One of the worst environmental disasters in history occurred when the supertanker *Exxon Valdes* ran aground on a reef in Prince William Sound, Alaska. Eleven million tons of oil spilled into the waters, fouling 700 miles of coastline and causing irreparable damage to flora and fauna.

March 25, 1990: A fire at the Happy Land Social Club in New York City was set by a disgruntled individual who was refused admission. Smoke inhalation killed 87 partygoers. There were only five survivors.

March 25, 1911: In New York City, a fire broke out in a rag bin at the Triangle Shirtwaist factory near Washington Square. The factory, located on the upper floors of the Asch Building, had only one small functional elevator, a rickety fire escape, and two exit doors, one of which was locked from the outside to prevent pilfering. For the immigrant female workers, it became their death trap. The death toll climbed to 146 as fire hoses could not maintain water pressure, safety nets were too fragile to save jumpers, and the fire ladders were not long enough to save those on the highest floors. The tragedy eventually ignited a series of fire prevention laws in the city and elsewhere.

March 26, 1993: A 1,200-pound terrorist bomb was detonated in the parking garage of the World Trade Center in New York City. It left a 60-foot crater, killed six people, and injured 1,000. Evacuating 50,000 workers from the Towers was a major enterprise that took all day.

March 27, 1977: Two 747 jumbo jets crashed into each other on the airport runway in Tenerife, Canary Islands, killing 583 souls. The disaster was caused by a combination of fog, unintelligible communication, and pilot error.

March 27, 1964: A 9.2M earthquake rocked the southern coast of Alaska. Anchorage sustained significant property damage and over 130 lives were lost. Thousands more sustained injuries. Most of the deaths were related to the tsunami that struck the shores of western North America and Hawaii. The tidal wave reached heights of 100 feet in some areas.

March 28, 1979: The nation's worst commercial nuclear accident occurred at Three Mile Island's Unit 2 Nuclear Generating Station. Radiation was released when part of the nuclear core was damaged. The core had overheated to 4,000°F. Had it heated to 5,000°F, there would have been a nuclear meltdown. The accident was a result of a technical malfunction combined with human error. No injuries or deaths resulted, but thousands of residents were evacuated as a precaution.

March 28, 2005: An 8.7M earthquake hit the Sumatran coastline, resulting in 1,300 deaths.

March 30, 1980: A floating apartment platform inhabited by oil workers in the North Sea was buffeted by gale-force winds during the early evening hours. Due to an unknown crack in one of the legs of the platform, the whole structure collapsed when a huge wave overwhelmed the structure. The disaster occurred suddenly and within minutes, preventing the workers from reaching the lifeboats. Poor weather prevented a timely rescue, and 123 oil workers perished.

April 2, 1979: Due to worker error, anthrax spores escaped out of the Ekaterinburg bioweapons plant in Soviet Russia and contaminated the surrounding countryside. By the time the situation was discovered and resolved, 62 people died and 32 sustained grave illnesses. It took 13 years before the rest of the world knew the true story behind this outbreak.

April 2, 2021: In Hualien, Taiwan, an unmanned construction truck rolled down a hill and into the path of a moving passenger train. The derailment occurred just as the train was entering a tunnel, making rescue difficult. Fifty people were killed and 178 were injured. This was the country's worst rail disaster in decades.

April 3, 1974: In the course of 18 hours, 148 tornadoes ravaged North America from Ontario, Canada, to the southern United States. The string of tornadoes encompassed 13 states and 900 square miles. Based on the Fujita Scale, there were 21 F0 tornadoes, 31 F1s, 30 F2s, 35 F3s, 24 F4s, and six F5s. The toll was devastating: 315 were killed, more than 6,000 were injured, and over 27,000 buildings were damaged. The greatest local impact fell upon Xenia, Ohio (population 25,000): An F5 tornado struck around 3 p.m., killing 34, injuring over 1,600, and destroying 1,300 buildings.

April 4, 1933: The dirigible *Akron* plummeted into the Atlantic off the New Jersey shore, killing 73. The cause of the crash was related to bad weather, miscommunications, and poor airmanship.

April 8, 1997: A 5,700-gallon hydrochloric acid (HCl) storage tank ruptured during filling activities at the Surpass Chemical Company in Albany, New York. Green-yellow fumes drifted across the area, ultimately sending eight workers and 32 others to the hospital. The toxic release, consisting of HCl, sodium hypochlorite, and chlorine, forced the evacuation of a 10-block area of businesses and homes.

April 9, 2021: La Soufrière volcano on the Caribbean island of St. Vincent began a series of eruptions that shot ash and gases into the air. The last time this active, 3,864-foot volcano had erupted was 1979. The toxic plume of volcanic ash in the current eruption climbed to thousands of feet into the air and forced the evacuation of thousands of islanders.

April 10, 1963: The USS *Thresher*, an atomic submarine, broke up off Cape Cod, killing 129 sailors and civilians. The breakup was the terminus of a series of events starting with a short circuit in critical electrical systems on board.

April 11, 1965: In this natural catastrophe known as the Palm Sunday tornadoes, six Midwestern states were overrun by 47 tornadoes that killed 271 people and injured 1,500. It is considered the fourth deadliest tornado outbreak in U.S. history, but it was the deadliest in Indiana's history, where 137 were killed and 1,200 were injured.

April 13, 1360: During the Hundred Years' War, English forces on their way from Paris to Chartres encountered severe weather. The lightning and hailstorm contributed to the overall panic of the English and, according to historical accounts, 1,000 troops died.

April 13, 1919: More than 350 unarmed demonstrators were mowed down by British and Gurkha troops in Amritsar, India, the holy city of the Sikh religion. Because of repeated demonstrations against the conscription of Indians into military service and the imposition of a war tax, the city was placed under martial law. The demonstration at the city park violated the ban on public gatherings, a ban that was not well publicized, despite the fact that April 13 was a day of religious celebration. Jallianwalla Bagh park was surrounded by troops who, without warning, opened fire. Besides the 379 dead, another thousand were wounded. This mass casualty incident is known as the Amritsar Massacre.

April 14, 1944: Along the docks of Bombay, India, a cargo ship exploded, killing 1,300 and injuring 3,000. Besides gold bullion and cotton, there was 300 tons of TNT in her hold.

April 15, 2013: Two bombings in quick succession turned the Boston Marathon from a traditional patriotic mass-gathering event into a terrorist mass casualty incident. Three spectators were killed and 260 were wounded.

April 15, 1912: The *Titanic*, the British ocean liner, sunk into the North Atlantic after striking an iceberg the evening before. Of the 2,200 passengers and crew, 1,500 lost their lives due to a shortage of lifeboats.

April 16, 1947: As ammonium nitrate fertilizer was being loaded on a ship in Texas City, Texas, an explosion occurred that killed nearly 600 people and injured thousands more. It was thought that it all started with a carelessly thrown cigarette that created an out-of-control fire that led to the igniting of the fertilizer. The sound of the explosion carried 150 miles.

April 16, 2007: A student from Virginia Tech killed 32 and wounded 25 in a rampage that lasted 10 minutes before the shooter took his own life. The mean Injury Severity Score for the survivors was 8.2.

April 16, 2021: A mass shooting occurred at the FedEx building in Indianapolis. Before the shooter took his own life, eight were dead and a number of others were wounded.

April 18, 1906: At 5:13 a.m. local time, an earthquake, estimated to have a magnitude of 8.0 on the Richter scale, devastated San Francisco.

The cause of the quake was a slippage of the San Andreas fault along a 250-mile span. Approximately 3,000 people died and 30,000 buildings were destroyed. It was not until April 23 that the city infrastructure was able to stem the fiery consequences of the tremors.

April 18, 1983: A suicide bomber destroyed the U.S. embassy in Beirut, Lebanon. The car-bomb explosion killed 63 people.

April 19, 1993: After a 51-day standoff between the FBI and the Branch Davidian compound, a fire broke out within one of the buildings defended by members of the religious cult. Eighty Branch Davidians were killed, including 22 children.

April 19, 1995: A massive truck bomb was detonated in front of the Alfred P. Murrah Federal Building in Oklahoma City, Oklahoma, by members of a radical-right survivalist group. Most of the north side of the edifice collapsed and 168 people lost their lives, including 19 children in the daycare center.

April 20, 1999: In Littleton, Colorado, two students went on a rampage at Columbine High School. Before killing themselves, Klebold and Harris killed one member of the faculty and 12 students. Twenty-one others were wounded.

April 20, 2010: A massive oil spill developed in the Gulf of Mexico when an explosion destroyed an oil drilling rig just 50 miles off the coast of Louisiana. Eleven people were killed and 17 were injured on the rig, and the nearly 5 million barrels of crude oil crippled the environment. It took 3 months for the leak to be capped, and the full environmental impact of the disaster has yet to be determined.

April 21, 1930: An accidental fire broke out at the Ohio State Penitentiary in Columbus. The prison was infamous for its decrepitude and overcrowding. Guards' efforts to rescue the prisoners were erratic. The disaster ultimately killed 320 inmates and seriously injured 130 more.

April 21, 2021: The Indonesian Navy's *KRI Nanggala 402* submarine sank off Bali. All 53 crew members were lost. It was found 4 days later in waters that were over 2,700 feet deep.

April 22, 1992: More than 200 people in Guadalajara, Mexico, were killed when a series of sewer explosions leveled part of the city. A few days earlier there were clues that a gas leak was developing underground, but they were ignored by federal agencies. The explosions decimated a

20-square-block area. About 1,500 residents required hospitalization and 25,000 more needed to be evacuated from the stricken zone.

April 23, 1940: A dance hall fire in Natchez, Mississippi, killed 209 and injured 200. The majority of the 24 windows in the nightclub were boarded up, thereby preventing escape. Most of the deaths were related to smoke inhalation and crush injuries.

April 25, 1980: Poor weather conditions and confusing communications between pilots and air traffic control caused a Danish Boeing 707 to plow into a mountain in Tenerife, Canary Islands. All 146 passengers and crew on board died on impact.

April 25, 2015: A 7.8M earthquake wreaked havoc in Nepal. Up to 9,000 people were killed and 16,800 were injured. Over 800,000 homes were destroyed and 2.8 million people were displaced.

April 25, 2021: An exploding oxygen tank ignited a fire that roared through a Baghdad hospital, claiming at least 82 lives. The hospital, over-whelmed with COVID-19 patients, lacked smoke detectors, fire hoses, and a sprinkler system.

April 26, 1986: At the nuclear power plant in Chernobyl, Ukraine, re-actor #4 exploded, exposing the core. This nuclear meltdown sent plumes of radioactive material into the air. The official death toll was 32, with dozens more sustaining radiation burns. Two hundred thousand inhabit-ants were evacuated. There is still a controversy about how many people were exposed to the radiation. There is expert opinion declaring that thou-sands died from radiation poisoning and about 70,000 were sickened by it.

April 28, 1996: A man went on a shooting rampage in Port Arthur, Tasmania. Thirty-five men, women, and children are killed, most of them enjoying lunch at the Broad Arrow Café.

April 29, 1992: Rioting broke out in Los Angeles after police officers were acquitted for beating an unarmed Black American without provo-cation. The 3-day rampage resulted in 60 dead, 2,000 injured, and the burning of 3,000 buildings.

April 29, 2021: In northern Israel, a religious mass gathering resulted in a crush-stampede at which at least 28 were killed and 50 were injured. Twenty casualties were described as critical.

April 31, 2019: A gunman hijacked a postal truck and, in a series of drive-by shootings in Midland and Odessa, Texas, killed seven and wounded 25.

It all began when the perpetrator sped away from the police after a routine traffic stop.

May 1, 1961: A fire broke out at the Top Storey Club in Bolton, outside of Manchester, England, killing 19, 14 by fire and five by jumping.

May 1, 2016: A wildfire began near Fort McMurray, Alberta, Canada. By May 3, 88,000 people were forced to evacuate. By the time the conflagration was brought under control, about 1.5 million acres were destroyed as well as 2,400 homes and buildings.

May 3, 1962: A double train mishap occurred near Tokyo. A freight train collided with a passenger train. Most of the passengers survived this first accident, but when a third train rammed into the primary incident, a boiler exploded and scalded many trapped victims. The second collision also pushed one of the trains down an embankment. The death toll ran up to 160 and the injured numbered over 400.

May 4, 1886: At Haymarket Square in Chicago, a labor demonstration got out of hand. A bomb was thrown at the police, police responded with gunshots, and a peaceful demonstration turned into a riot. More than 100 people were killed and 100 were injured.

May 4, 2002: Kano, Nigeria, was the site of a passenger plane crash that killed 149 people both in the plane and on the ground. Immediately upon takeoff from the local airport there was obvious signs of trouble with the Nigerian BAC 1-11-500 aircraft. It soon crashed, obliterating a working-class neighborhood and burning many of the townspeople to death.

May 6, 1937: Near Lakehurst, New Jersey, the German dirigible *Hindenburg* burst into flames. Out of 61 passengers and crew, 36 were killed.

May 7, 2014: Due to a chain-reaction multiple-vehicle accident, a tanker's storage compartment was breached, releasing hydrofluoric acid into the environment. Over 250 victims were injured, many of them contaminated with the caustic agent. Four of the most seriously burned and contaminated with HF required advanced airway management, extensive burn care, and antidotes such as calcium and magnesium to temper the effects of the acid. Despite the intensive care, three of the four died.

May 7, 2019: Two students shot at fellow students at a charter school in a Denver suburb. One student was killed attempting to save the others. Eight other students are wounded.

May 8, 1898: Food riots between the citizens of Italy and the Italian government reached its climax in Milan when barricades, rooftop tiles, and rifles were met with infantry, calvary, and cannon fire (known as the Bava Beccaris massacre). Estimates of the dead and wounded ranged from 300 dead and 1,000 wounded up to 400 killed and 2,000 wounded.

May 8, 1902: The city of St. Pierre in Martinique was wiped out as Mount Pelée continued its volcanic eruptions that had commenced the day before. The inhabitants were killed by suffocating gases that reached temperatures of 3,000°F and by avalanches of volcanic ash that swept down the mountain. The death toll was estimated at close to 30,000.

May 11, 1934: A massive storm swept the topsoil from the Great Plains agricultural lands and sent it as far as the East Coast. This event resulted from the drought conditions that crippled the Heartland in the early 1930s and created the periodic dust storms. Entire populations of the Great Plains were forced to abandon this "Dust Bowl" to seek new fortunes in the West.

May 11, 1985: A fire in the grandstands at the football stadium in Bradford, England, led to the deaths of 56 spectators. Hundreds more were injured.

May 12, 2008: Eastern Sichuan, China, was the epicenter of a 7.8M earthquake. Approximately 70,000 people died, 350,000 were injured, and 5 million were left homeless.

May 13, 1985: In Philadelphia, a governmental assault on the headquarters of MOVE, a Black liberation group, led to the deaths of 11, including two children. A police helicopter dropped C-4 plastic explosives onto the roof of the headquarters and the resulting fire not only killed the inhabitants but also destroyed 60 houses in the neighborhood.

May 14, 1991: Near Shigaraki, Japan, two commuter trains collided, killing 42 and injuring more than 400. Railway workers allowed one of the trains to depart the station without a green signal, declaring it was safe to do so. That human error plus a defective faulty-departure detector led to the collision.

May 15, 1929: A fire at the Cleveland Clinic killed 125 people, including seven physicians. The cause of the fire was the spontaneous combustion of used nitrocellulose radiographic film. The ignition of these X-rays caused the emission not only of carbon monoxide but also of toxic nitrous oxide. Deaths occurred early, but there was also evidence of late manifestations as respiratory compromise developed. Significant pulmonary edema was noted on autopsy of a number of the victims.

May 18, 1980: Mount St. Helens, Washington, erupted at 8:32 a.m. PDT. The massive eruption killed 57 and devastated 210 square miles of the surrounding territory.

May 18, 2018: A 17-year-old student, armed with a shotgun and a revolver, entered his Santa Fe High School in Texas and opened fire. He murdered 10 and wounded 10 more, many of them his fellow students.

May 19, 2016: EgyptAir Flight 804, with 66 souls on board, disappeared over the Mediterranean Sea. While initially it was thought that the event was caused by terrorism, it was later determined that a cockpit fire resulted in the disaster. It wasn't until June that the remains of the aircraft were discovered under water.

May 20, 2020: Cyclone Amphan made landfall in West Bengal. With sustained winds of 150 mph, it rampaged through India and into Bangladesh and killed 128 people. The relatively small number of deaths was related to the evacuation of more than 5 million people. The economic toll was significant: It is estimated that damage costs exceeded $13 billion.

May 21, 1960: A 7.6M earthquake rocked Valdivia, Chile, killing 5,000 and rendering 2 million homeless.

May 22, 1960: Southern Chile was crippled by an 8.5M earthquake whose epicenter was just offshore. Rockslides and a series of tsunamis followed. One tsunami measured 35 feet in height and was responsible for 1,000 deaths. The series of tsunamis traveled across the Pacific Ocean for about a week and caused hundreds of additional deaths in the Philippines and Japan.

May 22, 2017: At an Ariana Grande concert in Manchester, England, a suicide bomber detonated an explosion that killed 22 concertgoers and injured 116.

May 23, 1960: In Hilo, Hawaii, a tsunami created by a 9.5M earthquake off Chile's coast the day before killed 61 people. The waves reached the height of 35 feet and their force bent parking meters and swept trucks out to sea.

May 24, 1964: A soccer match in Lima, Peru, became a death trap when a riot developed after a disputed call by the referee. Three hundred fans were killed during the crush and stampede and 500 were injured.

May 25, 1979: American Airlines Flight 191 took off from Chicago's O'Hare Airport and almost immediately lost an engine. It rolled to the left, plunged to earth, and exploded, killing all 277 on board and a couple of bystanders on the ground. The fire was so intense that it took over an hour before firefighters could approach the scene. The cause of the engine loss was due to the maintenance crew's failure to comply with safety procedures.

May 26, 1991: A computer malfunction aboard a Boeing 767 caused the engines to go unexpectedly into reverse soon after departing Bangkok International Airport. The plane plunged into the Thai jungle and all 223 passengers and crew were killed.

May 26, 2021: A mass shooting in San Jose, California, left nine dead and several others wounded. The shooter, who worked at the shooting site, brought a bag filled with semiautomatic handguns and high-capacity magazines.

May 27, 2006: Five thousand people died after a 6.2M earthquake hit Yogyakarta (population of more than 433,000) on the island of Java.

May 28, 2010: Terrorists attacked two Ahmadiyya mosques in Pakistan. The attacks were coordinated, occurring just minutes apart. Armed with guns and grenades, the terrorists killed 94 and wounded more than 120.

May 31, 1889: In Johnstown, Pennsylvania, the South Fork Dam gave way due to a steady rain and a swollen water system. Water flowed at a speed of 40 mph and ultimately overwhelmed the community of 30,000 people in Johnstown. More than 2,200 people were killed by drowning or crushed by debris in the waters.

May 31, 1929: A race massacre occurred in Tulsa, Oklahoma. A White mob attacked the Black neighborhood called the Greenwood District. By the time the violence subsided, hundreds of African Americans were killed and the district, approximately 35 square blocks, was obliterated. More than 1,200 buildings, homes, churches, and a hospital were destroyed.

May 31, 2019: In Virginia, a disgruntled Virginia Beach public utilities engineer walked into the Virginia Beach Municipal Center and killed 12 people, wounding several more. Responding police fatally shot the assailant.

June 3, 2017: A van containing three terrorists mowed down pedestrians walking along London Bridge. Then, armed with steak knives, the assailants rampaged through a nearby market, entering bars and eateries and stabbing civilians out for a good time. Eight people were killed and 48 were injured.

The attack started a little before 10 p.m., and by 10:15 all three terrorists were killed by police.

June 4, 1989: The Tiananmen Square Massacre. Chinese troops stormed the famous square in Beijing in order to repel the thousands of youths trying to reclaim democracy. Gunfire from security forces resounded in the open spaces. Thousands fled and thousands fought back. Official estimates of the dead are difficult to ascertain, but reporters at the scene have stated that the numbers could be anywhere from 300 up to thousands.

June 5, 1870: A girl tripped as she was carrying hot coals into the kitchen. Her sudden loss of balance caused the charcoal to fly out the window and land on an adjacent roof. That set off a blaze throughout Constantinople that destroyed 3,000 homes and killed 900 people.

June 6, 1981: Along the Bagmati River in India, a train accident caused the deaths of 500 riders. The engineer of the train braked too hard in order to avoid a cow crossing the tracks. A number of cars derailed and slid into the monsoon-swollen river. Most of the victims drowned.

June 6, 1984: The Indian army poured into the Golden Temple in Amritsar in order to quell an insurrection. In the process, approximately 500 Sikh separatists and 100 Indian troops were killed.

June 11, 1955: During the 24-hour race at Le Mans, France, a Mercedes racing car went out of control and plowed into spectators, killing 82.

June 12, 2016: In the early morning hours, a 29-year-old gunman armed with an AR-15 assault rifle and a handgun entered the Pulse nightclub in Orlando, Florida, killing 49 and wounding scores more. It was finally over by 5 a.m. local time.

June 14, 2017: The Grenfell Tower, a 24-story apartment building in London, caught on fire and 72 inhabitants died. Partial blame for the morbidity and mortality was placed on the flammable cladding that was applied to the exterior of the building and the fact that the firefighters advised those caught in the building to remain where they were and await rescue.

June 15, 1904: The *General Slocum* riverboat traveled up the East River in New York with children, parents, and teachers on their annual Sunday School picnic. A fire in the storeroom went out of control and spread throughout the riverboat. Instead of heading toward the dock and safety, the captain attempted to beach on a nearby island. That action, coupled with lifeboats that couldn't be released and lifejackets that weighed down the children, resulted in over 1,000 deaths from burns, crush, and drowning.

June 16, 1896: An earthquake and its subsequent tsunami killed 27,000 in Japan.

June 17, 2015: Nine people were killed by a mass shooter at Emanuel African Methodist Episcopal Church in Charleston, South Carolina.

June 18, 1972: A BEA flight out of Heathrow Airport crashed just after takeoff, killing all 118 passengers and crew. The cause remains unknown, but the speculation is that the plane was carrying too much weight.

June 21, 1990: Fifty thousand people were killed and another 135,000 injured when a 7.7M earthquake struck Iran near the Caspian Sea. An estimated 400,000 were left homeless.

June 25, 1996: A truck loaded with 25,000 pounds of explosives devastated the U.S. Air Force military housing complex called Khobar Towers in Dhahran, Saudi Arabia. Nineteen U.S. airmen were killed and nearly 500 were wounded.

June 26, 1807: In a freak event of nature, lightning struck Napoleon's gunpowder factory in a commandeered castle in Kirchberg, Luxembourg. The massive explosion killed 300 people.

June 28, 1992: Two earthquakes rocked the area east of Los Angeles, one 7.3M and the other 6.3M. Three people were killed, 400 were injured, and the economic cost was about $92 million.

June 28, 2018: A man at war with a local newspaper chain invaded its newsroom in Annapolis, Maryland, and killed five of the staff and wounded two more.

June 29, 2020: In Alexandria, Egypt, a fire broke out in a private hospital, killing seven COVID-19 patients and injuring nine staff members. The accidental fire presumably spread as quickly as it did because of the high oxygen content in the room harboring the pandemic patients.

July 2, 1990: During Hajj, a stampede developed in a pedestrian tunnel in Mecca and caused more than 1,400 deaths due to crush injury and suffocation.

July 3, 1988: Over the Persian Gulf, the American warship *Vincennes* mistakenly shot down an Iranian passenger plane, causing the deaths of 290 passengers and crew.

July 3, 1990: A deadly stampede in a pedestrian tunnel in Mecca led to the deaths of 1,426 religious pilgrims. Most of the deaths were due to crush injuries and suffocation.

July 4, 1911: A deadly heat wave struck the northeastern region of the United States. It was as high as 106°F in Nashua, New Hampshire. Deaths mounted over an 11-day period. By the time the weather turned, 380 people were dead from the heat and heat-related maladies (e.g., train derailments due to bent rails and drowning while swimming to keep cool).

July 4, 2021: A Philippine Air Force plane crashed on the southern island of Jolo. It missed the runway as it was landing and crashed into a nearby village. Fifty military personnel on board, including the pilot in command, and three civilians on the ground died, while 46 occupants on board and four civilians on the ground were injured.

July 6, 1944: In Hartford, Connecticut, an arson fire broke out at the Ringling Bros. and Barnum & Bailey Circus during a show that was attended by 8,000 people. It killed 167 people and injured 682. Most of the victims were children. The whole episode lasted about 10 minutes.

July 7, 2005: During London's morning rush hour, a series of four bombings crippled the Underground at three subway locations and exploded a double-decker bus. The bombings began at 8:51 a.m. local time and ended at 9:47 a.m. Including the bombers themselves, 56 people were killed and over 700 were injured. London EMS deployed 100 ambulances with 250 personnel to respond to all four locations.

July 10, 1887: An 80-foot-high concrete dam in Zug, Switzerland, gave way. Seventy people were killed as floodwaters swept through the town.

July 11, 1978: Two hundred fifteen bathers were killed in San Carlos De La Rapita, Spain, when a truck carrying 1,500 cubic feet of liquid gas crashed into a vacation campsite. The massive explosion and fireball left a 20-foot-wide crater.

July 14, 2016: During Bastille Day celebrations in Nice, France, a white truck coursed through a closed-off main beachfront street crowded with revelers. The terrorist killed 86 and injured over 500. At the Lenval University Children's Hospital (LUCH), there were 47 casualties treated, including 12 adults. The relevant injuries that were recorded at LUCH were pelvic disruption, leg fractures, vascular trauma, and crush injures to the head and torso.

July 16, 1990: A 7.7M earthquake struck Luzon, Philippines, at 4:26 p.m. local time. It lasted only 45 seconds, but more than 1,000 people were killed and another 1,000 sustained severe injuries. Baguio City suffered the worst effects of the tremors.

July 17, 1996: TWA Flight 800 took off from Kennedy International Airport in New York City heading for Paris with 230 souls on board. Twelve minutes after takeoff, it exploded just south of Long Island. Controversy still remains as to whether this was a due to a terrorist attack or electrical failure.

July 17, 2014: Malaysia Flight 17 was shot down as it crossed over the Ukraine–Russia border during a time of conflict between the two countries. Which side committed the error remains in dispute, but the fact that 298 souls died is indisputable.

July 17, 1944: In Port Chicago, California, an ammunition ship exploded at the munitions pier, resulting in the deaths of 332 people, most of them African American Navy personnel. Most of them were killed instantly. The series of explosions were heard as far away as Nevada.

July 17, 2006: A 7.7M earthquake followed by a tsunami killed 550 people in West Java.

July 18, 1984: In San Ysidro, California, a mass shooter entered a crowded McDonald's armed with a 9mm Browning HP semiautomatic pistol, a 9mm Uzi carbine, and a Winchester 1200 12-gauge pump-action shotgun gunned down 21 people and wounded 19. The scene of horror lasted 77 minutes before the perpetrator was taken out.

July 18, 64: Rome burned while Nero allegedly fiddled. The fire burned out of control for 3 days. Hundreds perished and thousands became suddenly homeless.

July 20, 1977: A flash flood at Johnstown, Pennsylvania, killed 84 and caused $300 million in damages. The cause of the flood was the failure of an earthen dam after significant rainfall in the area (12 inches in 10 hours). Besides the first dam failure, five other dams burst, resulting in total release of 130 million gallons of water.

July 20, 2012: At a movie house in Aurora, Colorado, just outside Denver, a mass shooter killed 12 and wounded at least 70 as they were watching *The Dark Knight Rises*. Within a matter of 30 minutes, Anschutz Medical Center on the University of Colorado campus received 23 victims. All survived except for one, who was DOA.

July 21, 365: The city of Alexandria, Egypt, was devastated by an earthquake that was triggered off the Grecian coast. The tsunami that followed all but wiped out Alexandria, killed about 5,000 inhabitants, destroyed 50,000 buildings, and poisoned the surrounding farmland with salt water.

July 22, 1916: In San Francisco, during a Preparedness Day Parade in anticipation of America's entry into the war, a suitcase bomb was detonated. The explosion killed 10 bystanders and injured 40.

July 22, 2011: An individual with extremist views carried out attacks in Oslo and on the Norwegian island of Utoya. First, his van exploded in central Oslo, killing eight and wounding 200. Then, on Utoya, the perpetrator continued his killing spree, massacring 69 others, mostly teens.

July 23, 1967: An encounter between police and citizens grew to violent levels during a low point in race relations in the United States. The U.S. Army and the National Guard were called in. During the next week, stores were ransacked, 1,400 buildings were burned or ransacked, hundreds of people were injured, and 43 people were killed.

July 24, 1915: Over 800 passengers were killed when the *Eastland* tipped over in the Chicago River dockside. Hundreds were trapped in the hull of the steamer. Rescuers were able to save 40 or so by cutting through the hull, but the rest perished. The reason for the capsizing remains unclear.

July 25, 1956: The *Andrea Doria* collided with the *Stockholm* off Nantucket. The Italian liner eventually sank. A combination of fog and nautical errors contributed to the deaths of 51 people.

July 25, 2000: The Air France Concorde crashed on takeoff from Charles De Gaulle Airport, killing 105 passengers and four on the ground. The tragedy occurred when one of its tires was shredded by metallic debris on the runway from a plane that took off earlier.

July 27, 1996: In Atlanta, Georgia, during the XXVI Olympics, a pipe bomb was detonated. The explosion and the nails contained within the pipe tore through the crowd in Centennial Olympic Park, killing two and injuring hundreds.

July 28, 1945: In a heavy fog, a military plane slammed into the Empire State Building. Fourteen people were killed, three crew and 11 building occupants.

July 28, 1976: Tangshan, China, was the epicenter of an earthquake that measured somewhere between 7.8M and 8.2M. It's estimated that more than 240,000 people were killed. The fact that the quake occurred in the middle of the night explains the high mortality rate, since buildings collapsed as people were sleeping.

July 28, 2019: At annual Garlic Festival in Gilroy, California, a 19-year-old went on a rampage with a semiautomatic rifle. Three people were killed, including two children, and a dozen were wounded.

July 29, 1967: During the Vietnam War, a rocket from a plane aboard the carrier USS *Forrestal* was accidentally launched. It struck a plane, ignited a general fire on deck, and detonated a 1,000-pound bomb. The explosion and fires killed 134 servicemen and injured several hundred.

July 30, 1971: Over Japan, a Japanese F-86 Sabre jet collided with a Boeing 727 passenger plane, Nippon Airways Flight 58. The death toll was 162. The fighter jet was not equipped with radar.

July 31, 1715: Along the east coast of Florida, a hurricane decimated a Spanish convoy. Ten ships laden with treasure sank along with 1,000 crew.

August 1, 1943: A race riot broke out in Harlem, New York City, when a rumor spread that a White NYPD patrolman had shot and killed a Black MP from New Jersey during an encounter at the Braddock Hotel. The MP did not die but did sustain superficial wounds. Nevertheless, that ignited a situation where the Black population attacked White-owned stores, who allegedly practiced price gouging, in the immediate area. Eventually, the NYPD and the U.S. Army, at the request of Mayor LaGuardia, put down the riot. By the time the events settled down on August 2, six people had been killed and at least 500 were injured. This event is now known as the Harlem Riot of 1943.

August 1, 1966: At the 300-foot tower overlooking the University of Texas campus in Austin, an expert marksman armed with a stockpile of guns and ammo began a shooting spree that lasted 90 minutes. Before he was killed, he slaughtered 14 people and wounded 30.

August 2, 1973: A fire started on a small kiosk on the Isle of Man and extended to an adjacent building. The sheeting on the building was highly inflammable, and other architectural design flaws hastened the spread of the fire. Fire services were not called until 30 minutes after the fire was discovered. There were approximately 3,000 people in the building and the panicky rush to escape caused a significant amount of crush trauma. DOAs numbered 48. Of the 102 who survived at hospital, 32 required hospitalization. There were two in-hospital deaths.

August 2, 1985: Sudden wind shear during a thunderstorm caused a Lockheed L-1011 to crash as it was landing at Dallas/Fort Worth Airport. The total number of dead was 135.

August 3, 1975: A Boeing 707 crashed into the Atlas Mountains in Morocco. The plane was landing in heavy fog and in the process its wingtip and engine struck a mountain peak. All 188 souls on board perished.

August 3, 2019: In a Walmart in El Paso, Texas, a gunman shot and killed 23 people and wounded 27. Investigators believe that the incident was a hate crime directed at the Hispanic community.

August 4, 2019: In Dayton, Ohio, a man armed with an AR-15–style weapon targeted the entertainment center of the city, killing nine people and wounding 27 within 32 seconds. The shooter was fatally shot by police.

August 4, 2020: In Beirut, Lebanon, a cargo ship carrying more than 2,700 tons of ammonium nitrate exploded. Estimates vary, but when the dust settled, more than 190 people were dead, 6,500 were injured, and over 300,000 were rendered homeless. It is considered one of the worst non-nuclear explosions in history. It had the explosive power of between 500 tons and 1.1 kilotons of TNT.

August 7, 1956: In Cali, Colombia, seven military ammunition trucks exploded while parked for the night. Five hundred soldiers at a nearby barracks were killed immediately and another 500 lives were lost in the surrounding environs. There has been no definitive proof that this was caused by terrorists.

August 7, 1998: At 10:30 a.m. local time, in Nairobi, Kenya, a truck bomb leveled the American embassy. A few minutes later, another truck bomb was detonated outside the American embassy in Dar es Salaam, Tanzania. Between the two terrorist incidents, 224 people were killed and more than 4,500 people were injured.

August 11, 1965: During the 5-day Watts uprising, a result of increasing racial tension, 34 people died, more than 1,000 were injured, and over 4,000 were jailed. Property destruction was valued at $40 million.

August 12, 1985: A Japanese Airlines Boeing 747SR, JAL light 123, crashed into Mount Otsuka, killing over 500 souls. A structural explosion had occurred that severed the hydraulics, and the aircraft's "Dutch roll" directed it right into the mountainside. It took rescuers 12 hours to reach the crash site.

August 12, 2000: The Russian nuclear submarine *Kursk* sunk to the bottom of the Barents Sea following two explosions in the front hull. The crew of 118 died. No cause for the explosions was ever discovered.

August 14, 2003: A major power outage blacked out the eastern United States and parts of Canada. Twenty-one power plants were shut down in 3 minutes. The blackout impacted 50 million people. Cities from New York to Detroit to Toronto, Canada, were affected.

August 16, 1987: Northwest Flight 255 crashed on takeoff from Detroit Metro Airport when miscommunication between pilot and co-pilot caused a failure in extending the wing flaps. Additionally, the takeoff warning system was never turned on. Instead of reaching the necessary height of 600 feet, the aircraft was only 40 feet off the ground when it crashed into lampposts, a rental car agency, and a car with two people at the end of the runway. The two in the car perished. The only survivor out of the 156 on board was a 4-year-old girl.

August 21, 1986: A limnic eruption occurred at Lake Nyos in Cameroon. The sudden eruption of massive amounts of carbon dioxide from the depths of the lake formed a lethal cloud over the region, suffocating both people and animals. More than 4,000 people were forced to evacuate.

August 22, 1985: A fire started in the rear of a Boeing 737 as it was about to take off from Manchester Airport. Toxic smoke filled the cabin. Escape was possible for 85 of the 137 occupants, but the rest perished from the toxic gases and/or thermal trauma. Fifteen required hospitalization.

August 24, 79: Mount Vesuvius erupted on the Bay of Naples. Pompeii and Herculaneum, two Roman towns, were destroyed by lava, pumice stones, and hot ash. The eruption continued for 18 hours, and thousands perished.

August 24, 1992: Hurricane Andrew made landfall in southern Florida at 4:52 a.m., about 25 miles south of Miami. Andrew was a 175-mph behemoth that changed the way emergency management would be handled in the future. At the time, the Category 5 tropical cyclone resulted in fewer than 100 deaths, but it destroyed over 60,000 homes and damaged another 124,000. The economic loss was more than $23 billion.

August 24, 2020: Two suicide bombers detonated themselves in a populated area of Jolo in the south of the Philippines. At least 14 were killed and 75 wounded.

August 25, 2017: Category 4 Hurricane Harvey made landfall near Corpus Christi, Texas. Over a 5-day period, Texas and Louisiana were inundated by 51 inches of rain. About 150,000 residents evacuated, during which tens of thousands were stranded on roads and highways by floods. Thirty thousand water rescues were documented. During this time, over 330,000 residents were without power.

August 27, 1883: The volcano Krakatoa exploded, throwing 5 cubic miles of earth 50 miles into the air and creating tsunamis 120 feet high. It's estimated that 36,000 people died.

August 28, 1988: At the Ramstein Air Base air show in Germany, three Italian jets collided while executing an exacting stunt in midair and crashed into the spectator area containing 100,000 guests. Sixty-nine were killed and hundreds were injured.

August 29, 2005: Hurricane Katrina made landfall near New Orleans, Louisiana, as a Category 4 hurricane.

August 31, 2013: At a refrigerator workshop in Shanghai, China, a complex of pipelines dropped, releasing anhydrous ammonia to leak out and vaporize. Of the 58 workers at the site, 41 sustained burns from the leakage. Ten died at the scene due to inhalation of the noxious fumes and another five died en route to the hospital. Six of the most gravely injured patients (age range: 22 to 45 years) were transferred to the regional burn center at Changhai Hospital. Their cutaneous burn trauma ranged from 0.5% to 25% TBSA. They all sustained ocular trauma and their inhalation injuries were described as severe. Five survived but with severely compromised pulmonary function, glaucoma, and cataracts. Upon their discharge from the other hospital, the remaining casualties were described as having mild inhalation injury and minor burns.

August 31, 2019: An assailant initiated a series of drive-by shootings in Midland and Odessa, Texas. It started with a traffic stop and ended with the deaths of eight people, included the shooter, and the wounding of 25.

September 1, 1923: The Great Kanto earthquake. The initial quake, located in Sagami Bay just outside Tokyo, was followed by a 40-foot tsunami. Following the tremors and the tsunamis, fires blazed through the wooden homes and buildings of Tokyo and Yokohama. Approximately 140,000 people were killed.

September 1, 1983: A Korean Airlines passenger flight accidentally crossed into Russian airspace. It was shot down by Soviet jet fighters, killing 269 passengers and crew.

September 2, 1666: The Great London Fire. Within 4 days, 80% of London was destroyed. Firefighting in the medieval era consisted of bucket brigades, hand pumps, and pails of water.

September 3, 2004: A 3-day hostage standoff at a Russian school ended violently when 300 people were slaughtered, many of them children.

September 8, 1900: More than 6,000 people died on Galveston Island, Texas, when it was pummeled by one of the nation's deadliest hurricanes.

September 11, 2001: 9/11

September 12, 1988: Hurricane Gilbert slammed into Jamaica, killing hundreds.

September 16, 2013: A gunman killed 12 in the Washington, DC, Navy Yard.

September 20, 1929: A fire in a Detroit's Study Club speakeasy killed 22 and injured 50.

September 20, 2017: The Category 4 Hurricane Maria swept through Puerto Rico. In the aftermath, 44% of the 3.5 million residents lost access to potable water, cellphone towers and internet connectivity were lost, the entire island lost power, and only one of the 69 hospitals in Puerto Rico stayed operational.

September 21, 1999: A 7.6M earthquake in Taiwan killed thousands and caused billions of dollars in economic loss. One hundred thousand people were rendered homeless. Aftershocks were intense: Five of them registering a magnitude of at least 6 within 30 minutes of the initial quake.

September 21, 1938: A powerful Category 3 hurricane, dubbed the Long Island Express, slammed into Long Island and southern New England. Sustained winds measured 121 mph. Storm surges as high as 12 feet devastated coastal towns. As this tropical cyclone coursed through the United States, it was responsible for 600 deaths.

September 25, 1978: A Pacific Southwest Airlines jet collided in midair with a small Cessna over San Diego. The death toll was 153.

September 27, 1854: In a heavy fog, two ships, the *Arctic* and the *Vesta*, collided off Newfoundland, killing 322. When confronted with the fog, the

Arctic's captain did not reduce speed, sound the ship's horn to warn other ships, nor add extra lookouts.

September 27, 2012: In Gumi, South Korea, a hydrofluoric acid leak resulted in the deaths of five workers and first responders and injured 18. Poor scene management caused the dispersal of the caustic agent across the community of Gumi, exposing thousands to its effects. Complaints ranged from rash to chest pain to shortness of breath. Many of the symptomatic inhabitants who sought care received nebulized calcium gluconate.

September 28, 1994: In the Baltic Sea, the *Estonia*, a large car and passenger ferry, encountered extreme storms and waves 20 feet high. It sank with 852 deaths, one of the worst peacetime maritime disasters.

September 29, 1957: In the region around Kyshtym, USSR, a nuclear waste storage plant sustained a cooling failure and exploded. Radiation escaped containment and contaminated a 300-mile-square area. Soviet secrecy impeded the timely evacuation of nearby residents. It is estimated that 200 died from acute radiation syndrome.

September 29, 1999: At 1:47 a.m. local time, a 7.3M earthquake (known as the 921 earthquake or the Chi Chi earthquake) toppled buildings and killed more than 2,400 inhabitants of central Taiwan. Tens of thousands were injured and even more were left homeless in the freezing climate. The shock and aftershocks revealed how poorly the buildings had been constructed in the 1990s since so many toppled like a deck of cards.

September 30, 2009: A 7.6M earthquake struck Padang City, Sumatra (population 900,000). The quake occurred near where the Australian tectonic plate subducts beneath the Sunda plate. More than 1,000 people were killed, buried in the rubble, and hundreds were injured.

October 1, 2017: A gunman opened fire on a crowd attending the final night of a country music festival in Las Vegas, Nevada. Although the shooting rampage lasted only 10 minutes, it left 58 people dead and more than 800 wounded.

October 12, 2002: Three bombs, including a suicide bomber and a car bomb, were detonated in the tourist area of Bali, Indonesia. Over 200 people were killed and more than 200 were wounded.

October 8, 1871: The most devastating U.S. fire in terms of human death incinerated Peshtigo, Wisconsin. Twelve hundred people lost their lives and 2 billion trees were consumed by flames.

October 8, 1871: The Great Chicago Fire killed between 200 and 300 people, destroyed 17,450 buildings, left 100,000 homeless, and caused an estimated $200 million in damage (the equivalent of nearly $4.3 billion in 2021).

October 8, 2005: A 7.7M earthquake devastated northern Pakistan and parts of India and Afghanistan. Reportedly, 42,000 were killed and 60,000 injured. More than 3 million were suddenly homeless in freezing temperatures.

October 9, 1963: Heavy rains in the Vaiont Gorge region of Italy destabilized the mountainous Alpine terrain. A landslide from Mount Toc plunged into the reservoir below. The impact created a 300-foot tsunami that overwhelmed the dam and flooded the Piave River. This mass of water engulfed the riverside town of Longarone, killing about 1,000 residents and wiping out the town. Then it proceeded downstream to the town of San Martino, drowning hundreds more.

October 10, 1957: Workers at Windscale, Britain's first nuclear power plant, discovered that its nuclear core was on fire and had been on fire for a couple of days. This resulted in a release of radioactive contamination that spread across Great Britain and over Europe. No evacuations were ordered but the sale of milk from the surrounding region was prohibited. It is believed that the release was responsible for 240 cases of cancer.

October 12, 1918: The Moose Lake/Cloquet Fire raged through Minnesota, killing hundreds of people and leaving thousands more homeless.

October 16, 1996: A stampede of soccer fans before a World Cup qualifying match in Guatemala City killed 84 people and seriously injured more than 100.

October 16, 1991: In Killeen, Texas, a gunman drove his truck through the window of Luby's Cafeteria and proceeded to open fire on over 100 diners and staff during the lunch hour. Twenty-three people were killed and 20 were wounded.

October 17, 1989: The 6.9M Loma Prieta earthquake rocked the San Francisco Bay area, killing 67 people, injuring 3,757, and causing more than $5 to $6 billion in damage.

October 22, 1895: A passenger train in Paris, running late, was speeding to make up for lost time and failed to slow down as it was coming into the station because the crew had forgotten to engage the air brakes. The train plunged through the Gare Montparnasse and landed on a street. Only six of the 131 passengers were injured, but the train landed on and killed a pedestrian.

October 23, 1983: A suicide bomber drove a truck packed with explosives into the U.S. Marine barracks in Beirut, Lebanon, killing 241 military personnel. Two miles down the road, 58 French soldiers were killed in their barracks in a separate suicide attack.

October 23, 1989: Twenty-three people died in a series of explosions sparked by an ethylene leak at a Phillips petroleum factory in Pasadena, Texas.

October 26, 2002: A 57-hour hostage crisis ended when Russian special forces surrounded and raided a theater and, with the help of a narcotic gas, killed all the Chechen terrorists as well as 120 hostages.

October 27, 2018: At a Pittsburgh, Pennsylvania, synagogue, the Tree of Life congregation, a gunman armed with a semiautomatic rifle and three semiautomatic pistols killed 11 in the congregation and wounded six while yelling anti-Semitic slurs. He was captured alive.

October 29, 1998: A arson fire in the basement of an overcrowded discotheque in Gothenburg, Sweden, killed 63 and injured 213 young people. By all accounts, the prehospital response to this chaotic situation was exemplary. All the injured were hospitalized within 2 hours. The efficiency of this operation was even more spectacular given the fact that the disaster occurred late at night and the four local hospitals were operating with a limited number of personnel on night duty. Over the next 24 hours, the more seriously injured patients were transferred to receive care at other institutions in Sweden and Norway.

October 30, 1987: In Texas City, Texas, a hydrofluoric alkylation heater was dropped at the Marathon Oil refineries and 40,000 pounds of anhydrous HF was released. A toxic cloud drifted over the nearby population, forcing the evacuation of a 200-block area. One thousand people were seen at two local emergency departments and 95 were admitted for supportive and antidotal therapy.

October 31, 2020: In Chelyabinsk, Russia, a fire broke out in one of the area's temporary COVID-19 healthcare facilities. More than 150 patients required emergency evacuation. No one was killed or injured.

November 1, 1755: On All Saints' Day, a series of three devastating earthquakes hit Lisbon, Portugal, killing as many as 50,000 people. They occurred within 10 minutes of each other, with one estimated to be 8.0M. A 20-foot tsunami added to the death toll.

November 1, 1970: A discarded cigarette started a fire at the Club Cinq-Sept in Saint-Laurent-du-Pont, France. One hundred forty-six people perished. Investigators found that the fire laws in place at the time had been ignored, but those responsible, while found guilty, received suspended sentences.

November 2, 1982: A truck exploded in the Salang Tunnel in Afghanistan, killing an estimated 3,000 people.

November 3, 2020: Hurricane Eta made landfall near Puerto Cabezas, Nicaragua. At its peak it was classified as a Category 4 tropical cyclone. The number of fatalities exceeded 200 as it traveled up Central America, into the Gulf of Mexico, and slammed into the U.S. coastline.

November 5, 2009: Thirteen were killed and more than 30 other servicemen were wounded when a U.S. Army officer went on a shooting rampage at Fort Hood, Texas.

November 5, 2017: A mass shooting occurred at the First Baptist Church in Sutherland Springs, Texas. Armed with a Ruger AR-556 semiautomatic rifle, a Glock 19 semiautomatic pistol, and a Ruger SR 22 semiautomatic pistol, the shooter killed 25 worshippers and wounded 20. The shooter was also killed. Authorities estimated that 700 rounds were shot within 11 minutes.

November 7, 2018: At the Borderline Bar & Grill in Thousand Oaks, California, a Marine Corps veteran armed with a semiautomatic pistol and high-capacity magazines killed nine men and three women. The assailant died from a self-inflicted gunshot wound.

November 11, 1965: The Great Northeast Blackout.

November 13, 2015: Three allied groups of terrorists attacked six venues in Paris and its suburbs, including a football stadium, a theater, and several restaurants. One hundred thirty people died and 416 were wounded.

November 14, 2020: At the Piatra Neamț Regional Emergency Hospital in Romania, a fire broke out in the COVID-19 unit. Ten people were killed and four were injured.

November 17, 2020: Hurricane Iota made landfall in Nicaragua. At one point, it became a Category 5 tropical cyclone packing winds of more than 150 mph. The death toll across Central America was around 100; however, this hurricane, coming on the heels of Hurricane Eta, forced the evacuation and migration of hundreds of thousands as they lost their homes and livelihoods.

November 18, 1987: During rush hour in London, a fire broke out at the King's Cross Underground station. It was thought that the fire was started by a lit match dropped onto and through a wooden escalator. Thirty-one died and about 100 were injured. There were eight doctors at the scene providing triage, medical care, and death certification. Four hospitals received 58 casualties, mainly due to thermal trauma. In the aftermath, wooden escalators were phased out.

November 21, 1980: A fire started in the casino of the MGM Grand in Las Vegas, Nevada. Deadly smoke filled the hotel via stairwells, corridors, and elevator shafts and entered the guest rooms. There were 84 deaths. Multiple triage stations were established at the scene, and they processed about 3,000 people in 3.5 hours. School buses were drafted to transport the Green victims. As they were awaiting the arrival of patients, hospitals canceled elective surgeries, mobilized med/surg teams, and discharged in-house patients earlier than usual to free up bed space. By the fourth hour after the fire, the hospitals had received on average 150 victims each. Of the nearly 800 victims brought to the hospitals for evaluation, 322 required admission.

November 27, 2015: A Planned Parenthood clinic in Colorado Springs, Colorado, was attacked by a man with an assault rifle. Two civilians and a police officer were killed and two other civilians were wounded.

November 28, 1942: The Cocoanut Grove nightclub conflagration in Boston is considered one of the most noteworthy disasters in U.S. history. There were approximately 1,000 people in the building in anticipation of the big Holy Cross versus Boston College football game. Many of the revelers were servicemen about to embark for the war overseas. It is thought that a lit match dropped by an employee was the cause of the fire, which took off as it was fueled by the celebratory decorations around the rooms. There were nearly 500 deaths total. Two hundred people died at the scene. An investigation revealed that most of those deaths could have been prevented had the capacity not exceeded the legal limit and had the exit doors swung outward. Another 400 or so victims arrived at Boston City Hospital and Massachusetts General (MGH). Of those, 289 ultimately died. Some of the transported victims walked into the hospital only to collapse immediately and defied resuscitation. At MGH, it was decided to isolate all the burn patients in one of the general surgery wards—an improvisational burn unit. The strict isolation was maintained throughout and specialized teams were developed for dressing changes, wound care, and respiratory therapy. This tragedy prompted laws in multiple states requiring illuminated exit signs and outward-swinging exit doors, among other restrictions.

December 11, 1993: Heavy rains and mudslides caused the collapse of the hillside 12-story Highland Towers in Kuala Lumpur, Malaysia. Search-and-rescue teams were only able to pull three dwellers out alive, but 48 bodies were eventually recovered.

December 14, 2012: A former student entered the Sandy Hook Elementary School in Newtown, Connecticut, and shot 20 first graders and six employees before committing suicide. The rampage began at 9:30 a.m. and ended with his death at 9:40 a.m.

December 19, 2020: In Gaziantep, Turkey, a fire in the local hospital's ICU killed 10 COVID-19 patients. It was declared that the fire began with a high-flow-oxygen ventilation device.

December 24, 1971: A flight from Lima, Peru, flew into a violent thunderstorm, and the Lockheed L-188A Electra turboprop disintegrated when it was struck by lightning. It is considered the deadliest lightning strike in disaster history. All souls were lost save one.

December 26, 2004: In the early morning hours, a 9.1M undersea earthquake was recorded off Sumatra, setting off a series of tsunamis that crossed the Indian Ocean to the shores of East Africa. The waves were higher than 30 feet as they crashed onto shores. Deaths occurred across a dozen countries, but principally Indonesia, Sri Lanka, India Maldives, and Thailand. A final estimate was 225,000 dead. Casualties increased in the absence of food, potable water, and medical care.

Index

Tables, figures, and boxes are indicated by *t*, *f*, or *b* following the page number.

car, in disaster plan. *See* vehicle, in disaster plan

cardiac monitoring, for hydrofluoric acid victims, 104

Careflight triage, 28*t*

Cascade Mountains avalanche, 315

cash, in family disaster plan, 235

catastrophic disasters, 8

Category A biological/bioterror agents. *See also* botulism
anthrax, 302*f*, 303*f*, 320
incidents involving, 107–111, 110*b*
overview, 117*b*
pneumonic plague primary, 305*f*
ricin toxin, 306*f*
smallpox, 307*f*
trichothecene mycotoxin, 308*f*
tularemia, 309*f*
viral hemorrhagic fever, 310*f*

Category B biological agents, 117*b*

Category C biological agents, 117*b*

CDC (Centers for Disease Control and Prevention)
categories of biological agents, 117*b*
obtaining release of botulism antitoxin from, 114, 116

cells
outcomes after gamma ray radiation, 166–167
radiosensitivity of, 167*b*

Centennial Olympic Park bombing (Atlanta), 333

CESIRA triage, 28*t*

cesium-137 (Cs^{137}) exposure, 174*b*

Cessna collision with Pacific Southwest Airlines jet, 338

CG (phosgene), 294*f*, 295*f*

chain-reaction collisions
hydrofluoric acid incident after, 325
outside Fort Worth, Texas, 314
reacting to, 13, 14*f*, 15–16, 15*f*

Challenger explosion, 314

Chechen terrorist hostage crisis, 298*f*, 341

check-in phone numbers, in family disaster plan, 233

Chelyabinsk healthcare facility fire (Russia), 341

chemical release, in family disaster plan, 232

chemical terrorism, pediatric issues in, 92*f*. *See also* HAZMAT incidents

Chernobyl, Ukraine, 324

Chicago, Illinois
Great Chicago Fire, 340
Haymarket Square affair, 325

Chi Chi earthquake (Taiwan), 339

children
decontaminating, 91, 92*f*, 93
pandemic preparedness and response, 193
SALT triage, 33
triage considerations for, 25–28, 25*t*

Chile earthquake of 1960, 327

China
ammonium nitrate explosion in, 128*b*
anhydrous ammonia leak, 337
earthquake of 1556, 314
earthquake of 1976, 333–334
earthquake of 2008, 326
Tiananmen Square Massacre, 329

chlorine (CL), 293*f*

chloropicrin (PS), 299*f*

choking (pulmonary) agents, 293*f*, 294*f*, 295*f*

cholera in New York City, 1892, 205–206

Christchurch mosque attacks (New Zealand), 318

circulation, assessing during triage, 23–24

Circulation, Respiration, Abdominal and Thorax Exam, Motor Response, Speech (CRAMS) triage, 28*t*

Citizen's Health Committee (San Francisco), 208

civilian volunteerism, in past outbreaks, 203, 211, 213*b*

civil rights issues, in past outbreaks, 213*b*

CL (chlorine), 293f
Cleveland Clinic fire, 326–327
climate change, ix, 2, 8–9
clinical issues, in pandemic preparedness
and response, 193–194
closed points of distribution, 222b
closed spaces, blast mechanics in, 131, 134
clothes
removal after radioactive incident, 171,
171b
removal in decontamination procedures,
58, 59, 82, 85–86
Club Cinq-Sept fire (France), 342
CN (mace), 299f
coal mine explosion (Scotland), 314
Cocoanut Grove nightclub conflagration
(Boston), 343–344
"cocoon and mattress" technique, 154,
154b, 155f, 156f, 157, 157f, 158,
269b, 270f
Code Amber, 144
Code Black. See hospital evacuation
Code Disaster, 66–68, 129
Code Disaster-HAZMAT, 84–85
cold zone, HAZMAT, 59, 60f, 61, 90
Colorado Springs, Colorado shooting, 343
Columbine High School shooting
(Colorado), 323
command post, 35, 37, 38f
communication of victim status during
triage, 24
communications
in emergency department, 68–69
pandemic preparedness and response,
191–192
in regional incident command system, 217
community
hazards vulnerability analysis, 50, 51f,
52, 53b, 231–233
local nature of disasters, 4–5
mental impact of disasters, 8
pharmaceutical interventions in,
219–220

complex disasters, 5–7, 128
Consolidated School of New London
explosion (Texas), 318
Constantinople fire, 329
consultations, regarding hydrofluoric acid
victims, 105
contamination. See also decontamination;
HAZMAT incidents; radioactive
incidents
checking for after nuclear explosion, 179
complications in HAZMAT zones, 59,
61
minimizing exposure to, 58
radiological, 163–164, 163f, 170–172,
173b
self-contamination by staff, 191
of water, 238, 238b
contingency capacity (Stage 2), 190b
conventional capacity (Stage 1), 190–191,
190b
Courrières Colliery explosion (France), 317
covert assault clues, 110b
COVID-19 pandemic, 196, 216f
alternate care facilities, 224f
ethical issues, 195, 226, 227
identifying successes and challenges in
response to, 189, 191, 200
need for medical advisory committee in,
217–218, 219
points of distribution, 220, 220f
CRAMS (Circulation, Respiration,
Abdominal and Thorax Exam, Motor
Response, Speech) triage, 28t
credit cards, in family disaster plan, 235
crisis capacity (Stage 3), 190b
crisis leadership, in past outbreaks, 213b
crush syndrome, 136–137, 266b
Cs^{137} (cesium-137) exposure, 174b
CS/CR (tear gas), 299f
current ED patients, clearing, 70–72, 85,
145
cutaneous anthrax, 303f
cutaneous radiation syndrome, 170

CX (phosgene oxime), 282*f*
cyanides (AC), 287*f*, 288*f*
Cyclone Amphan, 327

D

Dale's Penthouse fire (Alabama), 314
Dallas/Fort Worth Airport Lockheed L-
    1011 crash, 335
Dan-Air crash (Canary Islands), 324
dangerous fallout zone (DFZ), 183, 184*b*
Dar es Salaam American embassy attack
    (Tanzania), 335
Dayton shooting (Ohio), 335
DC-10 crash (France), 316
decontamination
    ambulatory individuals, 85–87, 88*f*, 89*f*,
        90–91, 90*f*, 91*f*
    explosion victims, 129, 130*f*
    gross, 59, 61*f*
    "HAZMAT plus" incidents, 81, 85–86
    hospital decontamination area, 87, 88*f*,
        89*f*, 90*f*, 91*f*, 96–97, 129
    after organophosphate ingestion, 96–97
    pediatric patients, 91, 92*f*, 93
    potential threats to ED personnel, 82–83
    radiological, 164*f*, 165, 171–172, 173*b*
    special populations, 93
    of water, 238*b*
delayed radiation, 182–183
Denver charter school shooting (Colorado),
    325
Department of Transportation (DOT), 57
DFZ (dangerous fallout zone), 183, 184*b*
diazepam, 97
diphosgene (DP), 294*f*, 295*f*
dirigible disasters, 321, 325
dirty bombs, 143*b*
disaster admit team, 71
disaster code activation, 66–68, 129
disaster committees. *See* hospital disaster
    committees
disaster education. *See also* drills; mini-drills
    functional exercises, 256

gaming, 249, 251–252, 253*b*, 254, 255*f*,
    256
key points, 278
medical simulation centers, 257–258,
    258*f*
overview, 10, 247–248
seminars and workshops, 248
tabletop exercises, 249–250, 249*b*, 250*b*
disaster first-aid kit, 235, 236*t*
disaster kit, 240*b*
disaster magnitudes of severity, 5–8
Disaster Medical Assistance Teams
    (DMAT), 193
disaster medicine. *See also* hospital disaster
    committees; *specific disaster situations*;
    triage
    case histories, 2–4
    general discussion, 9–10
    impact of climate change, 8–9
    local nature of disasters, 4–5
    magnitudes of severity, 5–8
    mental impact of disasters, 8
    overview, ix–x, 2
    preparing for disasters, 4–8
disaster response and recovery cycle, 44, 45*f*
disaster vests, 67*f*, 69
discharging current ED patients, 70–71
discrimination, in past outbreaks, 213*b*
discussion-based exercises, 248, 251–252.
    See also disaster education
distillation of water, 238*b*
DIY potty, 239*b*
DM (adamsite), 299*f*
DMAT (Disaster Medical Assistance
    Teams), 193
DNA outcomes, after gamma ray radiation,
    166–167
documents, in family disaster plan,
    233–234
Domodedovo International Airport
    bombing (Moscow), 314
doors, blocking in active assailant situations,
    122–123, 123*f*

DOT (Department of Transportation), 57
DP (diphosgene), 294*f*, 295*f*
drills. *See also* mini-drills
  active assailant blitz, 259*b*
  blast injuries, 265*b*, 266*b*, 267*f*
  hydrofluoric acid scenario, 263*b*, 265*f*
  overview, 256
drive-by shootings, 324–325, 337
drones, 66*f*
Dust Bowl, 326
dynamic triage, 35, 39–40

E

earthquakes, 150, 231–232. *See also specific*
    earthquakes
EAS (Emergency Alert System), 235
Eastland steamer capsize, 333
education. *See* disaster education
egress, pre-hospital management, 38*f*, 39
EgyptAir Flight 804, 327
Ekaterinburg bioweapons plant (USSR),
    320
electricity, in family disaster plan, 234
electric vehicles (EVs), in disaster plan, 245
electromagnetic pulse (EMP), 181
electromagnetic radiation, 162, 165–166,
    166*f*, 179, 181–182. *See also* acute
    radiation syndrome
El Paso, Texas shooting, 335
Emanuel African Methodist Episcopal
    Church shooting (South Carolina), 330
Emergency Aid Society (Philadelphia), 210,
    211
Emergency Alert System (EAS), 235
emergency evacuations. *See also* hospital
    evacuation
  of emergency department, 150–152
  key points, 158
  mini-drill, 269*b*, 270*f*
  overview, 149–150
  vehicular issues during, 244–246
Emergency Management Institute (EMI),
    FEMA, 47, 48, 50

emergency medical services. *See* EMS; pre-
    hospital care
emergency medicine. *See also* disaster
    education; hospital disaster
    committees; regional pandemic plan;
    specific emergency situations; triage
  aftermath of disasters, 75–77
  blood products and services, 75
  case histories, 2–4
  clearing current ED patients, 70–72, 85
  Code Disaster-HAZMAT activation, 84–85
  communications in, 68–69
  disaster code activation, 66–68
  disaster vests, donning, 67*f*, 69
  first wave and second wave victims, 69–70
  general discussion, 9–10
  imaging, 73–74
  impact of climate change, 8–9
  key points, 78
  laboratory services, 74–75
  local nature of disasters, 4–5
  magnitudes of severity, 5–8
  mental health in, 77
  mental impact of disasters, 8
  need for disaster education in, 248
  overview, ix–x, 2
  pandemic preparedness and response,
    190–193, 192*f*
  preparing for disasters, 4–8
  radioactive incident response, 161–162,
    171–172, 171*b*, 173*b*
Emergency Severity Index (ESI) Triage, 28*t*
EMI (Emergency Management Institute),
    FEMA, 47, 48, 50
EMP (electromagnetic pulse), 181
Empire State Building plane crash, 333
EMS (emergency medical services). *See also*
    pre-hospital care
  biological incidents, etiology unknown, 108
  HAZMAT incident response, 58–59, 58*b*
  hydrofluoric acid incidents, 101–102
  roles and responsibilities, 35, 36*t*, 39–40
  SALT versus START triage use by, 34

hospital incident command system (HICS), 45, 46f, 48f, 67f, 75–76
hospital lockdown, 143b, 145, 178
hospital pandemic preparedness and response. *See* pandemic preparedness and response
hospital shootings. *See* active assailant situations
hostage standoff at Russian school, 338
hot zone
    active assailant situations, 125
    ambulatory individuals and, 85–86, 96
    biological incidents, etiology unknown, 109
    HAZMAT scene, 58, 59, 60f, 61
    after nuclear explosion, 182
    and Red zone, 87
HS (hydrogen sulfide), 291f, 292f
Hundred Years' War, 322
Hurricane Andrew, 6–7, 6f, 336
Hurricane Eta, 342
Hurricane Gilbert, 338
Hurricane Harvey, 16, 337
Hurricane Iota, 342–343
Hurricane Irma, 8, 245
Hurricane Katrina, 3, 223, 227, 337
Hurricane Maria, 9, 338
Hurricane Sandy, 2
HVA. *See* hazards vulnerability analysis
hybrid vehicles, in disaster plan, 245
hydrochloric acid (HCl) incidents, 321
hydrofluoric acid (HFA) incidents, 10, 103f
    after chain-reaction multiple-vehicle accident, 325
    drill, 263b, 265f
    general discussion, 101–106
    Gumi, South Korea leak, 339
    toxic cloud in Texas City, Texas, 341
hydrogen sulfide (HS), 291f, 292f
hydroxocobalamin, 288f
hyperkalemia, 103, 137
hypocalcemia, 102, 103–105
hypomagnesemia, 103

I

IISC (Interprofessional Immersive Simulation Center), 257–258, 258f
imaging, ED use of after disaster, 73–74, 76
immigration, and past outbreaks, 204–206
improvised explosive devices, 317–318
improvised weapons, in active assailant situations, 123–124, 271b
incapacitating agents, 296f, 297f, 298f
incident commander
    in emergency department, 66–68
    HAZMAT incident response, 58–59, 58b
    pre-hospital care roles and responsibilities, 35, 36t
incident command systems (ICSs), 48f, 49f. *See also* regional pandemic plan
    for full-scale exercises, 257
    overview, 47–48, 50
    regional, 215, 216f, 217, 218f
Indianapolis shooting, 322
infection control issues, 194
infectious disease threats, 107–111, 110b, 142
influenza pandemics, 3–4, 208–211
ingress, pre-hospital management, 38f, 39
inhalational anthrax, 302f
Inland Regional Center shootings (California), 121–122
inoculation, during smallpox outbreaks, 200–201
intentional biological assaults, 107–111, 110b
intentional bombings. *See* bombing events
intentional HAZMAT incidents, 82. *See also* HAZMAT incidents
intergovernmental cooperation during outbreaks, 212–213, 213b
internal perimeter, pre-hospital management, 38f, 39
Interprofessional Immersive Simulation Center (IISC), 257–258, 258f
intra-arterial treatment for hydrofluoric acid victims, 104

intradermal treatment for hydrofluoric acid victims, 104
intraosseous infusions (IOs), 86–87, 97
intravenous treatment for hydrofluoric acid victims, 104
intubated-ventilated patients, evacuation of, 157
intubations, after organophosphate ingestion, 97
ionizing radiation, 162. *See also* nuclear explosions; radioactive incidents
Iran earthquake of 1990, 330
Iranian passenger plane shooting, 330
iridium-192 (^{192}Ir) exposure, 174*b*
irradiation. *See* radioactive incidents
IS-100.C: Introduction to the Incident Command System, ICS 100 course (EMI), 47
IS-700.B: Introduction to the National Incident Management System (NIMS) course (EMI), 48, 50
Iserson "cocoon and mattress" technique, 154, 154*b*, 155*f*, 156*f*, 157, 157*f*, 158, 269*b*, 270*f*
Isle of Man fire, 334
isolation
    biological incidents, etiology unknown, 108–109
    during cholera outbreaks, 206
    public health characteristics of past outbreaks, 213*b*
    during smallpox outbreaks, 200, 201, 207
Israeli religious gathering stampede, 324

J

Japan Air Lines Flight 123, 335
Japan Atomic Power Company, 317
Japan earthquake of 1896, 330. *See also* Tokyo, Japan
Japanese F-86 Sabre jet collision, 334
Java earthquake of 2006, 328, 332
Johnstown disasters (Pennsylvania), 328, 332

joint command, 35, 36*t*
Jolo bombings (Philippines), 314, 336
jumbo jet crash in Canary Islands, 320
Jump-START triage, 26, 26*f*

K

Kano plane crash (Nigeria), 325
Karlslust dance hall fire (Berlin), 314
Kathmandu soccer stadium stampede (Nepal), 318
Kempster, Walter, 207
Khobar Towers bombing (Saudi Arabia), 330
Killeen shooting (Texas), 340
King's Cross Underground station fire (UK), 343
King Soopers grocery store shooting (Colorado), 319
Kirchberg explosion (Luxembourg), 330
Korean Airlines plane shooting, 338
Krakatoa volcano, 337
KRI Nanggala 402 submarine, 323
Kursk submarine, 336
Kyshtym nuclear incident (USSR), 339

L

laboratory services
    ED use of after disaster, 74–75
    for hydrofluoric acid victims, 104
    after radioactive incident, 173*b*
Lake Nyos limnic eruption (Cameroon), 336
Lakeview Elementary School fire (Ohio), 316
language barriers in disaster response, 77
large liquid exposure to nerve agents, 286*f*
Larrey, Dominique Jean, 21
La Soufrière volcano, 321
Las Vegas, Nevada
    country music festival shooting, 68, 339
    MGM Grand fire, 70, 343
latent stage of acute radiation syndrome, 168*f*, 169

latrine, creating, 239*b*

lava lake rupture (Democratic Republic of Congo), 313

law enforcement, in pre-hospital care, 35, 36*t*, 37

LDZ (light damage zone), nuclear detonation, 183, 184*b*

Lebanese ammonium nitrate explosion, 128, 128*b*

Le Mans race accident (France), 329

Level A PPE, 59

Level B PPE, 59, 84, 85*f*, 87*f*, 96–97

Level C PPE, 62*t*, 84

Level D PPE, 62*t*

levels of capacity, 190, 190*b*

Lewisite, 281*f*

life-saving interventions in triage, 22, 23*f*, 24, 32*f*, 33

light damage zone (LDZ), nuclear detonation, 183, 184*b*

lightning, 322, 344

Lima soccer match riot and stampede (Peru), 327

liquid exposure to nerve agents, 285*f*, 286*f*

liquid spills, HAZMAT events, 58

Lisbon earthquakes (Portugal), 341–342

Litvinenko, Alexander, 174*b*

Lloyd A. Jacobs Interprofessional Immersive Simulation Center (IISC), 257–258, 258*f*

"load-and-go" strategy, 41, 61, 151

local health department, obtaining release of botulism antitoxin from, 114

local nature of disasters, 4–5

local public health authorities, 108, 110

location
ensuring safety of in suspected HAZMAT event, 57
providing to 911 operator, 20*t*

lockdown, hospital, 143*b*, 145, 178

Lockheed L-1011 crash (Dallas/Fort Worth Airport), 335

Loma Prieta earthquake of 1989, 340

London, UK
bombings of 2005, 147*b*, 331
Grenfell Tower fire, 329
King's Cross Underground station fire, 343
London Bridge terrorist attack, 328–329
radioactive incident in, 174*b*

Long Island Express hurricane, 338

Los Angeles, California
earthquakes of 1992, 330
riots in, 324

low-energy explosions
blast wind, 134–138, 134*f*, 135*f*, 136*f*, 137*f*
factors contributing to blast injuries, 131–132, 132*f*
schematic representation of, 132*f*

low-energy explosives, 131*t*

low vapor exposure to nerve agents, 283*f*

Luby's Cafeteria shooting (Texas), 340

lungs, impact of blast wave on, 133

lysergic acid diethylamide (LSD), 297*f*

M

mace (CN), 299*f*

Madrid terrorist bombings, 67, 147*b*, 317–318

magnesium levels, hydrofluoric acid effect on, 103

magnitudes of severity for disasters, 5–8

Maine explosion, 315

Malaysia Airlines Flight 17, 332

Malaysia Airlines Flight 370, 316–317

manifest illness stage of acute radiation syndrome, 168*f*, 169

Marathon Oil refineries (Texas), 341

Marjory Stoneman Douglas High School shooting (Florida), 315

MASS (Move, Assess, Sort, Send) triage, 28*t*

mass casualty incidents (MCIs). *See* disaster medicine; *specific incidents*; *specific incident types*

mass decontamination after explosions, 129, 130*f*

N

nailbed examinations during triage, 24

Nairobi American embassy attack (Kenya), 335

Natchez dance hall fire (Mississippi), 324

National Incident Management System (NIMS), 48, 49f, 50

natural gas explosion, 318

Navy Yard shooting (Washington, DC), 338

nebulization treatment for hydrofluoric acid victims, 105

needle thoracostomy, in SALT triage, 33

negative-pressure environment, 108–109

Nepal
  earthquake of 2015, 324
  Kathmandu soccer stadium stampede, 318

nerve agents
  HAZMAT incidents related to, 95–97, 98f, 99
  high vapor exposure, 284f
  large liquid exposure, 286f
  low vapor exposure, 283f
  small liquid exposure, 285f
  Tokyo sarin attacks, 68, 82–83, 97, 318–319

neurovascular syndrome, in acute radiation syndrome, 168f, 169

neutrons, 162, 182

New Madrid Fault, 231

New Orleans Convention Center, 223

Newtown shooting (Connecticut), 344

New York City
  cholera outbreak in 1892, 205–206
  Happy Land Social Club fire, 319
  Harlem Riot of 1943, 334
  smallpox outbreak in 1947, 211–213, 220
  Triangle Shirtwaist factory fire, 319–320
  yellow fever outbreak in 1858, 204–205

New Zealand earthquake of 2011, 315

Nice terrorist attack (France), 331

NIMS (National Incident Management System), 48, 49f, 50

911 calls
  information to provide to operator, 19, 20t
  multiple vehicular accidents, 15–16
  suspected HAZMAT events, 56–57

921 earthquake (Taiwan), 339

Nippon Airways Flight 58, 334

NOAA Weather Radio All Hazards (NWR), 235

non-ambulatory patients, evacuation from hospital, 151, 152–154, 153f, 157–158

non-pharmaceutical interventions, 218

Normania ship, 206

North Sea oil platform collapse, 320

Northwest Flight 255, 336

Novichok organophosphate agent, 99

nuclear explosions
  considerations when evaluating victims, 185b
  key points, 186
  overview, 177–179
  planning response, 183–185, 184b
  types of injuries from, 180–183, 180b

nuclear incidents
  Chernobyl, 324
  in Japan, 317
  in Kyshtym, USSR, 339
  Three Mile Island, 320
  Windscale, 340

NWR (NOAA Weather Radio All Hazards), 235

O

OC (pepper spray), 299f

Odessa drive-by shootings (Texas), 324–325, 337

odors, in HAZMAT events, 57–58

off-gassing, 82–83, 90–91, 143b

Ohio State Penitentiary fire, 323

oil platform collapse in North Sea, 320

oil spills, 319, 323
Oklahoma City bombing, 323
Olive View-UCLA Medical Center
    (California), 150
open points of distribution, 222*b*
Operation Iraqi Freedom, 75
operations-based exercises, 256. *See also*
    drills
organophosphate HAZMAT incidents,
    95–97, 98*f*, 99
Orlando Regional Medical Center, 3
Oslo terror attacks (Norway), 333
Oso mudslide (Washington), 319

P

Pacific Southwest Airlines collision, 338
packed red blood cells (PRBCs), 75
pain control, for hydrofluoric acid victims,
    104
Pakistan
    earthquake of 2005, 340
    mosque attacks, 328
Palm Sunday tornadoes, 321
pandemic preparedness and response. *See
    also* regional pandemic plan
    challenges occurring during outbreaks,
        215
    cholera in New York City, 1892,
        205–206
    clinical issues, 193–194
    emergency department, 190–193, 192*f*
    ethical issues, 195–196
    infection control issues, 194
    influenza pandemic in Philadelphia,
        1917–1918, 208–211
    key points, 196
    lessons learned from past outbreaks,
        214–215
    levels of capacity, 190, 190*b*
    next pandemic, preparing for, 196
    overview, 189–190
    past epidemics and pandemics, studying,
        200

personnel issues, 194–195
    public health characteristics of outbreaks,
        213*b*
    resource issues, 194
    structural issues, 195
pandemic subcommittee, hospital disaster
    committee, 193–196
Paris, France
    terrorist attacks of 2015, 7, 147*b*, 342
    train accident in, 340–341
particulate radiation, 162, 163–165, 163*f*,
    164*f*, 179, 182
Pasadena explosions (Texas), 341
patient scenario cards, 252, 253*b*
pediatric disaster kit, 236*t*
pediatric patients
    decontaminating, 91, 92*f*, 93
    pandemic preparedness and response, 193
    SALT triage, 33
    triage considerations for, 25–28, 25*t*
penetrating trauma, from blast wind, 134–135,
    134*f*
pepper spray (OC), 299*f*
pericardial tamponade, 265*b*
peritonitis, in blast victims, 135
perpetrators
    in blast injury exercises, 267*f*
    of intentional HAZMAT incidents, 82
personal disaster plans. *See* family disaster
    plan
personal hazards vulnerability analysis
    (HVA), 52
personal non-pharmaceutical interventions,
    218
personal protection while on the road, 245*t*
personal protective equipment. *See* PPE
personnel issues in pandemics, 194–195
Peru, radioactive incident in, 174*b*
Peshtigo fire (Wisconsin), 339
pesticides, HAZMAT incidents related to,
    95–97, 98*f*, 99
pet safety, 237*b*
pharmaceutical interventions, 219

Philadelphia, Pennsylvania
  governmental assault on MOVE, 326
  influenza pandemic, 1917–1918,
    208–211
  yellow fever outbreak in 1793, 202–204
Philippine Air Force plane crash, 331
Philippines earthquake of 1990, 332
phone apps, in family disaster plan, 235
phone numbers, in family disaster plan, 233
phosgene (CG), 294f, 295f
phosgene oxime (CX), 282f
photographer, for ED triage process, 73
Piatra Neamţ Regional Emergency Hospital
    fire (Romania), 342
Piave River flooding (Italy), 340
PIO (public information officer), 46f, 47
Pittsburgh synagogue shooting
    (Pennsylvania), 341
plague
  bubonic, in San Francisco, 1907,
    207–208
  pneumonic, as bioterror agent, 305f
plane disasters. See specific disasters
Planned Parenthood clinic shooting
    (Colorado), 343
pneumonic plague primary, 305f
points of distribution (PODs), 222f
  generic considerations, 223b
  overview, 220
  personnel issues and, 194
  public health characteristics of past
    outbreaks, 213b
  during smallpox outbreak in New York
    City, 1947, 212
  types of, 222b
  vaccination, 220f, 221f
police, in pre-hospital care, 35, 36t, 37
polonium-210, 174b
Port Arthur shooting (Tasmania), 324
Port Chicago ammunition ship explosion
    (California), 332
potassium levels
  crush syndrome, 136–137
  hydrofluoric acid effect on, 103

potty, DIY, 239b
PPE (personal protective equipment)
  biological incidents, etiology unknown,
    108, 109
  botulism, 114
  for HAZMAT incidents, 59, 61, 61f,
    62t, 84–85, 85f
  hydrofluoric acid incidents, 102
  mini-drills, 277b
  for organophosphate incidents, 96–97, 99
  pandemic preparedness and response, 191
  for radiological decontamination, 165
  for radiological incidents, 171
  in RTR response system, 184b
pralidoxime chloride, 97, 99
PRBCs (packed red blood cells), 75
pregnant victims, triage considerations for,
    25t, 26–27
pre-hospital care, 35, 36t, 37, 38f, 39–41,
    40f. See also EMS; triage
Preparedness Day Parade bombing (San
    Francisco), 333
preparedness strategies, 44, 45f. See also
    pandemic preparedness and response
preparing for disasters, 4–8
primary blast injuries, 132–134, 133f, 265b
primary surveys
  hydrofluoric acid incidents, 102, 104
  after radioactive incident, 171–172
  radiological contamination, 173b
prison, botulism outbreak in, 113–114
prodromal stage of acute radiation
    syndrome, 168f, 169
prompt radiation, 181–182
prophylactic pharmaceutical interventions,
    219
pruno, 113
PS (chloropicrin), 299f
public fears during past outbreaks, 213b
public health
  characteristics of outbreaks, 213b
  and medicine, 218, 219
public information officer (PIO), 46f, 47
pulmonary (choking) agents, 293f, 294f, 295f

pulse, assessing during triage, 23–24, 23f, 26f
Pulse Nightclub shooting (Orlando), 3, 329

Q

quarantine
  biological incidents, etiology unknown, 109
  in cholera outbreaks, 206
  public health characteristics of past outbreaks, 213b
  in smallpox outbreaks, 200, 201, 207
  in yellow fever outbreaks, 204
quaternary blast injuries, 135–136, 136f, 266b
quinary blast injuries, 137f, 138, 181
quinuclidinyl benzilate (BZ), 296f

R

race massacre in Tulsa, Oklahoma, 328
race riots of 1967, 333
radial pulse, assessing during triage, 23f, 24, 26f
radiation caution zone (RCZ), 183
Radiation Injury Treatment Network (RITN), 183–184
radiation safety team, 171, 179
radiation sources, common, 165t
Radiation Triage, Treat, Transport System (RTR response system), 183, 184b
radiation units of measure, 163b
radioactive incidents. See also nuclear explosions
  acute radiation syndrome, 166–167, 168f, 169–171, 170b, 170t
  alpha and beta particles, 163–165, 163f, 164f
  Chernobyl, 324
  common radiation sources, 165t
  emergency department response, 171–172, 171b, 173b
  in family disaster plan, 232
  gamma rays, 165–166, 166f
  historical examples, 174b
  in Japan, 317

  key points, 175
  in Kyshtym, USSR, 339
  overview, 161–162
  radiation units of measure, 163b
  Three Mile Island, 320
  Windscale, 340
radiology, ED use of after disaster, 73–74, 76
radiosensitivity of human cells, 167b
railcars, HAZMAT events involving, 57
Ramstein Air Base air show (Germany), 337
rats, and plague outbreak in San Francisco, 208
RCZ (radiation caution zone), 183
recovery, disaster, 44, 45f, 125
Red-tagged patients/victims
  evacuation from disaster scene, 41
  evacuation from hospital, 151
  first wave and second wave victims, 70
  pregnant women as, 27
  SALT triage, 32f, 33
  START triage, 22–25, 22t, 23f
  tagging children as, 25, 26
redundancy in communications, 68–69
Red zone
  botulism incidents, 114
  hospital decontamination area, 87, 90
  hospital disaster plan, 45, 46f
  imaging in, 74
  intentional bombings, 143b
  when activating disaster code in hospital, 71
regional pandemic plan. See also pandemic preparedness and response
  allocation of scarce resources, 226–228, 227b
  alternate care facilities, 223–226, 224f
  community pharmaceutical interventions, 219–220
  key points, 228
  medical specialist role, 215, 216f, 217–219, 218f
  overview, 199–200
  points of distribution, 220, 220f, 221f, 222b, 222f, 223b
registrar, for ED triage process, 73

severe damage zone (SDZ), nuclear detonation, 182, 184*b*

severity, disaster magnitudes of, 5–8

sewer explosions, Guadalajara, Mexico, 323–324

SFGH (San Francisco General Hospital), 76

Shaanxi earthquake of 1556 (China), 314

Shanghai anhydrous ammonia leak (China), 337

Sharpeville shootings (South Africa), 319

Sheffield stampede (UK), 83–84

sheltering in place after nuclear explosion, 178, 182, 186

shielding, radiation, 166

Shigaraki train accident (Japan), 326

shootings. *See* active assailant situations; *specific shootings*

Sichuan earthquake of 2008 (China), 326

sieve triage, 28*t*

significant liquid exposure to nerve agents, 286*f*

simple disasters, 5, 13, 75, 78

Simple Triage and Rapid Treatment triage. *See* START triage

simulation centers, 257

sliding doors, blocking in active assailant situations, 123

small liquid exposure to nerve agents, 285*f*

smallpox
    as bioterror agent, 307*f*
    outbreak in Boston, 1775, 200–202
    outbreak in Milwaukee, 1894, 207
    outbreak in New York City, 1947, 211–213, 220

Smart triage, 28*t*

smiling death syndrome, 137

smoke, clues to identify HAZMAT events, 57

societal non-pharmaceutical interventions, 218

Sort—Assess—Life-saving interventions—Treatment/transport (SALT) triage, 31, 32*f*, 33–35, 41, 271*b*

SORT triage, 28*t*

South Fork Dam disaster (Pennsylvania), 328

Spanish convoy sinking (1715), 334

special populations, decontaminating, 93

SS *Normania* ship, infection control on, 206

Stage 1 (conventional capacity), 190–191, 190*b*

Stage 2 (contingency capacity), 190*b*

Stage 3 (crisis capacity), 190*b*

staging area
    in hospital, 46*f*, 47
    pre-hospital management, 37, 38*f*

staging officer, 36*t*

staircases, marking during hospital evacuation, 152

stampedes
    during Hajj, 83, 330, 331
    at Israel religious mass gathering, 324
    related to HAZMAT events, 81, 83–86
    at soccer game in Guatemala City, 340
    at soccer match in Lima, Peru, 327
    in soccer stadium in Kathmandu, Nepal, 318

Stardust nightclub fire (Dublin), 314–315

START (Simple Triage and Rapid Treatment) triage
    algorithm used for, 23*f*
    combining with medical experience and knowledge, 27, 31
    general discussion, 21–25
    key points, 41
    mini-drills, 271*b*
    versus SALT triage, 33–34
    victim categories, 22*t*

Station nightclub fire (Rhode Island), 315

Steffens, Lincoln, 209

STM (Sacco Triage Method), 28*t*

Stockholm collision, 333

stockpiling, 191

storing water, 237

structural issues, in pandemic preparedness and response, 195

first wave and second wave, 69–70
getting ready, 66–68, 67f
imaging, 73–74
key points, 78
laboratory services, 74–75
mental health, 77
overview, 65
triage, 72–73
tornadoes, historical examples of, 318, 321
tourniquet mini-drill, 268b, 268f, 269f
train disasters
along Bagmati River, India, 329
caused by avalanche in Washington, 315
derailment in Taiwan, 321
double train mishap near Tokyo, 325
freight train disaster in Italy, 315–316
Madrid terrorist bombings, 67, 147b,
317–318
near Shigaraki, Japan, 326
in Paris, 340–341
training, 10, 191. *See also* disaster
education; drills
transport officer, 36t, 38f, 41
trauma management
Asiana Airlines Flight 214 crash, 76
in "HAZMAT plus" incidents, 83, 84
pandemic preparedness and response,
194
after radioactive incident, 161–162, 172
traumatic rhabdomyolysis, 136–137
treatment officer, 36t, 38f
Tree of Life congregation shooting
(Pennsylvania), 341
triage. *See also* START triage
active assailant situations, 125
botulism victims, 114
considerations in mass casualty incidents,
25–27, 25t
of current ED patients, 71
dynamic nature of, 35, 39–40
early example of, 203
in emergency department, 72–73
by EMTs, 39

first responder victims, 25t, 27
first wave and second wave victims, 70
"HAZMAT plus" incidents, 85
information to provide to 911 operator,
19, 20t
intentional bombings, 143b, 145
Jump-START for children, 26, 26f
key points, 41
mini-drills, 271b
overview, 19, 21
pandemic preparedness and response,
192–193
pregnant victims, 25t, 26–27
pre-hospital management diagram, 38f
pre-hospital personnel, 36t
re-triage, 35, 39–40
reverse, 28t, 151, 152
role of medical knowledge and
experience, 27, 31, 34–35
SALT, 31, 32f, 33–35, 41, 271b
tools used around the world, 27, 28t
Triage Early Warning Score (TEWS), 28t
triage officer, 36t, 72–73
Triangle Shirtwaist factory fire (New York
City), 319–320
trichothecene (T2) mycotoxin, 308f
Tri-State Tornado, 318
tropical diseases, 107–111, 110b
truck bombs, 335
tsunamis
from Alaska earthquake of 1964, 320
in Alexandria, Egypt, 333
from Chile earthquake of 1960, 327
Great Kanto earthquake, 337
in Hawaii, 320, 327
in Japan in 1896, 330
in Japan in 2011, 317
in Java in 2006, 330
from Krakatoa explosion, 337
in Piave River, Italy, 340
from Sumatra earthquake of 2004, 344
tularemia, 309f
Tulsa, Oklahoma race massacre, 328

Turkish Airlines crash (France), 316
turnpike crashes, 249*b*. *See also* multiple
vehicular accidents
TWA Flight 800 explosion, 332
2-pralidoxime chloride, 97, 99
type 1 complex disasters, 5–7
type 2 complex disasters, 7

U

unified command, 35, 36*t*
United Kingdom (UK). *See also* London,
England
Ariana Grande concert bombing, 327
Boeing 737 fire at Manchester Airport,
336
Bradford football stadium fire, 326
Glasgow coal mine explosion, 314
Hillsborough Stadium stampede, 83–84
Top Storey Club fire, 325
units of measure, radiation, 163*b*
University of Texas shooting, 334
unmanned aerial vehicles (UAVs), 66*f*
"uphill, upwind, upstream" adage, 15, 56
urgency, disaster code activation and, 67–68
U.S. Department of Transportation
(DOT), 57
USS *Forrestal* disaster, 334
USS *Maine* explosion, 315
USS *Thresher* submarine disaster, 321
utilities, in family disaster plan, 234
Utoya terror attacks (Norway), 333

V

vaccination, smallpox, 207, 212
vapor exposure to nerve agents, 283*f*, 284*f*
variolation, 200–201
vascular access, after organophosphate
ingestion, 97
vehicle, in disaster plan. *See also* multiple
vehicular accidents
electric and hybrid vehicles, 245
emergency evacuations, 244–246
key points, 246

overview, 234, 243–244
personal protection while on the road,
245*t*
preparing vehicle, 244*t*
ventilators, when evacuating hospital, 151
vesicants, 280*f*, 281*f*, 282*f*
Vesta ship collision, 338–339
vests, disaster, 67*f*, 69
Vincennes warship, 330
violence, during past outbreaks, 213*b*
viral hemorrhagic fever (VHF), 310*f*
Virginia Beach Municipal Center shooting,
328
Virginia Tech shooting, 322
volcanoes
Krakatoa, 337
La Soufrière, 321
Mount Etna, 317
Mount Nyiragongo, 313–314
Mount Pelée, 326
Mount St. Helens, 327
Mount Vesuvius, 336
Volendam café fire (Netherlands), 313
vulnerability assessment. *See* hazards
vulnerability analysis
vulnerable populations, decontaminating, 93

W

waiting room, HAZMAT incidents in,
95–96, 97
Walmart shooting in El Paso, Texas, 335
warm zone, HAZMAT, 59, 60*f*, 61, 90
warning phase of disasters, 44, 45*f*
Washington, DC Navy Yard shooting, 338
Washington, George, 201
water
decontamination, 238*b*
in family disaster plan, 233, 236–238
sources of uncontaminated, 238*b*
supply, shutting off, 234
Watts uprising, 335
weapons, improvised in active assailant
situations, 123–124, 271*b*

weather information, providing to 911
    operator, 20*t*
wildfires, 150, 325, 339, 340
Windscale nuclear incident, 340
winter driving, 243–244
Wireless Emergency Alerts (WEA), 235
withdrawal of care, ethics of, 195–196, 227,
    227*b*
workshops, 248
World Trade Center bombing of 1993, 320

X

X-rays, 73–74

Y

Yanango, Peru radioactive incident, 174*b*
yellow fever outbreaks

in New York City, 1858, 204–205
in Philadelphia, 1793, 202–204
Yellow-tagged patients/victims
    evacuation from disaster scene, 41
    evacuation from hospital, 151
    first wave and second wave victims, 70
    SALT triage, 32*f*, 33
    START triage, 22–25, 22*t*, 23*f*
Yellow zone
    hospital decontamination area, 90
    hospital disaster plan, 45, 46*f*
    imaging in, 74
    when activating disaster code in hospital,
        71

Z

Zug, Switzerland dam disaster, 331